Medical Implications of Elder Abuse and Neglect

Editors

LISA M. GIBBS
LAURA MOSQUEDA

CLINICS IN GERIATRIC MEDICINE

www.geriatric.theclinics.com

November 2014 • Volume 30 • Number 4

ELSEVIER

1600 John F. Kennedy Boulevard • Suite 1800 • Philadelphia, Pennsylvania, 19103-2899

http://www.theclinics.com

CLINICS IN GERIATRIC MEDICINE Volume 30, Number 4
November 2014 ISSN 0749–0690, ISBN-13: 978-0-323-32373-4

Editor: Jessica McCool
Developmental Editor: Yonah Korngold

Clinics in Geriatric Medicine (ISSN 0749-0690) is published quarterly by Elsevier Inc., 360 Park Avenue South, New York, NY 10010-1710. Months of issue are February, May, August, and November. Business and Editorial Offices: 1600 John F. Kennedy Blvd., Suite 1800, Philadelphia, PA 191023-2899. Periodicals postage paid at New York, NY, and additional mailing offices. Subscription prices are $280.00 per year (US individuals), $498.00 per year (US institutions), $145.00 per year (US student/resident), $370.00 per year (Canadian individuals), $632.00 per year (Canadian institutions), $195.00 per year (Canadian student/resident), $390.00 per year (foreign individuals), $632.00 per year (foreign institutions), and $195.00 per year (foreign student/resident). Foreign air speed delivery is included in all *Clinics* subscription prices. All prices are subject to change without notice. POSTMASTER: Send address changes to *Clinics in Geriatric Medicine,* Elsevier Health Sciences Division, Subscription Customer Service, 3251 Riverport Lane, Maryland Heights, MO 63043. Telephone: 1-800-654-2452 (U.S. and Canada); 314-447-8871 (outside U.S. and Canada). Fax: 314-447-8029. E-mail: journalscustomerservice-usa@elsevier.com (for print support) or journalsonlinesupport-usa@elsevier.com (for online support).

Reprints. For copies of 100 or more, of articles in this publication, please contact the Commercial Reprints Department, Elsevier Inc., 360 Park Avenue South, New York, New York 10010-1710. Tel.: 212-633-3874; Fax: 212-633-3820, E-mail: reprints@elsevier.com.

Clinics in Geriatric Medicine is covered in *MEDLINE/PubMed (Index Medicus), EMBASE/Excerpta Medica, Current Contents/Clinical Medicine (CC/CM),* and the *Cumulative Index to Nursing & Allied Health Literature.*

Contributors

EDITORS

LISA M. GIBBS, MD
Chief, Division of Geriatric Medicine and Gerontology, Department of Family Medicine; Clinical Professor, Center of Excellence on Elder Abuse and Neglect, University of California, Irvine, Orange, California

LAURA MOSQUEDA, MD
Chair and Professor, Family Medicine and Geriatrics, Keck School of Medicine at the University of Southern California, Los Angeles, California

AUTHORS

W. ANDREW ACHENBAUM, PhD
Deputy Director of the UT Health, UT Health Consortium on Aging, Texas Elder Abuse and Mistreatment Institute (TEAM); Gerson and Sabina David Professor of Global Aging; Professor of Social Work and History, Graduate School of Social Work, The University of Houston, Houston, Texas

TRIMIKA BOWDRE, PhD, MPH
University of Tennessee Health Science Center College of Nursing, Memphis, Tennessee

JASON BURNETT, PhD
Division of Geriatric and Palliative Medicine, Department of Internal Medicine, Assistant Professor, UT Health, Medical School-Houston; UT Health Consortium on Aging, Texas Elder Abuse and Mistreatment Institute (TEAM); Harris Health System, Houston, Texas

TESSA DEL CARMEN, MD
Assistant Professor, Division of Geriatrics and Palliative Medicine, New York Presbyterian Hospital, Weill Cornell Medical College, New York, New York

AMY Y. CARNEY, PhD, APRN, FNP-BC, FAAFS
School of Nursing, California State University San Marcos, California

CLAUDIA COOPER, PhD, MSc, BM
Division of Psychiatry, University College London, London, United Kingdom

JILL CRUM, BSN, RN, SANE-A
Eisenhower Medical Center Emergency Department, Rancho Mirage, California

CARMEL BITONDO DYER, MD, FACP, AGSF
Division of Geriatric and Palliative Care, Department of Internal Medicine, University of Texas Medical School; Texas Elder Abuse and Mistreatment Institute (TEAM); Harris Health System, Houston, Texas

RACHELL A. EKROOS, MSN, ARNP-BC, AFN-BC, DF-IAFN
Center for Forensic Nursing Excellence International, Henderson, Nevada

ERIKA FALK, PsyD
Clinical Psychologist, Institute on Aging, San Francisco, California

DIANA K. FAUGNO, MSN, RN, CPN, SANE-A, SANE-P, FAAFS
Consultant, Eisenhower Medical Center Emergency Department, Rancho Mirage, California

DAVID V. FLORES, PhD, LMSW, MPH, CPH
Division of Geriatric and Palliative Care, Department of Internal Medicine, University of Texas Medical School; Texas Elder Abuse and Mistreatment Institute; Harris Health System, Houston, Texas

LISA M. GIBBS, MD
Chief, Division of Geriatric Medicine and Gerontology, Department of Family Medicine; Clinical Professor, Center of Excellence on Elder Abuse and Neglect, University of California, Irvine, Orange, California

JOHN M. HALPHEN, MD
Division of Geriatric and Palliative Care, Department of Internal Medicine, University of Texas Medical School; Texas Elder Abuse and Mistreatment Institute; Harris Health System, Houston, Texas

MARGARET T. HARTIG, PhD, APN, FNP-BC, FAANP
University of Tennessee Health Science Center College of Nursing, Memphis, Tennessee

RON HAUGEN, DNP, FNP-BC, PMH-BC
Synergy LLC, New Mexico

NANCY HOFFMAN, PsyD
Geriatric Forensic Neuropsychologist, Assessment and Psychotherapy, San Rafael, California

DIANA HOMEIER, MD
Associate Professor of Clinical Family and Internal Medicine, Keck School of Medicine at the University of Southern California, Los Angeles, California

WENDY LIKES, PhD, DNSc, APN, FNP-BC
University of Tennessee Health Science Center College of Nursing, Memphis, Tennessee

GILL LIVINGSTON, MD
Professor of Psychiatry of Older People, Division of Psychiatry, University College London, London, United Kingdom

VERONICA M. LoFASO, MS, MD
Associate Professor of Clinical Medicine, Division of Geriatrics and Palliative Medicine; Roland Balay Clinical Scholar, Weill Cornell Medical College, New York, New York

KATHLEEN PACE MURPHY, PhD
Assistant Professor, Division of Geriatric and Palliative Medicine, UT Health, Medical School-Houston; UT Health Consortium on Aging, Houston, Texas

JAMES S. POWERS, MD
Associate Clinical Director, Tennessee Valley Health System Geriatric Research, Education and Clinical Center; Associate Professor of Medicine, The Center on Aging, Vanderbilt University School of Medicine, Nashville, Tennessee

CARLOS A. REYES-ORTIZ, MD, PhD
Division of Geriatric and Palliative Care, Department of Internal Medicine, University of Texas Medical School, Houston, Texas

TONY ROSEN, MD, MPH
Instructor in Medicine, Department of Emergency Medicine, Weill Cornell Medical College, New York, New York

PATRICIA M. SPECK, DNSc, APN, FNP-BC, FAAFS, FAAN
Associate Professor, The University of Alabama at Birmingham School of Nursing, Birmingham, Alabama

PAMELA TRONETTI, DO, AGSF
Medical Director, Parrish Senior Consultation Center, Titusville, Florida

MARY S. TWOMEY, MSW
Co-director, Division of Geriatric Medicine and Gerontology, Center of Excellence on Elder Abuse and Neglect, University of California, Irvine, Orange, California

LIDIA VOGNAR, MD
Assistant Professor, Division of Geriatric and Palliative Medicine, Alpert School of Medicine, Brown University; Staff Geriatrician, Providence VAMC, Providence, Rhode Island

CHRISTINE WEBER, MSG
Community Health Program Representative, Division of Geriatric Medicine and Gerontology, Center of Excellence on Elder Abuse and Neglect, University of California, Irvine, Orange, California

LISA M. YOUNG, MD, MBA
HealthCare Partners, Torrance, California

Contents

> Elder abuse is a public health problem that is growing more pervasive despite being grossly underreported and underdetected. Annually, many vulnerable older adults suffer various forms of abuse threatening their overall health, quality of life, and survival. To better protect our aging population, we must overcome obstacles such as ageism, lack of geriatric health professional training, and low screening practices in clinical settings. Addressing these challenges is not sufficient for eliminating the abuse of older adults, but it is necessary for diminishing the potential for abuse and the associated negative health outcomes.

> Physical abuse of the elderly is a significant public health concern. The true prevalence of all types is unknown, and under reporting is known to be significant. The geriatric population is projected to increase dramatically over the next 10 years, and the number of abused individuals is also projected to increase. It is critical that health care providers feel competent in addressing physical elder abuse. This article presents cases illustrating the variety of presenting symptoms that may be attributed to physical elder abuse.

> Because neglect is the most common form of elder abuse, identifying patients who are vulnerable to neglect allows clinicians to intervene early and potentially prevent situations that can escalate and lead to harm or even death. Health care workers have a unique opportunity to uncover these unfortunate situations and, in many cases, may be the only other contact that isolated, vulnerable patients have with the outside world. Responding appropriately and quickly when neglect is suspected and using a team approach can improve the health and well-being of older victims of neglect.

> In this article, sexual assault of older persons is analyzed in a literature review and case series, and exemplar pseudocases of suspected older person sexual assault are discussed.

> Self-neglect, the most common form of elder mistreatment seen by Adult Protective Service Agencies across the United States, is an often unrecognized geriatric syndrome characterized by squalor and unsafe living

circumstances. It is a result of medical, neurologic, or psychiatric disorders coupled with lack of capacity for self-care and self-protection in the absence of necessary services or medical care, and it leads to increased morbidity and mortality. Clinicians should evaluate self-neglecters and plan interventions based on comprehensive geriatric and capacity assessment. State and federal policies are needed in order to address the pressing needs of this vulnerable population of seniors.

For patients with dementia, abuse ranges from subtle scams to outright physical violence. As dementia progresses, abuse escalates. The stages of dementia—mild cognitive impairment, mild dementia, moderate dementia, and severe dementia—lend themselves to varied presentations of abuse. Knowing which types of abuse are more prominent at each stage aids the clinician in anticipating risk of abuse and patient and caregiver needs. Interviewing the victim is crucial in uncovering, documenting, and intervening in an abuse situation. A clinician who is skilled in drawing out the facts while remaining supportive of the patient is key in ending the victimization.

Elder abuse may be defined as a violation of a vulnerable older person's human and civil rights. Psychiatric illness is an important cause of vulnerability to abuse, especially when it is comorbid with other risk factors, such as physical frailty, sensory impairment, social isolation, and physical dependency. Health care providers are likely to encounter elder abuse regularly, and therefore have an important role in its detection and management, and in the treatment of subsequent psychiatric illness. This article reviews the relationships between psychiatric illnesses and elder abuse and neglect, examines the psychiatric consequences, and discusses how these may be treated.

Capacity evaluations of older adults assist in determining whether a situation should be considered elder/dependent adult abuse and which type of intervention is warranted. Capacity evaluations must integrate multiple sources of data and focus on functional abilities. Understanding the legal standard underlying the capacity needed for a specific decision is key in making a clinical opinion relevant in legal settings. Capacity evaluations for guardianships help to identify preserved abilities and make recommendations to enhance decisional and functional capacities that promote the dignity and independence of older adults.

The number of elder abuse cases is expected to rise as the number of persons older than age 65 doubles over the next 20 years. Patients affected by elder abuse present in all care settings, including inpatient and outpatient clinical care, emergency rooms, long-term care facilities, and home care. Victims experience significant medical consequences, both physical and psychological, and often need additional resources, including legal guidance. Health care professionals need additional training in order to be effective advocates for survivors of elder abuse. Care of the victim must also be recognized as an equally important topic for research and education.

Health care professionals play a vital role in addressing elder abuse by identifying and reporting elder abuse and caring for survivors. However, most are unaware of the opportunities to work with allied professionals in elder abuse intervention. This article discusses the various roles of interdisciplinary members and the contribution of health care professionals in these teams. Terminology used in elder abuse teamwork is discussed.

CLINICS IN GERIATRIC MEDICINE

NOW AVAILABLE FOR YOUR iPhone and iPad

Erratum

In the August 2014 issue of *Clinics in Geriatric Medicine*, author Susan Merel should have been listed as Susan E. Merel in the article "Palliative care in advanced dementia." The corrected article listing should be:

Merel SE, DeMers S, Vig E. Palliative care in advanced dementia. Clin Geriatr Med 2014;30(3):469-92.

http://dx.doi.org/10.1016/j.cger.2014.09.003
0749-0690/14/$ – see front matter **geriatric.theclinics.com**

Preface

Medical Implications of Elder Abuse and Neglect

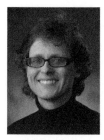 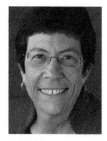

Lisa M. Gibbs, MD   Laura Mosqueda, MD
Editors

Our world is experiencing an unprecedented population growth, and the older adult populace is the fastest-growing segment in many countries. While many people are enjoying good health into their old age, many find these years attended by changes and illnesses that result in vulnerability to abuse or neglect.

Health care professionals are often in a unique position of trust and may be among the first, and perhaps the only, sources of help for older adults victimized by abuse. All who care for older adults must learn to identify the signs and symptoms of elder abuse, whether this abuse takes the form of physical abuse, emotional abuse, sexual abuse, financial abuse, neglect, or self-neglect. All types of abuse result in poorer medical and psychological outcomes. Although reporting a case of suspected abuse is not as obviously dramatic as a life-saving surgery, it may be the one action that relieves suffering and prevents the downward spiral of a victim.

Despite this, health care professionals are among the least likely to report suspected abuse. Many factors interfere with our ability to adequately address abuse, including lack of knowledge and awareness. This issue seeks to address some of these factors by providing information needed to effectively recognize and intervene when persons under our care are affected or are likely to be affected by elder abuse.

Elder abuse is not only a medical issue, but it is also a social, legal, and ethical one. The complexities inherent in addressing elder abuse require the work of multiple agencies. Many articles in this issue illustrate how health care providers are an integral part of a greater team of allied professionals.

We are indebted to the authors of these articles, leaders and experts in their fields, who generously gave of their knowledge and time to produce a timely and comprehensive issue on the medical implications of elder abuse. In addition, we appreciate the invaluable assistance from Chelsea Lenard, who helped make this edition possible. We are also grateful to Yvette Warner, Nancy Brown, Cordula Dick-Muehkle, and Cher Hill. We are indeed thankful to Jessica McCool and Yonah Korngold at Elsevier

Clin Geriatr Med 30 (2014) xv–xvi
http://dx.doi.org/10.1016/j.cger.2014.08.015
0749-0690/14/$ – see front matter

for the opportunity to edit this issue and for their continuing support and encouragement throughout this project.

Lisa M. Gibbs, MD
Chief, Division of Geriatric Medicine and Gerontology
Center of Excellence on Elder Abuse and Neglect
Department of Family Medicine
University of California, Irvine
Orange, CA 92868, USA

Laura Mosqueda, MD
Chair and Professor
Family Medicine and Geriatrics
Keck School of Medicine at the University of Southern California
Los Angeles, CA 90089, USA

E-mail addresses:
lgibbs@uci.edu (L.M. Gibbs)
laura.mosqueda@usc.edu (L. Mosqueda)

Aging

Physiology, Disease, and Abuse

Diana Homeier, MD

KEYWORDS

• Aging • Physiology • Disease • Abuse

KEY POINTS

- There are physiologic changes associated with aging.
- There are medical conditions that occur more commonly with advancing age.
- These physiologic changes and medical conditions increase an older adult's vulnerability to and injuries from abuse or neglect.
- An older adult may have more difficulty recovering from an abuse incident.
- The investigation of abuse or neglect may be more difficult because of aging changes.

With advancing age, an interplay of multiple factors places the older adult at increased risk for abuse and neglect. Consider the following scenario:

*A 70-year-old man was brought to the emergency room by paramedics after his daughter called 911 when she found him on the floor in his home without his caregiver. The emergency room doctor reported that the patient was dehydrated and confused; he could not provide his own medical history and did not know the date. You were the admitting physician; you were told that the patient had probably fallen at home. As you examined this patient's injuries, you began to wonder if the injuries were consistent with a fall. When you met the patient, he was receiving a fluid bolus and was still confused. On review of his chart, you found that he had a history of macular degeneration, hypertension, coronary artery disease, severe arthritis, depression, incontinence, and mild Alzheimer disease. His medications included donepezil, aspirin, clopidogrel, hydrochlorothiazide, metoprolol, and sertraline. On examination, he had multiple bruises along his right shoulder, a large bruise on his left upper arm, and a large confluence of bruises scattered across his chest. There was also an unusual linear pattern bruise on the left side of his chest (**Figs. 1** and **2**). After seeing him and reviewing the chart, you considered the following questions: were these injuries consistent with the history of a fall? Where was the patient's caregiver when he fell? Was the severity of the bruising caused by aspirin and clopidogrel? Could these injuries have been caused by physical abuse?*

Disclosures: none.

Division of Geriatrics, Keck School of Medicine of USC, 2020 Zonal Avenue, IRD 620, Los Angeles, CA 90033, USA

E-mail address: dianasch@usc.edu

Clin Geriatr Med 30 (2014) 671–686

http://dx.doi.org/10.1016/j.cger.2014.08.001

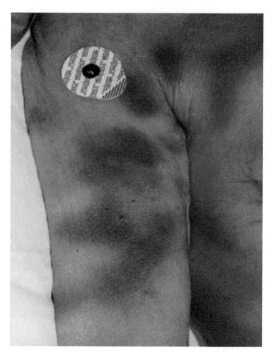

Fig. 1. Right shoulder.

The proportion of the population in the United States that is considered elderly (aged ≥65 years) has increased dramatically in the past 50 years and will continue to do so in the next 50 years as the baby boomers age. According to US Census bureau data, in 2010, 40 million Americans were 65 years or older. This number is expected to increase to more than 80 million by 2050.[1] This demographic imperative means that health care providers must understand the medical conditions that occur commonly with age as well as the psychological issues, social factors, and changes in function that may accompany these conditions.

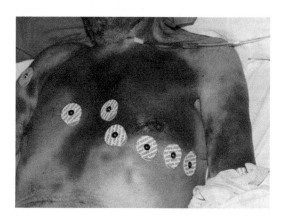

Fig. 2. Chest.

Aging is associated with many physiologic changes that are common to all persons. In addition to these changes, there are medical conditions (diseases) that occur more commonly with age. These changes and conditions increase an older adult's vulnerability to abuse or neglect.

OVERVIEW OF AGING PHYSIOLOGY

As a human body ages, there is a progressive decline in physiologic functioning, which affects all organ systems. These changes place an older adult at increased susceptibility to illness; they also create a disadvantage in recovering from illness. Although these changes are common to everyone, they progress at different rates in each individual and, even in the same person, progress at different rates in each organ system. **Table 1** denotes the physiologic changes that can be significant in considering a diagnosis or even a suspicion of elder abuse.

Body Composition

From young adulthood to old age, the percentage of body fat increases from 15% to 30%. This increase is accompanied by a decrease in muscle mass, total body water, and bone mass. These changes are important when considering the metabolism of medications and are part of the reason that some medications (eg, benzodiazepines) are more dangerous in older adults than younger adults.

Skin

Skin is an important organ, which provides a protective, thermoregulatory, and sensory function. The effects of aging on the skin can be divided into intrinsic and extrinsic changes.[2] The epidermal cells have a slower turnover rate, causing thinning of the epidermis. This thinner epidermis also has fewer melanocytes and Langerhans cells, decreasing the barrier and immune function of the skin and increasing risk for sunburn and cancer. In the dermis, there is a decrease in fibroblasts, collagen, and elastin, causing skin wrinkling and a loss of elasticity. A diminution of subdermal fat tissue in combination with capillary fragility leaves an elder more prone to bruising from seemingly minor trauma. In addition, several medications and conditions could increase an older adult's risk for bruising. For example, aspirin, clopidogrel, and warfarin may increase bleeding time and propensity for bruising. Diseases such as cirrhosis or myelodysplasia could cause disruptions in the clotting mechanism and predispose to bruising or bleeding. Chronic sun exposure, the predominant extrinsic factor in age-related changes, contributes to wrinkling and loss of tone in the skin.

Bone

With aging, there are changes in the architecture of both trabecular and cortical bone, as well as changes in the bone marrow. There is a reduction in trabecular and cortical bone volume, caused by an imbalance between bone formation and resorption. There is also an increase in adiposity of the bone marrow.[3] These changes result in a decline in bone mineral density (BMD), poorer bone structure and quality, and enhanced fragility and fracture risk. In women, the BMD begins to decrease about 0.5% per year after the third decade. This decrease accelerates to 3% to 5% per year during menopause. In men, the decline in BMD is more gradual until later, when the risk for fractures increases substantially.[4]

Aging also affects joint tissue and function. Within the joints, cartilage becomes more brittle, and there is increased stiffness of tendons and ligaments. These

Table 1
Physiologic changes that occur with normal aging; considerations for elder abuse

System	Physiologic Change	Considerations for Elder Abuse
Body composition	Increased fat Decreased water and muscle mass	Increased side effects of lipophilic medications
Skin	Thinning epidermis Decreased elasticity Decreased subdermal fat tissue	Increased bruising, skin tears, pressure sores
Bone	Decreased bone mineral density Stiffer joints	Increased fragility and fracture risk More prone to musculoskeletal injuries from minor trauma
Eyes	Decreased tear production Presbyopia Miosis	Increased risk for falls Difficulty reading documents Difficulty identifying abuser
Ears	Cerumen more tenacious Sensorineural hearing loss	Impaired ability to understand surrounding circumstances Difficulty communicating in investigation
Cardiovascular	Decreased carotid baroreceptor sensitivity Decreased maximal heart rate Arterial wall stiffness Increased left ventricle thickness	Difficulty recovering from illness/trauma More severe outcome from injuries
Pulmonary	Increased residual volume Decreased FEV_1, vital capacity Weaker respiratory muscles Stiffer chest wall	Increased likelihood of respiratory failure Increased risk for pneumonia
Muscle	Decreased muscle mass and strength Increased stiffness of tendons and ligaments	Loss of independence Difficulty rising from the floor Difficulty regaining independence after an injury
Renal	Decreased functioning glomeruli Decreased renal blood flow Glomerular filtration rate declines	Increased susceptibility to medications
Gastrointestinal	Decreased salivation Slowed esophageal peristalsis Delayed colonic transit time	
Neurologic	Decreased white matter Loss of synapses Mild cognitive changes Decreased proprioception and vibratory sense	Slower information processing Balance problems Increased risk for falls
Reproductive	Vaginal atrophy Narrowing of the vaginal introitus	Increased risk for injury from sexual assault More difficult sexual assault examination

changes, in addition to changes in bone and muscle tissue, can predispose joints to osteoarthritis, particularly when there has been previous trauma, obesity, or other risk factors. Joints may become stiffer, less flexible, and more easily prone to injury. The amount of force required to produce an injury may be less than that of a younger individual. There may also be a decrease in range of motion (as much as 20%–25%).[5]

Eyes

Many structures within the eye show changes with aging. The eyelids become more lax and the lower lid may be prone to eversion (ectropion) or inversion (entropion). There is a decrease in tear production, causing dry eyes. There is a progressive miosis.[6] The cornea becomes less transparent. The lens becomes thicker and more rigid, and there is less elasticity in the lens capsule. This process leads to presbyopia (a difficulty accommodating to near objects).[7] Vision deteriorates with age, and there is a decline in visual acuity, visual fields, and contrast sensitivity. There may also be a reduction in depth perception and color vision. Older adults may note more glare with lights and have difficulty adapting to bright light. These changes increase risk for accidents, falls, and injuries. An older adult may have difficulty reading a document that they are asked to sign (a possible mechanism for financial abuse). An older adult who has been in an abuse situation may have difficulty identifying the abuser.

Ears

There are numerous changes in the auditory system, which often lead to functional problems. The external auditory canal atrophies, and the cerumen becomes more tenacious and is more likely to become impacted. Although the tympanic membrane thickens and the ossicles undergo some degenerative changes, transmission of sound is fairly well preserved. Changes in the inner ear include a loss of sensory cells, loss of cochlear neurons, and vascular changes in the cochlea, which lead to age-related hearing loss (presbycusis).[8] The hearing loss generally begins in the high frequencies. Presbycusis may first affect the ability to understand speech and progress to impair the ability to detect and identify sounds.[9] The use of hearing aids may improve communication and quality of life for older adults with hearing impairment. However, only a few of those with hearing loss use hearing aids.[10] Impaired hearing can affect an older adult's ability to understand everything going on around them. It may also impair an elder abuse victim's ability to communicate with investigators and examiners.

Cardiovascular

The heart increases in size with age, mostly caused by an increase in left ventricular wall thickness. The myocardium and endocardium both thicken and the valves become thick and calcified. These changes can increase the risk for diastolic dysfunction and atrial fibrillation with age. Central arterial wall thickness increases with age and is accompanied by an increase in stiffness, leading to an increase in blood pressure.[11] Resting heart rate remains unchanged, but maximal heart rate decreases with age. Ejection fraction and resting cardiac output are not affected by age in the absence of disease. Systolic function is relatively preserved at rest, but exercise capacity significantly declines with age. The elderly have a limited ability to respond to physiologic stress, because cardiovascular reserve declines.[12] The cardiovascular responses to any stress (eg, trauma, catecholamine stimulation, fluid shifts) are markedly impaired in the older person. This impairment is associated with an increase in vulnerability, morbidity, and mortality. For example, an older adult who sustains an open fracture from an abuse incident may suffer shock, intensive care unit resuscitation, and death, whereas a younger adult might survive the injury, because the younger cardiovascular system has a more robust response. Not only survival but recovery from injury may also be significantly affected. The recovery time may be longer and fraught with complications.

Pulmonary

The chest wall becomes stiffer and less compliant with age. The elastic recoil of the lung tissue decreases with age. Although total lung capacity remains unchanged, there is an increase in residual volume and a decrease in vital capacity. FEV_1 (forced expiratory volume in first second of expiration) declines with age at a rate of about 0.33 L per decade.[13] There is a decrease in lower respiratory muscle strength and a weaker cough with age.[14] This factor may predispose older individuals to diaphragmatic and ventilatory failure when there is increased load on the respiratory system, which can occur with pneumonia or congestive heart failure.[15] All of these changes can result in decreased exercise tolerance, decreased pulmonary reserve, and increased risk for pneumonia. The aging lung is more vulnerable to respiratory or systemic stress than the respiratory system of young adults.

Muscle

Muscle mass decreases with age and the type II fibers (fast twitch) are selectively lost. Lipofuscin and fat are deposited in muscle tissue, and lost muscle tissue may be replaced with fibrous tissue. Water content decreases and cross-linking increases in tendons and ligaments, causing stiffness. There is a decline in joint range of motion, partly because of changes in tendons and ligaments. The amount of trauma required to produce an injury to one of these structures is decreased in an older individual compared with a younger individual. Muscles show a decrease in contractile force. Although some of this weakness can be mitigated with regular exercise, there is still some loss of strength that occurs with aging. Muscle weakness can cause limitations in activities of daily living, which can lead to loss of independence and increased risk for falls.[5] Weakness can also increase vulnerability to injury from trauma. For example, an older adult who has fallen or been pushed to the ground may not be able to rise from the floor. A long lie on the floor may then complicate any injuries that they sustained from the initial fall. In addition, an older adult who has sustained an injury may have more difficulty recovering from an injury, because of muscle weakness. An older adult who is being threatened may have more difficulty fleeing the threat.

Renal

There is a progressive decrease in renal blood flow and renal mass with age, along with a decrease in the number of functioning glomeruli. The glomerular filtration rate declines.[16] Although the creatinine clearance rate decreases, there is also a decrease in creatinine production (decreased muscle mass), and consequently, serum creatinine does not increase as much as expected. Serum creatinine may appear falsely normal. These changes make older adults more susceptible to the development of clinical conditions in response to stimuli that younger adults compensate for (such as acute kidney injury, dehydration).[17] Age-related conditions and medications can aggravate these changes. The renal system may retain function fairly well until it is challenged. Older adults may have more difficulty handling medications and are more susceptible to further kidney injury from stress. Medications can also be used as a form of abuse to harm an older adult. For example, an older adult may be more susceptible to toxic dosages of medication (eg, digitalis).

Gastrointestinal

Although aging does affect the gastrointestinal system in many ways, there is great reserve in the gastrointestinal tract when compared with other organ systems.[18] Loss of teeth, dental decay, and decreased salivation can cause problems with chewing and swallowing food. There is an increased risk for dysphagia and aspiration with aging. Peristalsis is slowed through the esophagus, and there is delayed transit time through the colon.[19] The liver preserves its function well with aging, and although there are changes that occur with hepatic function, the basic liver function remains normal. The liver does decrease in size with age, and this can lead to a decline in hepatic drug metabolism, making an older individual more prone to an adverse drug reaction.[20]

Neurologic

Cerebral atrophy and diminished cerebral perfusion are common age-related changes. There is a significant loss of white matter and, to a lesser extent, loss of neuronal tissue. There are some changes to neurotransmitters, receptors, and enzymes in the brain. These changes in the brain can cause older adults to experience minor slowing and change in cognition. The cognitive changes associated with normal aging include mild impairment in working memory (active manipulation and processing of information), task switching, mental rotation (visuospatial), and word finding (tip of the tongue).[21]

Aging is also associated with changes in the peripheral nervous system. The older adult may have impaired distal lower extremity proprioception, vibration, and discriminative touch as well as impaired balance.[22] These changes predispose older adults to falls. An older adult who is pushed off balance, even with a minor force, may fall in a situation in which a younger adult would not.

Reproductive

With aging, low estrogen results in vaginal dryness, shortening of the vagina, and narrowing of the introitus. In addition, the labia are thinned and the fat pad under the mons pubis is diminished. There is atrophy of the vaginal mucosa.[23] The genital examination may be difficult in an older woman because of these changes as well as arthritis and problems with positioning. Traumatic injuries could indicate sexual abuse. A sexual assault response team should be consulted when there is consideration for possible sexual abuse, so that evidence can be preserved and collected.

OVERVIEW OF COMMON CONDITIONS OF AGING (GERIATRIC SYNDROMES)

On top of the age-related changes described in the preceding section, there are certain diseases or conditions that occur more commonly with increasing age. For example, there is an increase in the frequency of hypertension, diabetes, cancer, stroke, heart disease, and neurocognitive disorders. With most of these conditions, there is an increased vulnerability to abuse and neglect. **Table 2** lists common conditions and their possible impact in elder abuse. Several of the more common geriatric conditions are discussed in detail.

Delirium

Delirium is an acute decline in cognitive functioning, which affects nearly 50% of older adults in hospital. This acute change in cognition is typically multifactorial. In an elderly patient with predisposing factors (dementia, multiple medical problems), an insult (such as a medication or procedure) that might otherwise be fairly benign can cause delirium. Key diagnostic features include inattention, impaired consciousness, and disturbance in cognition (disorientation, memory impairment, language changes).[24] Older patients who are delirious are at risk for falling. They may have behavioral problems, such as restlessness, agitation, and hallucinations, which could be difficult for

Table 2
How common geriatric conditions may affect risk and detection of elder abuse

Condition/Syndrome	Effect on Risk and Detection of Elder Abuse
Delirium	Difficulty obtaining history Poor decision making If documents signed, did the patient have capacity at that time? Behaviors (agitation, hallucinations) may increase risk for abuse
Dementia	Difficulty obtaining history Poor decision making If documents signed, did the patient have capacity at that time? Behaviors (agitation, sleep problems, hallucinations) known to increase risk for abuse
Depression	Poor concentration Effect on decision making Less reporting of abuse
Urinary incontinence	Increased risk for skin wounds/pressure ulcers Increased burden of care Social isolation Increased risk for falls
Falls	Increased risk for injuries Possible long lie on floor Possible fear of falling
Osteoporosis	Increased risk for fracture with less force
Vision/hearing impairment	Increased risk for falls Difficulty communicating Social isolation Unable to read a document; forced to sign without reading May be assumed to have dementia
Substance abuse	Increased risk for falls Possible depression Social isolation May not recognize poor care
Polypharmacy	Increased risk for falls Possible confusion (high-risk medications)
Frailty	Increased risk for falls Increased risk for injuries Higher morbidity/mortality when stressed (injury, pain)
Decreased physical function	Increased risk for falls Dependency
Social issues	Social isolation: increased risk for abuse Loneliness Depression

caregivers to manage. In addition, patients who are delirious could be coerced into making decisions or signing documents that they cannot understand. Delirium may be a marker of elder abuse (eg, in an elder who is purposefully overmedicated).

Dementia/Neurocognitive Disorder

Dementia is a progressive neurodegenerative condition, which is estimated to affect 3.4 million Americans and 35 million persons worldwide.[25] Dementia (known as major neurocognitive disorder in the *Diagnostic and Statistical Manual of Mental Disorders*,

Fifth Edition) is characterized by a decline in cognitive function that is severe enough to cause functional decline (problems performing activities of daily living or instrumental activities of daily living). Alzheimer disease is the most prevalent cause of dementia, accounting for about 60% of all dementias. Other types of dementia include vascular dementia, dementia with Lewy bodies, and mixed types of dementia. Mild cognitive impairment (MCI, known as mild neurocognitive disorder) is defined as cognitive impairment not affecting function. Many patients with MCI progress to having dementia. Although the hallmark of dementia is cognitive impairment, noncognitive manifestations are common and can cause functional disability and distress for both the patient and the caregiver. These manifestations include changes in mood, affect, and psychotic symptoms.[26] Because they are unable to perform daily functions, elders with dementia are dependent on others for care. This situation places them at risk for multiple forms of abuse and neglect.

Lower levels of cognitive functioning, mini-mental state examination scores, episodic memory, and perceptual speed have been found to be associated with an increased risk for elder abuse.[27] Older adults with cognitive impairment, neurocognitive disorder (dementia), depression, and delirium may have behavioral manifestations. Behavioral disturbances such as agitation, aggression, disinhibition, hallucinations, and sleep problems are common in people with dementia[28] and are associated with abuse in several studies.[29–31] A possible mechanism of this situation is that disruptive or aggressive behaviors could cause caregiver stress and potentially provoke retaliation.[32] If a caregiver is unable or unwilling to provide care, they may be neglecting the person whose care has been entrusted to them. Even MCI makes an elder susceptible to financial abuse and undue influence.

Depression

Up to 10% of older adults seen in primary care clinics have depression. Major depressive disorder may present differently in older adults compared with younger adults, and risk factors change as well. Somatic complaints of pain, change in weight/appetite, irritability, agitation, fatigue, headache, insomnia, cognitive changes, and weakness can all be presenting symptoms of depression in older patients.[26] Older patients with depression can also present with psychotic symptoms. Because of cognitive or concentration problems, these patients may be vulnerable to many forms of abuse, neglect, or self-neglect. In addition, feelings of worthlessness or apathy could affect decisions and create a high risk for undue influence. In addition, older adults who are abused may have depressive symptoms. Depression could either make a person susceptible to abuse or be the result of an abusive situation.

Urinary Incontinence

Urinary incontinence (UI) is the involuntary leakage of urine, which may affect up to 55% of women and 34% of men older than 65 years.[33] Older adults with UI report worse quality of life and more social isolation than those without UI. It is associated with an increased risk for falls and fractures, as well as admission to nursing homes. UI may also be associated with dermatitis and pressure ulcers. It can be a source of frustration for caregivers. Older adults with UI may be vulnerable to multiple forms of abuse: neglect (being left on toilet too long, pressure ulcers), psychological abuse (name calling or inappropriate caregiver responses), and physical abuse (inappropriate use of catheters). Because the incontinent older adult may isolate themselves, they are at higher risk for other forms of abuse. Incontinence is one of the common health problems found in older people who neglect themselves.[34]

Falls

One-third of older persons living in the community have at least 1 fall per year. Among nursing home residents or persons older than 80 years, this figure increases to one-half. There are many factors that can predispose an older adult to a fall: intrinsic changes in the individual (medications, illness), environment (slippery floor, rug), and situation (change in position, risky behavior).[35] The sequelae of falls can be serious. Injuries include soft tissue damage, fractures, and subdural hematomas and can lead to chronic pain or even death.[36] An older adult who falls may have significant fear of falling and may restrict their own activities out of fear. This situation can lead to social isolation or dependency, both of which may increase vulnerability to abuse.

Clearly, it is often difficult to differentiate whether an injury seen in an older adult was caused by a fall versus intentionally inflicted. For example, when a confused older adult presents to the emergency room with facial bruising and a humerus fracture, a fall may be in the differential diagnosis, because falls are common. Why did the fall occur? Did the person fall or were they pushed? Without a history or a witness to the event, a clinician must evaluate the individual, the environment, the situation, and the injuries in making a determination of abuse versus a fall.

Osteoporosis

Osteoporosis is a common disease that is characterized by low bone mass, changes in bone structure, and bone fragility, resulting in an increased risk for fracture.

The National Osteoporosis Foundation has estimated that more than 10 million Americans have osteoporosis and an additional 33.6 million have low bone density of the hip. About 1 of every 2 white women experience an osteoporosis-related fracture at some point in their lifetime, as do approximately 1 in 5 men.[37] This is a common problem for older adults (men and women) and confounds elder abuse issues. It is clear that an older adult who falls or is pushed and falls may more easily fracture a hip, vertebrae, or wrist. In addition, an older adult who has experienced inflicted trauma may more easily suffer a fracture than a younger adult. The confounding factor is that so many older adults suffer fractures from an accidental fall that identifying the elder who has suffered a fracture from abuse or neglect (being left alone when requiring 24-hour care) can be difficult.

Conditions That Affect Sensory Systems

Vision and hearing loss are common among older adults. Hearing loss affects at least 25% of patients older than 50 years and more than 50% of those older than 80 years.[38] In the elderly, hearing loss can impair the exchange of information, thus significantly affecting everyday life, causing loneliness, isolation, dependence, and frustration, as well as communication disorders.[39] Vision impairment caused by cataracts, macular degeneration, or glaucoma is estimated to affect 1 in 2 senior Americans by the year 2030.[40] Older people with visual impairment participate in activities less than their peers, have less social interaction, feel lonelier, and are at risk for developing depressive symptoms.[41]

Sensory impairment can lead to impairment in function: less ability to keep track of finances, keep the home clean, and take medications. Older adults with sensory impairment may be more dependent on a caregiver. Impairment in hearing or vision could make it more difficult for an older adult to be aware of everything going on around them. For example, they may be unable to read a document they are to sign or to hear a full discussion about their wishes or needs. Because vision and hearing impairment are so common, many victims of elder abuse or neglect are affected by one of these conditions and some have both. Sensory impairment can affect the elder's ability to report an abusive situation and the health care provider's ability to interview the victim. When investigating a case of abuse and neglect, hearing or vision impairment can make the interview and evaluation process more difficult. Assistive devices, such as a voice amplifier, may be useful in working with these victims.

Substance Abuse

Alcohol abuse is a major issue among older adults. A 2012 National Survey on Drug Use and Health found that 8.3% of adults 65 years and older reported binge drinking, defined as having 4 or 5 drinks on 1 occasion in the past month, whereas the rate of heavy drinking was 2%.[42]

Abuse of other substances and prescription drugs is less prevalent in today's older population, but it is thought that the baby boomers will bring an increase in illicit drug use with them as they age.[43] Abuse of alcohol and other substances is dangerous enough in itself. Adding aging-related physiologic changes and common medical conditions may increase the older adult's sensitivity to the effects of the substance used. Medications can also interact with alcohol or other substances.[44] Substance abuse may impair an older adult's ability to perform their activities of daily living, affecting function as well as relationships with others. There has also been evidence that elder mistreatment is associated with substance abuse, either in the victim or the abuser. Substance abuse may contribute to a risky living environment for an older adult and may hamper the reporting and investigation of abuse or neglect.[45] For example, an older adult using an illicit substance may not be aware of a lack of care from caregivers (neglect) or self (self-neglect).

Polypharmacy

Polypharmacy is often defined as the use of 5 or more medications.[46] Studies have shown that polypharmacy is common in the older population, estimating that 50% of individuals aged 65 years or older receive an average of 5 or more medications.[47] These medications may or may not be appropriate, but the risk for adverse drug events in patients 65 years and older increases as more medications are prescribed. The risk for adverse drug events increases exponentially with the number of medications, from 13% in people who take 2 medications to 58% in people who take 5 medications and to 82% in people who take 7 medications.[48] Adverse drug events are responsible for approximately 100,000 hospitalizations among older persons each year.[49] In addition, an increase in exposure to high-risk medications (such as benzodiazepines, opiates, antidepressants, and antipsychotics) has been associated with outcomes such as falls, fractures, impaired physical function, impaired cognition, and increased mortality in older people.[50] These outcomes can in turn increase the older individual's risk for abuse or neglect. Medications can also be used as a tool to abuse or neglect an older adult: overmedicate, undermedicate, or mismedicate. An example is to give a drug originally prescribed for neuropathy and use it at a higher dose to sedate. Another example is a caregiver who threatens not to give an older adult their pain medicine unless they sign over the house.

Frailty

Frailty is a clinical state of increased vulnerability resulting from aging-associated decline in reserve and function across multiple physiologic systems such that the ability to cope with stressors is compromised.[51] Fried and colleagues[52] developed 5 criteria for frailty: low grip strength, low energy, slowed walking speed, low physical activity, or unintentional weight loss. It is thought that as many as 40% of adults aged 80 years and older are frail, and most of the 1.6 million elderly nursing home residents in the United States are frail.[53]

Frail elders have difficulty in maintaining function when faced with stressors (illness, injury, environmental stressors). Frailty is closely associated with falls, hospitalization, comorbidity, functional limitations, disability, and death[52]; it has also been shown to be a risk factor for elder abuse.[30] Frailty can be a confounding factor in assessing older adults with injuries. The frailty has placed the older adult at a higher risk for injuries and has placed them at a higher risk for abuse. In addition, when a frail older adult is abused or neglected, they may have more severe injuries and less ability to recover.

Conditions That Affect Physical Function

There are multiple medical conditions more common in aging that affect physical function in older adults. Arthritis is common (one of the most common reasons for outpatients visits by older adults) and can be responsible for alteration in function, increased risk for falls and injuries, and decreased quality of life. Heart conditions such as congestive heart failure (the most common cause of hospitalization in older adults) can significantly impair functioning, increase risk for falls, and increase medication use. Neurologic conditions such as Parkinson disease and stroke can certainly impair function and increase risk for falls and injury as well as causing cognitive impairment. Functional dependency has been shown to be a risk factor for elder abuse in multiple studies.[30] In addition, many of these conditions are treated with multiple medications, which can increase risk for falls or injuries. Certain conditions may require the use of anticoagulant medications, aspirin, or antiplatelet agents, which can affect bleeding and bruising. These factors can be confounding in investigating possible abuse.

Functional impairment causes an older adult to be dependent on others for care. This situation could increase the opportunities for abuse. Regardless of age group, having a disability or a long-term physical, mental, or other health problem increases the likelihood of reporting emotional/financial or physical/sexual abuse.[54] The normal physiologic changes of aging compounded by a medical problem, or several chronic medical problems, increase the functional dependence. In addition, when older adults are dependent on others, the persons who come into the home to help them may have easier access to the elder and their finances and they may not be adequately scrutinized.[55] The older adult may feel less in control and more at the mercy of a caregiver, potentially setting the stage for abuse or neglect.[56]

Social Issues Affecting Older Adults

The older adult is faced with multiple social issues that can affect function and increase risk for abuse, neglect, or self-neglect. Aging is associated with changes in work, relationships, sexuality, social support, health, and at times, environment. Loss and bereavement are common issues among older adults and predispose to depression or isolation. Loneliness has been defined as a subjective negative feeling associated with a perceived lack of a wider social network or the absence of a specific desired companion. Rates of severe loneliness among adults aged 65 years and older range from 2% to 16%.[57] Social isolation has been defined as the objective lack or paucity of social contacts and interactions with family members, friends, or the wider community.[57]

Both loneliness and social isolation have been linked to elder abuse.[30,58,59] Low level of social support was found in 1 study to be a risk factor, with one of the highest odds ratios.[30] Social isolation could be the result of loss of loved ones but could also result from any impairment in function. Social isolation could be disease imposed (stroke, dementia) or self-imposed (depression, hearing impairment). Social isolation and lack of support may also impair an elder abuse victim's ability to recover from the abuse or neglect.

ELDER MISTREATMENT: DIFFICULTY IN DIAGNOSIS AND RECOVERY

The physiologic changes of aging as well as the common conditions associated with aging discussed earlier increase vulnerability to abuse, neglect, and self-neglect. When an older adult is a victim of abuse, the likelihood of injury is higher, and the severity of the injury may be greater. In addition, there are many factors that make their ability to recover from abuse more difficult. Elders who experienced abuse or self-neglect have shorter survival after adjusting for other factors associated with increased mortality in older adults.[60] Bruises, lacerations, and abrasions may take longer to heal. Fractures may also take longer to heal because of compromised bone regeneration capacity in the elderly patient.[61] Older adults are more likely to have compromised reserve because of the physiologic changes of aging. They may also have diseases that specifically affect their heart, lungs, and kidneys and restrict their ability to maintain homeostasis when faced with a stressor such as blood loss, severe injury, or pain. In these cases, if the victim sustains an injury that requires surgery, for example, the injury itself may be survivable, but the surgery may cause a stress that the elder cannot survive. Another example is that an injury may exacerbate underlying illness, which could lead to more severe illness or death.[62] Certainly, in cases of frailty, the elder who is victimized may suffer severe consequences from a seemingly minor injury.

For older adults, the psychological effects of being victimized can be severe. Victims of elder abuse have significantly higher levels of psychological distress than older adults who have not been victimized. Social support seems to be protective to some degree.[63] If an older victim does not have an adequate social support network, it may be more difficult for them to recover from the psychological effects of the abuse.

A health care provider who is evaluating an older adult with signs of abuse, neglect, or self-neglect must attempt to determine the likelihood that abuse or neglect occurred. This can often be a difficult task, because the same conditions that make an older adult vulnerable to abuse can sometimes cause or exacerbate injuries or signs that can appear to be abuse related. Confounding this problem is that many of the victims may have some degree of cognitive impairment and the inability to tell the story of how an injury occurred. The consideration of these underlying conditions must be balanced with the realization that these patients are vulnerable to abuse and neglect. History obtained from several sources, review of records, and careful examination of patterns of injuries can be useful in evaluating these cases.

Consider further the earlier scenario:

The patient was more alert after fluid boluses were given. He still could not tell you the year and did not remember a fall. His caregiver never arrived at the emergency room, but his daughter (who usually resided in another state) explained that his caregiver was his daughter-in-law and that she had not been allowing his daughter to visit or speak with him on the telephone. When you spoke with his daughter-in-law on the telephone, she said that she was the caregiver. She stated that he was confused, incontinent, and agitated and that he fell frequently. She admitted that she was frustrated with how much work it was to care for him and that she did not think she should have to be his caregiver because she was not his daughter. She did not plan to come to the emergency room because she was "too busy."

In evaluating this case, there were many physiologic changes, medical conditions, and medications that increased this patient's risk for a fall and also placed him at higher risk for abuse. He had the skin of a 70-year-old man (thin, less subcutaneous fat, more prone to bruising) and was on several medications that can increase bruising (aspirin and clopidogrel). He had cognitive impairment with agitation reported by his caregiver, who sounded frustrated and overwhelmed. He also had visual impairment, depression, and incontinence. He was not able to give a clear history, but the injuries on his shoulder, arm, and chest appeared to be significant and difficult to explain from a fall or even several falls. Although this patient was clearly at risk for falls (medications, visual impairment, dementia, balance problems), the injuries and his risk factors for abuse suggested a high likelihood for abuse in this case. Adult Protective Services and law enforcement were contacted. Careful documentation and photographs were undertaken.

REFERENCES

1. Available at: http://www.census.gov/compendia/statab/2012/tables/12s0009.pdf. Accessed February 1, 2014.
2. McCullough JL, Kelly KM. Prevention and treatment of skin aging. Ann N Y Acad Sci 2006;1067:323–31.
3. Chan GK, Duque G. Age-related bone loss: old bone, new facts. Gerontology 2002;48:62–71.
4. Duque G, Troen BR. Osteoporosis. In: Halter JB, Ouslander JG, Tinetti ME, et al, editors. Hazzard's geriatric medicine and gerontology. 6th edition. New York: McGraw Hill Medical; 2009. p. 1421–34.
5. Loeser RF, Delbono O. Aging of the muscles and joints. In: Halter JB, Ouslander JG, Tinetti ME, et al, editors. Hazzard's geriatric medicine and gerontology. 6th edition. New York: McGraw Hill Medical; 2009. p. 1355–68.
6. McNabney MK, Fedarko NS. Biology. In: Durso SC, Sullivan GM, editors. Geriatrics review syllabus: a core curriculum in geriatric medicine. 8th edition. New York: American Geriatrics Society; 2013. p. 9–19.
7. Salvi SM, Akhtar S, Currie Z. Ageing changes in the eye. Postgrad Med J 2006; 82:581–7.
8. Howarth A, Shone GR. Ageing and the auditory system. Postgrad Med J 2006; 82:166–71.
9. Gates GA, Mills JH. Presbycusis. Lancet 2005;366:1111–20.
10. Chien W, Lin FR. Prevalence of hearing aid use among older adults in the United States. Arch Intern Med 2012;172(3):292–3.
11. Laurent S. Defining vascular aging and cardiovascular risk. J Hypertens 2012; 30(Suppl 1):S3–8.
12. Dai D, Chen T, Johnson SC, et al. Cardiac aging: from molecular mechanisms to significance in human health and disease. Antioxid Redox Signal 2012;16(12): 1492–526.
13. Enright PL. Aging of the respiratory system. In: Halter JB, Ouslander JG, Tinetti ME, et al, editors. Hazzard's geriatric medicine and gerontology. 6th edition. New York: McGraw Hill Medical; 2009. p. 983–6.
14. Enright PL, Kronmal RA, Manolio TA, et al. Respiratory muscle strength in the elderly. Correlates and reference values. Cardiovascular Health Study Research Group. Am J Respir Crit Care Med 1994;149(2 Pt 1):430.
15. Sharma G, Goodwin J. Effect of aging on respiratory system physiology and immunology. Clin Interv Aging 2006;1(3):253–60.
16. Presta P, Lucisano G, Fuiano L, et al. The kidney and the elderly: why does the risk increase? Int Urol Nephrol 2012;44:625–32.
17. Musso CG, Oreopoulos DG. Aging and physiological changes of the kidneys including changes in glomerular filtration rate. Nephron Physiol 2011;119(Suppl 1):1–5.

18. Hall KE. Effect of aging on gastrointestinal function. In: Halter JB, Ouslander JG, Tinetti ME, et al, editors. Hazzard's geriatric medicine and gerontology. 6th edition. New York: McGraw Hill Medical; 2009. p. 1059–64.
19. Salles N. Basic mechanisms of the aging gastrointestinal tract. Dig Dis 2007;25: 112–7.
20. Anantharaju A, Feller A, Chedid A. Aging liver. Gerontology 2002;48:343–53.
21. Drag LL, Bieliauskas LA. Contemporary review 2009: cognitive aging. J Geriatr Psychiatry Neurol 2010;23(2):75–93.
22. Shaffer SW, Harrison AL. Aging of the somatosensory system: a translational perspective. Phys Ther 2007;87:193–207.
23. Lindau ST. Sexuality, sexual function, and the aging woman. In: Halter JB, Ouslander JG, Tinetti ME, et al, editors. Hazzard's geriatric medicine and gerontology. 6th edition. New York: McGraw Hill Medical; 2009. p. 567–81.
24. Inouye SK, Westendorp RG, Saczynski JS. Delirium in elderly people. Lancet 2013. http://dx.doi.org/10.1016/S0140-6736(13) 60688-1.
25. Available at: http://careforyou.us/latest-dementia-statistics-from-the-world-health-organization/. Accessed February 1, 2014.
26. Downing LJ, Caprio TV, Lyness JM. Geriatric psychiatry review: differential diagnosis and treatment of the 3 Ds: delirium, dementia and depression. Curr Psychiatry Rep 2013. http://dx.doi.org/10.1007/s11920-013-0365-4.
27. Dong X, Simon M, Rajan K, et al. Association of cognitive function and risk for elder abuse in a community-dwelling population. Dement Geriatr Cogn Disord 2011;32:209–15.
28. Gauthier S, Cumming J, Ballard C, et al. Management of behavioral problems in Alzheimer's disease. Int Psychogeriatr 2010;22(3):346–72.
29. Friedman LS, Avila S, Tanouye K, et al. A case-control study of severe physical abuse of the elderly. J Am Geriatr Soc 2011;59(3):417–22.
30. Johannesen M, LoGiudice D. Elder abuse: a systematic review of risk factors in community-dwelling elders. Age Ageing 2013;42:292–8.
31. Wiglesworth A, Mosqueda L, Mulnard R, et al. Screening for abuse and neglect of people with dementia. J Am Geriatr Soc 2010;58(3):493–500.
32. Lachs MS, Pillemer K. Elder abuse. Lancet 2004;364:1263–72.
33. Couture JA, Valiquette L. Urinary incontinence. Ann Pharmacother 2000;34(5): 646–55.
34. Ernst JS, Smith CA. Adult protective services clients confirmed for self-neglect: characteristics and service use. J Elder Abuse Negl 2011;23: 289–303.
35. Berry SD, Kiel DP. Falls. In: Durso SC, Sullivan GM, editors. Geriatrics review syllabus: a core curriculum in geriatric medicine. 8th edition. New York: American Geriatrics Society; 2013. p. 261–9.
36. Karlsson MK, Magnusson H, von Schewelov T, et al. Prevention of falls in the elderly–a review. Osteoporos Int 2012. http://dx.doi.org/10.1007/s00198-012-2256-7.
37. National Osteoporosis Foundation. Clinician's guide to prevention and treatment of osteoporosis. 2010. Available at: http://www.nof.org/files/nof/public/content/file/344/upload/159.pdf. Accessed February 1, 2014.
38. Walker JJ, Cleveland LM, Davis JL, et al. Audiometry screening and interpretation. Am Fam Physician 2013;87(1):41–7.
39. Ciorba A, Bianchini C, Pelucchi S, et al. The impact of hearing loss on the quality of life of elderly adults. Clin Interv Aging 2012;7:159–63.
40. Eichenbaum JW. Geriatric vision loss due to cataracts, macular degeneration and glaucoma. Mt Sinai J Med 2012;79:276–94.

41. Renaud J, Bédard E. Depression in the elderly with visual impairment and its association with quality of life. Clin Interv Aging 2013;8:931–43.

42. Available at: http://www.samhsa.gov/data/NSDUH/2012SummNatFindDetTables/NationalFindings/NSDUHresults2012.htm#ch3.1.1. Accessed March 16, 2014.

43. Wang YP, Andrarde LH. Epidemiology of alcohol and drug use in the elderly. Curr Opin Psychiatry 2013;26(4):343–8.

44. Wu LT, Blazer DG. Illicit and nonmedical drug use among older adults: a review. J Aging Health 2011;23(3):481–504.

45. Jogerst GJ, Daly JM, Galloway LJ, et al. Substance abuse associated with elder abuse in the United States. Am J Drug Alcohol Abuse 2012;38:63–9.

46. Salazar JA, Poon I, Nair M. Clinical consequences of polypharmacy in elderly: expect the unexpected, think the unthinkable. Expert Opin Drug Saf 2007; 6(6):695–704.

47. Linton A, Garber M, Fagan NK, et al. Examination of multiple medication use among TRICARE beneficiaries aged 65 years and older. J Manag Care Pharm 2007;13(2):155–62.

48. Budnitz DS, Lovegrove MC, Shehab N, et al. Emergency hospitalizations for adverse drug events in older Americans. N Engl J Med 2011;365(21):2002–12.

49. Hitzeman N, Belsky K. Appropriate use of polypharmacy for older patients. Am Fam Physician 2013;87(7):483–4.

50. Hilmer SN, Gnjidic D. The effects of polypharmacy in older adults. Clin Pharmacol Ther 2008;85(1):86–8.

51. Xue Q. The frailty syndrome: definition and natural history. Clin Geriatr Med 2011;27(1):1–15. http://dx.doi.org/10.1016/j.cger.2010.08.009.

52. Fried LP, Tangen CM, Walston J, et al. Frailty in older adults: evidence for a phenotype. J Gerontol A Biol Sci Med Sci 2001;56:M146–56.

53. Fried LP, Ferrucci L, Darer J, et al. Untangling the concepts of disability, frailty, and comorbidity: implications for improved targeting and care. J Gerontol A Biol Sci Med Sci 2004;59(3):M255–63.

54. Yon Y, Wister AV, Mitchell B, et al. A national comparison of spousal abuse in mid- and old age. J Elder Abuse Negl 2014;26:80–105.

55. Hafemeister TL. Financial abuse of the elderly in domestic settings. In: Bonnie RJ, Wallace RB, editors. Elder mistreatment: abuse, neglect, and exploitation in an aging America. Washington, DC: National Academies Press; 2003. p. 382–445.

56. Doyle S. The impact of power differentials on the care experiences of older people. J Elder Abuse Negl 2014. http://dx.doi.org/10.1080/08946566.2013.875970.

57. Valtorta N, Hanratty B. Loneliness, isolation and the health of older adults: do we need a new research agenda? J R Soc Med 2012;105:518–22.

58. Dong X, Simon MA, Gorbien M, et al. Loneliness in older Chinese adults: a risk factor for elder mistreatment. J Am Geriatr Soc 2007;55:1831–5.

59. Bonnie RJ, Wallace RB, editors. Elder mistreatment: abuse, neglect, and exploitation in an aging America. Washington, DC: National Academies Press; 2003.

60. Lachs MS, Williams CS, O'Brien S, et al. The mortality of elder mistreatment. JAMA 1998;280(5):428–32.

61. Gruber R, Koch H, Doll BA, et al. Fracture healing in the elderly patient. Exp Gerontol 2006;41:1080–93.

62. Paranitharan P, Pollanen MS. The interaction of injury and disease in the elderly: a case report of fatal elder abuse. J Forensic Leg Med 2009;16(6):346–9.

63. Comijs HC, Penninx BW, Knipscheer KP, et al. Psychological distress in victims of elder mistreatment: the effects of social support and coping. J Gerontol 1999; 54(4):240–5.

Understanding the Medical Markers of Elder Abuse and Neglect: Physical Examination Findings

Lisa M. Gibbs, MD

KEYWORDS

- Elder abuse • Elder neglect • Medical markers • Physical injury

KEY POINTS

- Physical examination is a foundation for detecting many types of abuse, including physical abuse, neglect, self-neglect, and sexual abuse.
- Knowledge of traumatic injuries, including patterns of injury, is important for health care providers who care for older adults.
- Physical findings suggestive of abuse must be evaluated within the context of the history, including functional status.
- Elder abuse should be included in the differential diagnosis for all injury evaluations in older adults.

INTRODUCTION

Incidents of elder abuse often involve physical examination findings. Evaluating these signs frequently requires knowledge of the physiology of normal aging as well as the pathophysiology of the injuries or abnormal findings. Physical findings that are suggestive of abuse must be placed within the context of history, including functional status, to be evaluated. Often, physical signs of elder abuse are mistaken for expected sequelae of aging, medications, or disease, as in the cases of bruising and ulcers, or accidental events, such as falls. Types of elder abuse associated with visible physical examination findings include physical abuse, neglect, self-neglect, and sexual abuse. Major physical findings of abuse are reviewed, along with patterns of injury and associated mechanisms, including those for bruises, burns, rashes, ulcers, head injuries, strangulation, and fractures. A thorough skin examination along with vague or inconsistent histories often provide the clues needed to identify abuse.

Division of Geriatric Medicine and Gerontology, Department of Family Medicine, University of California, Irvine, 101 The City Drive, Orange, CA 92868, USA
E-mail address: lgibbs@uci.edu

Clin Geriatr Med 30 (2014) 687–712
http://dx.doi.org/10.1016/j.cger.2014.08.002
0749-0690/14/$ – see front matter © 2014 Elsevier Inc. All rights reserved.

PHYSICAL FINDINGS ASSOCIATED WITH ELDER ABUSE
Trauma Involving Skin

Accidental skin injuries are common in older adults because of normal physiologic changes and skin damage from the sun. In normal aging, multiple changes in skin structure and function occur. Connections between the dermis and epidermis decrease, and, as a result, there is less nutrient transfer and an increase in fragility.[1] Also, there are fewer fat cells in the epidermis, and skin tends to be drier. The turnover of epidermal cells slows, so there is a decrease in healing rates.[1,2] In addition to normal changes, a lifetime of exposure to the sun accounts for changes known as dermatoheliosis in sun-exposed areas. These changes include dilation of small blood vessels and decrease of the integrity of the connective tissue. Uneven pigmentation and solar elastosis result.[1]

Because of the physiologic changes in aging skin, skin integrity is disrupted more easily, and there is a tendency to dismiss injuries as normal or expected events. This category includes injures such as bruises, contusions, tears, lacerations, and abrasions. Traumatic injuries caused by elder abuse are often missed because of these assumptions. However, skin findings from abuse can often be distinguished from accidental causes by applying forensic knowledge to an awareness of the possibility of abuse.

Bruising Characteristics

Knowledge of bruising is required to separate potential cases of elder abuse from accidental causes. Bruising, by definition, is the disruption of blood vessels caused by blunt force trauma. Bruising that is common in aging and sun-exposed skin occurs on the dorsal aspects of hands and arms and is referred to as senile purpura.[3] Steroid purpura occurs in areas of skin chronically treated with topical steroids, and systemic steroids increase purpura in areas of sun exposure and mild trauma.[4] Factors such as these make aging skin susceptible to bruising, even from mild trauma. Another example is atrophy in the skin and mucosa of menopausal women as a result of the decrease in estrogen levels.

By definition, hematomas result when the bleeding, or bruising, produces a raised surface. Bruises can also be complicated by abrasions and are then referred to as contusions.[5] Depending on the force and location of the trauma, bruises may occur in skin, soft tissues, muscle, and bone. Blood tracking is another characteristic of bruising that is important to the evaluation of injuries. Depending on the laxity of the tissues involved, extravasated blood follows gravity and flows through fascial planes so that the bruising appears at a site distal to the point of impact. Common areas include the face, where injury on the scalp or above the eye may result in bruises forming below the eye (**Fig. 1**).[6] Other examples, common in abuse, involve a subgaleal hematoma, in which blood travels to the forehead after traumatic hair pulling, and tracking in the perineum after genital trauma.[7] Basilar skull fractures are also associated with blood tracking, producing the Battle sign or raccoon eyes, discussed in the section on head trauma (**Fig. 2**).[6] In addition, in some cases, the extent of bleeding may be evident only after a delay, after blood tracks through fascial planes.

One of the most important aspects of traumatic bruises is their location. In 1 study,[8] the occurrence, progression, and resolution of accidental bruises were studied to compare accidental and traumatic bruising. Results of this observational study showed that 90% of accidental bruises occurred on the extremities. No accidental bruises were found on the neck, ears, genitalia, buttocks, or soles. In addition, 15% of the bruises were yellow within the first 24 hours of onset. Many bruises did not

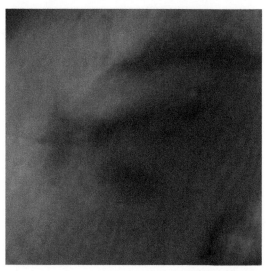

Fig. 1. Blood tracking inferior to eye. Point of impact is seen as yellow bruising lateral to the eye. (*Courtesy of* Center of Excellence on Elder Abuse and Neglect, University of California, Irvine, CA; with permission.)

follow the standardly accepted notions of color progression, in which, as the hemoglobin is broken down, the color of the bruising changes from red to blue and purple and then yellow and green.

This study was followed by another observational study,[9] which chronicled the appearance of bruises known to result from physical elder abuse. Not only did the locations differ significantly, but the inflicted bruises were larger, more than 5 cm (**Fig. 3**).

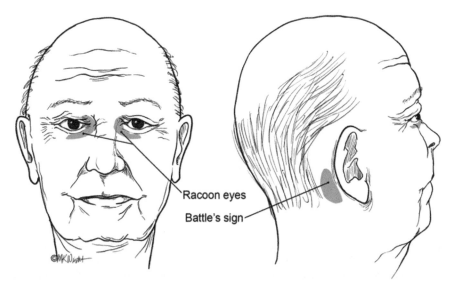

Racoon eyes

Battle's sign

Fig. 2. Signs of basilar skull fractures. (*Courtesy of* Center of Excellence on Elder Abuse and Neglect, University of California, Irvine, CA; with permission.)

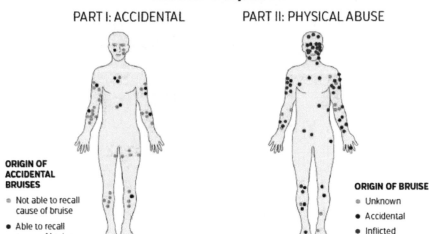

Anterior Comparison

PART I: ACCIDENTAL   PART II: PHYSICAL ABUSE

ORIGIN OF ACCIDENTAL BRUISES
- Not able to recall cause of bruise
- Able to recall cause of bruise

ORIGIN OF BRUISE
- Unknown
- Accidental
- Inflicted

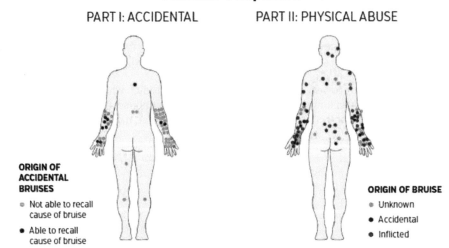

Posterior Comparison

PART I: ACCIDENTAL   PART II: PHYSICAL ABUSE

ORIGIN OF ACCIDENTAL BRUISES
- Not able to recall cause of bruise
- Able to recall cause of bruise

ORIGIN OF BRUISE
- Unknown
- Accidental
- Inflicted

Fig. 3. Locations of accidental bruising and bruising associated with physical elder abuse. (*Adapted from* Mosqueda L, Burnight K, Liao S. The life cycle of bruises in older adults. J Am Geriatr Soc 2005;53:1339–43. This study was supported by National Institute of Justice Grant 2001-IJ-CX-KO14; and *Data from* Wiglesworth A, Austin R, Corona M, et al. Bruising as a marker of physical elder abuse. J Am Geriatr Soc 2009;57:1191–6.)

Also, almost 90% of abused seniors recalled the cause of at least 1 bruise compared with only 25% of their peers with accidental bruises. In this study, bruises associated with abuse occurred on the lateral right arm, and to the head and neck. Other research has shown that the most severe injuries in elder abuse occur on the head (61%) and torso (31.7%).[10] A literature review of 9 studies, including 839 injuries, found that two-thirds occurred on the upper extremities and maxillofacial regions. Torso injuries accounted for 10% of the total. Compared with the previous study, many of the 839 injuries were milder in nature.[11] Suspicious or traumatic bruises may occur in atypical locations, such as the head, neck, chest, abdomen, genitalia, buttocks, palms, soles, and ears (**Figs. 4–8**). Bruising from sexual abuse is often located on the labia majora, labia minora, or posterior fourchette.[12] Bruises may show the pattern of the striking object if the bruise is superficial in nature and are then referred to as intradermal. However, if the bruise is in the deeper dermis, or subcutaneous tissues, then, the borders are poorly circumscribed or hazy. Pattern bruises may include, but are not limited to, fingertip or pad bruises, shoe stamps, belt buckles, and tramline bruises (**Figs. 9–11**). Tramline bruises are formed from cylindrical objects and appear as a pale linear central area bordered on both sides by linear bruises.[6] Other marks that may be associated with bruising include bite marks and abrasions from identifiable material.

Each bruise must be evaluated within context, especially those in atypical locations. For instance, common scenarios for chest bruising, aside from blunt trauma, may include the use of restraints (**Fig. 12**). Rough handling may result in bilateral bruises from fingertips on the upper extremities, on the neck from strangulation, or the inner thighs from sexual abuse.[13] Also, bruises in older adults may not follow the standard color progression, so dating the time of assault from appearance of the bruise may not be reliable in the elderly.[8] If multiple bruises of varying ages are found, they may indicate chronic physical abuse. In addition, experience has shown elder abuse experts that if innocuous or accidental bruising occurs in atypical areas, there is usually a convincing and logical history to explain its presence.

Other Skin Injuries

Other skin findings seen both with and without bruising include skin tears, avulsions, and lacerations. Skin tears also occur more commonly in aging skin, often on the outer proximal arms. Skin tears occur when there is separation of skin layers by shearing, friction, or blunt trauma and are classified as partial or full thickness. Abrasions involve scraping damage to the epidermis; avulsions are deep abrasions affecting all layers of the skin. Lacerations are irregular tearlike wounds from blunt trauma, such as to the elbow, knee, or eyebrow during a fall against a hard surface (**Fig. 13**).[14] Incised wounds are clean wounds caused by a sharp-edged object, such as a knife or razor, and are less likely to be accidental. Defensive stab wounds are found on the inner (volar) side of the wrist or forearm and are consistent with individuals trying to protect themselves by raising their arms in front of the body.[14] Although none of these skin

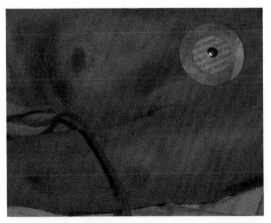

Fig. 4. Atypical bruising of the chest in a case of substantiated abuse. (*Courtesy of* Center of Excellence on Elder Abuse and Neglect, University of California, Irvine, CA; with permission.)

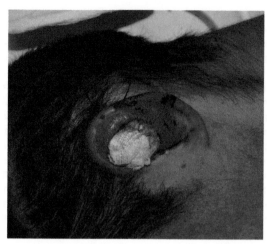

Fig. 5. Bruising of the ear, called boxer ear, in a case of substantiated abuse of a dependent adult. (*Courtesy of* L. Gibbs, MD, Orange, CA.)

findings is pathognomonic for elder abuse, understanding the injury in context may lead to a conclusion of abuse. However, some injuries occur commonly with certain acts of abuse. When lacerations and abrasions are noted in the genital area, for instance, sexual abuse must be considered, and explanations such as botched catheterization or rough perineal care recognized as excuses.[15]

Burns

A burn is a skin injury caused by heat, chemicals, electricity, or radiation. Burns are classified as first, second, or third degree. A first-degree burn is defined as heat damage to the epidermis, a second-degree burn to the dermis, and a third-degree burn to the deeper subcutaneous tissue. Although second-degree burns, also called partial-thickness burns, usually heal spontaneously, many third-degree, or full-thickness, burns require skin grafting.

Burn injuries from elder abuse are underreported, at times, with dire consequences. Missing a diagnosis of elder abuse caused by burns, as with other injuries, may result in continued abuse and mortality,[16] both from coexisting types of abuse and the burn injuries themselves. The mortality in burn patients older than 65 years is higher than that in the overall population with burns.[17] Most burn facilities do not have formal guidelines for abuse and neglect screening.[18]

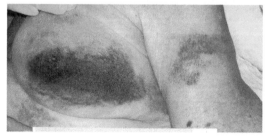

Fig. 6. Bruising across the breast and upper arm from blunt trauma. (*Courtesy of* L. Gibbs, MD, Orange, CA.)

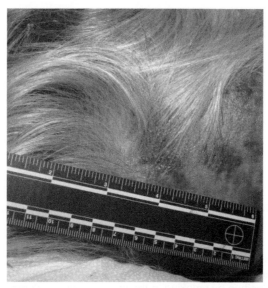

Fig. 7. Atypical bruising on the scalp. (*Courtesy of* Center of Excellence on Elder Abuse and Neglect, University of California, Irvine, CA; with permission.)

Some evidence suggests that elder abuse accounts for at least 10% of burns caused by battery and assault. In 1 review,[19] 4 of 41 victims of burns from assault were older adults residing in nursing homes. The abusers were caregivers. In a 1-year retrospective review,[20] 14% of burns in older adults (n = 28) resulted from neglect and physical abuse, and an additional 25% were caused by self-neglect. Total body surface area (TBSA) burned was highest in the neglected patients, all of whom died. Another retrospective study reported that almost 20% of geriatric patients with burns were residents of facilities, many with severe dementia. These burns covered a higher TBSA and resulted in higher mortality. The most common causes of burns were hot water scalds and radiator contact. Lack of appropriate supervision was noted as a contributing cause.

Adults older than 60 years have a significantly higher death rate for any given extent of burn.[21] Comorbid conditions such as diabetes, chronic obstructive pulmonary disease, and coronary artery disease worsen outcomes.[22] Of the burns caused by elder abuse, the most common precipitant seems to be neglect,[20,23] in which a caregiver negligently allows high-risk situations. In these cases, burns are most frequently

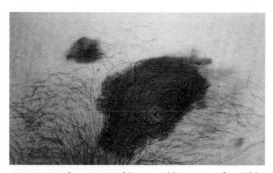

Fig. 8. Atypical hematoma on the suprapubic area. (*Courtesy of* L. Gibbs, MD, Orange, CA.)

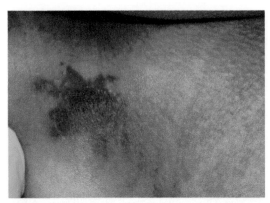

Fig. 9. Pattern bruise on the left buttock from unknown object. (*Courtesy of* L. Gibbs, MD, Orange, CA.)

caused by flames, scalding, and contact with hot surfaces (**Fig. 14**). Contact burns may be from heaters or radiators, scalding burns from hot water in the bathtub, and flame burns from ignition by smoking in the presence of supplemental oxygen.

Persons with dementia may lack the judgment necessary to avoid unsafe situations and depend on caregivers for ensuring safety. For those who lack safety judgment and do not have caregivers, a burn may be the first physical finding of self-neglect. Medical conditions may increase the risk of burns. For examples, older adults who suffer from peripheral neuropathy with lack of feeling in the lower extremities may not recognize a burning heat source until they have been burned. Intentional burn injuries may be inflicted by angry caregivers. In 1 case, a woman with advanced dementia suffered extensive second-degree burns to her back and buttocks after being dipped into a hot tub (**Fig. 15**).

Some burn injury findings studied in child abuse are applicable to elder victims. Such findings include scalds from hot water with or without the presence of splash marks. If one is able to struggle, burns likely include splash marks.[16] When victims, such as older adults who are immobile and unable to struggle because of movement disorders or contractures, suffer burns, they may not have splash marks. Uniformity of

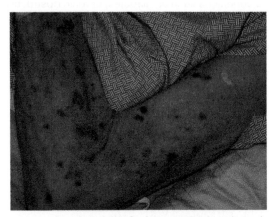

Fig. 10. Distinct bruising pattern from lying for hours on bird seed on a hard floor. (*Courtesy of* L. Gibbs, MD, Orange, CA.)

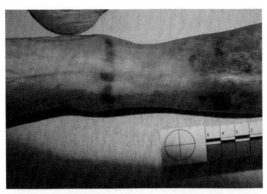

Fig. 11. Pattern bruising on lower leg from a ligature. (*Courtesy of* L. Gibbs, MD, Orange, CA.)

burn depth throughout the injury is believed to indicate that the victim was held still in the water. Bilateral, or stocking and glove injuries, imply that one has been forcibly immersed. Skin sparing with a surrounding burn area may be evident in flexed surfaces, palms, soles of the feet, or buttocks when in contact with a surface, such as a bath or sink. Burns from objects, such as cigarettes, heated metal objects, such as irons, and electrical shocks may leave recognizable pattern injuries.[16]

SKIN FINDINGS ASSOCIATED WITH NEGLECT AND SELF-NEGLECT
Rashes

The skin may harbor the first signs of neglect and poor hygiene by oneself or others. Findings often include unkempt fingernails and toenails, often thickened, long and dirty with onychogryphosis, dirty appearance of the skin, unkempt hair, poor oral dentition (**Fig. 16**), untreated skin cancers (**Fig. 17**), and rashes. Although many types of rashes occur frequently in the general population, persistent, recurrent, and severe rashes may indicate a delay in medical care. Moisture-associated skin damage (MASD) describes a group of rashes that includes incontinence-associated dermatitis (IAD), intertriginal dermatitis, and periwound maceration, among others. MASD is a common finding in neglect (**Fig. 18**). In the setting of IAD, the skin becomes irritated

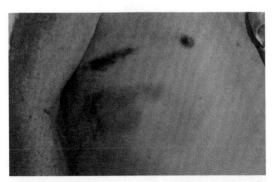

Fig. 12. Atypical bruising on the chest in a tramline fashion, possibly from the use of a restraint belt. (*Courtesy of* the Center of Excellence on Elder Abuse and Neglect, University of California, Irvine, CA; with permission.)

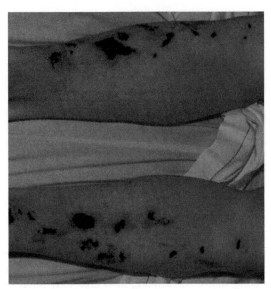

Fig. 13. Lacerations and abrasions cause by blunt trauma from steel-toed boots. (*Courtesy of* the Center of Excellence on Elder Abuse and Neglect, University of California, Irvine, CA; with permission.)

with prolonged exposure to urine and stool. Urea, from urine, damages the stratum corneum layer of the skin, making it vulnerable to friction and erosion. Wet skin, under pressure, has less blood flow than dry skin, which may contribute to infection and the formation of erosions and ulcers. Fecal enzymes are also damaging to the skin, and fecal bacteria may cause a secondary infection. Bacterial infection may cause abscesses or cellulitis, which may evolve into a life-threatening infection necessitating intravenous antibiotics and hospital care. In addition to bacterial infections, fungal infections often complicate IAD. Adults requiring containment devices such as incontinence pads, diapers, or other products are at increased risk. These are absorbent products that create an environment of heat and moisture, which predisposes skin

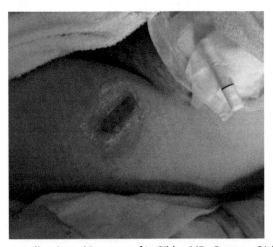

Fig. 14. Burn from a curling iron. (*Courtesy of* L. Gibbs, MD, Orange, CA.)

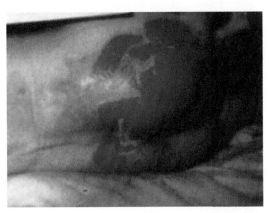

Fig. 15. Burn injuries on the back and buttocks from scalding water. (*Courtesy of* the Center of Excellence on Elder Abuse and Neglect, University of California, Irvine, CA; with permission.)

to damage.[24] Neglectful caregivers have been known to place multiple layers of adult diapers on care recipients to lessen their workloads, further exacerbating these conditions.

Intertrigo is a condition of skin inflammation between skin folds, which are prone to moisture and friction. Normally, skin folds, such as in the groin, axilla, and inframammary areas, are exposed to air and stay dry. However, adults with obesity, immobility, or contractures are particularly susceptible to intertriginal dermatitis. As with IAD, secondary infections from bacteria and fungus are common.[25] When rashes persist or worsen despite appropriate treatment, neglect should always be considered. This advice also includes rashes from dermatophytes, which cause lice and scabies.

Patients with dermatitis and skin infections suffer from itching and pain. Patients with dementia or expressive aphasia may lack the ability to voice their concerns about these symptoms. Others, dependent on the care of a threatening caregiver, may be fearful of complaining about their discomfort. Still others, such as those with severe dementia, may not understand the source of their pain. A routine thorough skin evaluation is indicated in the care of vulnerable adults.

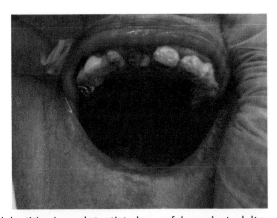

Fig. 16. Poor oral dentition in a substantiated case of dependent adult neglect. (*Courtesy of* L. Gibbs, MD, Orange, CA.)

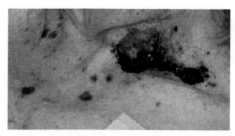

Fig. 17. Untreated skin cancer in a case of neglect of an older man with dementia. (*Courtesy of* the Center of Excellence on Elder Abuse and Neglect, University of California, Irvine, CA; with permission.)

Ulcers

Ulcers affect the integument and deeper structures and are associated with neglect and self-neglect rather than physical abuse. Ulcers are common, often preventable, and always treatable. All types of ulcers, including decubitus ulcers as well as venous, arterial, and diabetic ulcers, are common. Venous, arterial, and diabetic ulcers are not a direct result of immobility, but stem from underlying chronic medical conditions. Decubitus ulcers, or pressure sores, occur with medical conditions that lead to immobility. Timely and appropriate medical care of all ulcers is imperative, and lack of care, either by self or caregivers, may be considered neglect.

Venous ulcers make up 80% of all lower extremity ulcers.[26] Venous ulcers occur in the setting of chronic venous insufficiency, which may stem from incompetent valves, venous thrombosis, or calf-muscle pump failure. Risk factors include obesity, immobility, inflammatory conditions, and neuropathies. Venous ulcers usually occur in the gaiter area (between the midcalf and ankle). Increased venous pressures lead to inadequate oxygen perfusion to tissues, which then decompose, forming shallow ulcers, with irregular shapes and ragged borders. The surrounding skin becomes hardened with dyspigmentation. Elevating the legs above the level of the heart improves the edema.[26] Delays in care decrease the probability of healing, with the size and duration of venous ulcers portending prognosis. Almost two-thirds (64%) of ulcers are present for less than 1 year compared with 48% present for 1 to 3 years and 24% present for

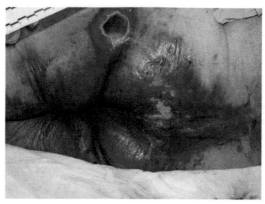

Fig. 18. Case of elder abuse neglect showing MASD and ulcers in the sacrum, buttocks, and thighs. (*Courtesy of* L. Gibbs, MD, Orange, CA.)

more than 3 years. Only 40% of ulcers larger than 5 cm heal.[26] Successful treatment requires specific medical expertise.

Arterial ulcers are a consequence of peripheral arterial disease and occur on the lower leg. The most common areas include the pretibial, supramalleolar (typically lateral), toes, and areas of minimal trauma to the foot. Arterial ulcers are painful and often worse when legs are elevated.[27] They appear as punched-out lesions with well-demarcated borders. Surrounding skin is pale and mottled. Peripheral arterial disease and consequent ulcers, if left untreated, place the patient at risk for infection, gangrene, and sepsis. In severe cases, amputation is required. Appropriate treatment includes wound care and evaluation by a vascular specialist.

Diabetic ulcers occur on the plantar surface of the foot over bony prominences, usually on the great toe and sole, over the first, second, or fifth metacarpophalangeal joints and heels. Ulcers are punched out, surrounded by a ring of callus, and may extend to underlying joint and bone.[28] Often, neuropathy is present, combined with impaired circulation. Routine care of diabetes is important, as is routine care of the feet. Ulcers, including diabetic ulcers, may be complicated by soft tissue infections, osteomyelitis, and sepsis. In 1 case series of fatal neglect, the cause of 8 deaths was sepsis as a result of severe decubitus ulcers and dehydration.[29]

Decubitus ulcers, also called pressure sores, or pressure ulcers, are a common finding in elder neglect. These pressure sores develop as a consequence of immobilization and prolonged pressure over bony prominences. Any condition which affects one's mobility, including advance stage dementias, Parkinson disease, stroke, frailty, and deconditioning, places an older adult at risk of developing ulcers. In addition, impairment of the microcirculatory system from diabetes, sepsis, and hypotension increase the risk.[30] Other contributing factors include moisture, nutrition, activity, friction, and shearing forces.[31]

Decubitus ulcers are staged in 4 levels, from the least to most severe, depending on the depth of the ulcer (**Fig. 19**). In addition, a decubitus ulcer may be categorized as unstageable or suspected deep tissue injury. Although the earliest sign of an impending ulcer is a blanchable erythematous area, a stage 1 ulcer is a nonblanchable and reddish section of intact skin. A stage 2, or partial-thickness, ulcer presents as a shallow open ulcer with a clean red wound base. A stage 3, or full-thickness, ulcer appears as a deeper ulcer with subcutaneous fat and may include undermining and tunneling. A stage 4 ulcer is deepest, exposing tendons, muscles, and, if progressive, the bone.[32] Unstageable ulcers represent areas covered with slough and eschar, which cannot be staged until the more superficial covering is removed and the true depth is determined. Suspected deep tissue injury occurs in cases in which the injury begins at the bony prominence or deep tissue layer and spreads to the skin. In this case, discolored intact skin may hide soft necrotic tissue underneath.[32,33] Common areas for decubitus ulcers include the sacrum, ischial tuberosities, trochanters, and heels, although ulcers can occur on almost any bony prominence, including the scapula and auricula, for those who lie on their sides, and the forehead from pressure bands (**Figs. 20–22**).

Even in the setting of immobility and risk factors, care management techniques are successful in preventing the development of most ulcers. The most well studied involves repositioning of pressure-sensitive areas of the body and support surfaces. Ideal repositioning increments vary from 2 to 3 hours.[34,35] Turning every 2 hours remains the most-cited standard, although 1 study evaluated repositioning every 4 hours with a specialized foam mattress.[36] Pressure-reducing surfaces are either static, standard mattresses and mattress overlays, or dynamic, such as alternating pressure mattresses.

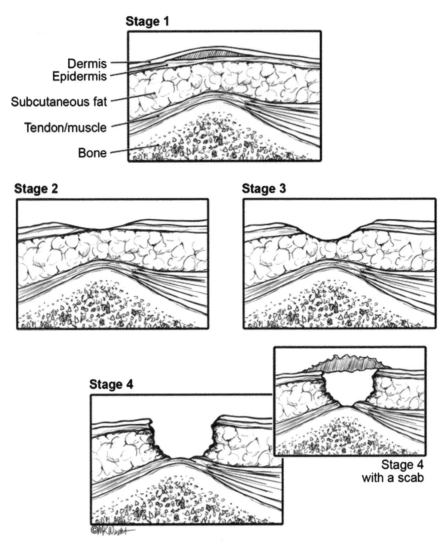

Fig. 19. Stages of decubitus ulcers. (*Courtesy of* the Center of Excellence on Elder Abuse and Neglect, University of California, Irvine, CA; with permission.)

The duration of time for ulcer development depends on many factors, including the habitus of the individual, area of pressure, extent of pressure (eg, prolonged), and underlying medical conditions. Ulcers can take hours[31] to days to develop and there is no standard formula for determining this period. The suffering that pressure ulcers cause is underappreciated. Pressure ulcers are painful, and medical professionals should pay attention to pain control, because it is typically undertreated.[32] In 1 study,[32] 87% of patients noted pain with dressing changes, and 84% reported pain at rest. Ongoing medical care by health care professionals, including wound care nursing, is integral to preventing and treating pressure ulcers. **Fig. 23** shows the many options for treating pressure ulcers.

Caregiver neglect is often evident when pressure ulcers are discovered in the absence of medical care, or when medical advice is not followed (**Figs. 24** and **25**).

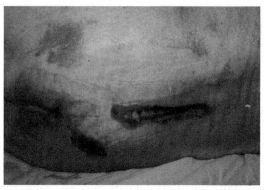

Fig. 20. Stage I and II ulcers on the buttocks and stage II to III on the lower back. Developed within 18 hours on a hard surface. (*Courtesy of* L. Gibbs, MD, Orange, CA.)

Investigators can check history for medical appointments, home health nursing visits, and for supplies, including dressing changes and mattresses. Neglectful caregivers may place the burden for lack of improvement on medical professionals. Therefore, a well-documented care plan with instructions for follow-up care by the health care team counters these assertions. Physicians should be cognizant of the home health care certification and recertification forms and examine the patient at regular intervals. If an ulcer is not improving, a new plan of care should be clearly documented. The medical record may be the key to confirming cases of caregiver neglect by investigators. Also, nursing home providers should be highly skeptical when a family member requests a home discharge for a patient with extensive care needs. In many cases of severe neglect, the motive is financial, and the caregiver is ill equipped to provide the high level of care needed, including frequent positioning, for pressure ulcer prevention and treatment as well as general care.

Medical professionals are often consulted to evaluate cases involving pressure ulcers. There is a long-standing controversy as to whether all pressure ulcers are preventable. One survey of experts in decubitus ulcer care[37] found that 62% of respondents believed that not all pressure ulcers occurring in nursing homes were preventable. Most agreed that pressure sores were not pathognomonic for neglect.

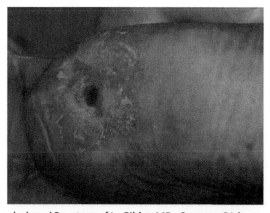

Fig. 21. Stage II heel ulcer. (*Courtesy of* L. Gibbs, MD, Orange, CA.)

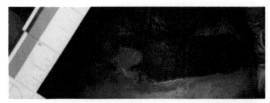

Fig. 22. Forehead ulcer with eschar from a gauze pressure dressing. The texture of the gauze is visualized. (*Courtesy of* L. Gibbs, MD, Orange, CA.)

Many experts believe that, given the multiple risk factors present in the development of ulcers, pressure ulcers can develop, even with the best care. As with all physical signs of abuse and neglect, pressure ulcers must be evaluated within medical, functional, and historical contexts.

Head, Face, and Neck Findings

Many older patients may present for health care with visible injuries on the head, face, and neck. Physical injuries in these areas may be the result of head trauma, including

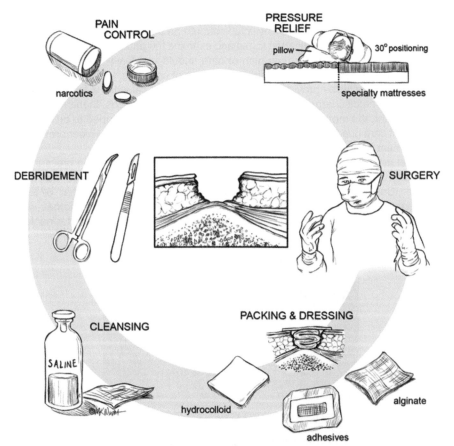

Fig. 23. Accoutrements for decubitus ulcer treatment. (*Courtesy of* the Center of Excellence on Elder Abuse and Neglect, University of California, Irvine, CA; with permission.)

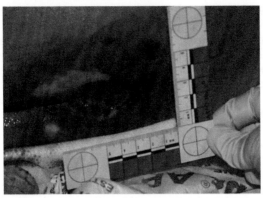

Fig. 24. Stage 3 sacral ulcer in a case of elder neglect. (*Courtesy of* L. Gibbs, MD, Orange, CA.)

skull fractures, traumatic brain injury (TBI), facial fractures, and strangulation. The head, neck, and face are the most common areas of injury in intimate partner violence (IPV) and elder abuse. In a study of 67 confirmed elder abuse cases,[38] 14.9% of the victims suffered significant injures to the head and neck region. Victims with head and neck injuries had 6, 8, and 14 times greater odds of endorsing that the abuser "beat me up," "choked me," and "punched me," respectively. Older adults are particularly vulnerable to injuries of the head and neck causing asphyxia and TBI, because of comorbid conditions such as stroke and dementia.

Strangulation

Strangulation is a well-recognized type of physical abuse in IPV, and the severity of episodes increases over time.[39] It is less well studied in elder abuse; however, there are many case reports of strangulation in older adults. In 1 study, older adults made up 7.4% of 134 victims who survived strangulation.[40] In another, older adults made up 7.4% of strangulation deaths by caregivers.[41] Consistent with other age groups, women older than 65 years were more likely to die from strangulation than men of

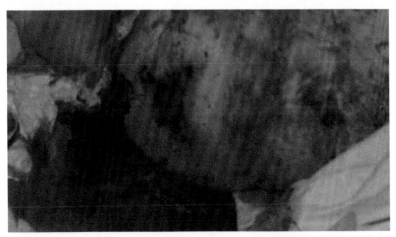

Fig. 25. Sacral decubitus ulcer embedded with feces in a case of elder neglect. (*Courtesy of* the Center of Excellence on Elder Abuse and Neglect, University of California, Irvine, CA; with permission.)

the same age (33% women vs 7% men).[42] Older adults are more susceptible to some injuries, including bleeding, fracture, and cerebral injury.

Strangulations have been categorized as light, moderate, and severe. Cases of light strangulation include superficial skin lesions. Moderate cases cause injuries to the soft tissues or the neck, pharynx, or larynx, and severe cases include signs of cerebral hypoxia, loss of consciousness, and loss of urine.[40] Some signs of injury, such as swelling to the neck, may be absent in the initial assessment.[43] Progressive, irreversible encephalopathy and neurologic sequelae caused by cerebral artery infarcts may present after strangulation.[44] External markings do not necessarily reflect the severity of the strangulation, and even in cases of fatal strangulation, there may be no external evidence.[45]

Physical signs of strangulation include patterned abrasions or contusions of the anterior neck (**Fig. 26**). These signs may be caused by fingernails, finger pads, ligatures, or clothing. Hand marks may be the victim's, produced while trying to get free. Alternatively, there may be no physical evidence of injury on the neck.[45] Alternative light sources used for evidence collections have been used to detect intradermal injuries in 98% of those victims who had no visible sign of external injury.[46]

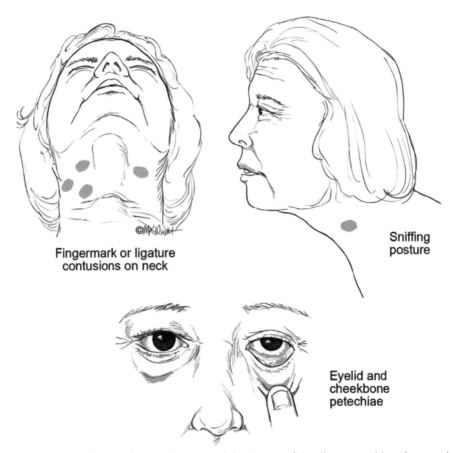

Fingermark or ligature contusions on neck

Sniffing posture

Eyelid and cheekbone petechiae

Fig. 26. Signs of strangulation. (*Courtesy of* the Center of Excellence on Elder Abuse and Neglect, University of California, Irvine, CA; with permission.)

Physical findings often include petechiae on the neck, head, face, forehead, eyes, ears, conjunctive, and buccal mucosa.[44] On autopsy, petechiae may be found on the undersurface of the scalp and internal organs. Petechiae are a sign of asphyxia from multiple causes, including strangulation,[45] and are also noted to occur with increased vascular congestion.[44] Hoarseness occurs in roughly half of strangulation cases,[43] and some victims may present with difficulty swallowing, dyspnea, and stridor[44] as well as assuming a sniffing position to assist with breathing (see **Fig. 26**). The hyoid bone and thyroid cartilage are more susceptible to fracture in older adults compared with younger victims.[43]

Although death from the carotid sinus reflex is uncommon, older patients may be more susceptible to cardiac arrest from sustained pressure on the carotid body caused by atherosclerosis.[47] Neurologic sequelae may include cerebral artery infarct, encephalopathy, and mental status changes caused by cerebral hypoxia and intracranial injury.[44] Although uncommon, damage to the intimal layer of the carotid artery may induce thrombosis of the artery or an embolus to distal cerebrovascular circulation.[43] Older adults, because of aging physiology, comorbid conditions, history of cognitive impairment, dementia, or stroke are even more susceptible to cerebral injury. One study[48] reported that 34% of strangulation victims had been strangled multiples times, increasing the risk of recurrent hypoxia.

One's choice of words is important when questioning alleged strangulation victims about what occurred. Asking whether a victim was choked rather than strangled, or whether someone placed their hands around their neck, may yield more information.[44] Many patients demonstrate what happened if asked. In addition, if the victim is an older adult with cognitive impairment, it is especially important to ask open-ended questions in a nonpressured setting to allow the individual to communicate to the best of their ability.

Head and Face Findings

Older adults are more prone to serious injury and mortality from trauma to the face and head than younger adults. This situation is true even with low mechanism injuries.[49] In addition, many older adults are taking anticoagulants, such as warfarin, which increase the risk of bleeding. The rate of intracranial bleeding is estimated to be between 7% and 14% in blunt trauma victims who are anticoagulated, even in the absence of symptoms.[50] Also, internal head injuries may be missed if signs of cognitive impairment are assumed to stem from age or underlying dementia. Brain injury may be missed if facial bruising that indicates deeper injury is not recognized. TBI is also a frequent sequela from head trauma and is common in older patients.[49] Studies[51] show that 72% of victims with brain injury from IPV reported multiple episodes of TBI. The impact of elder abuse related to head injuries in older adults is unknown, because many injuries are ascribed to accidental falls.

Basilar skull fractures are common. The bruising patterns in the head and face regions occur when the dura mater lining over the brain is torn, allowing fluid to leak into the ears or nose. Basilar skull fractures are often missed, because the bruising appears near the eyes and ears and can be mistaken for facial trauma. Understanding the mechanism of injury is paramount to placing the history into an accurate context. Two major types of basilar skull fractures affect the lower part of the skull near where the olfactory nerve exits to the nasal passages, and where facial nerves and those affecting balance and hearing exit into the ear canal. Cerebrospinal fluid discharge from the nares with periorbital bruising around both eyes (raccoon eyes) occurs with fractures of the anterior cranial fossa. Cerebrospinal fluid discharge from the ear with bruising over the mastoids (Battle sign) occurs with petrous temporal bone fractures (see **Fig. 2**).[52]

Bruising from direct trauma to the eye region must be distinguished from anterior basilar skull fractures (raccoon eyes). Trauma directed to the eye causes a classic black eye, at the site of the injury. Trauma to the periorbital area causes blood vessels to rupture, and the blood flows through connective tissue and downward with gravity around the eye(s) affected (**Fig. 27**). On the other hand, Battle sign may be mistaken for direct trauma directed behind the ear. However, basilar skull fractures may occur concomitantly with facial fractures in older patients. Five percent of patients older than 60 years with facial fractures in 1 study[53] had an associated basilar skull fracture. Falls accounted for 51% and trauma accounted for 8.8% of facial fractures in this study.

A scalp injury may indicate serious intracranial disease. Both coup and contrecoup injuries result from head trauma, including assault and falls. One incident of blunt trauma injury to the head may cause 2 sites of brain contusion. A brain contusion may occur inside the head under the point of impact, the coup injury, and another contusion, contrecoup, opposite to the site of contact, as the brain rebounds from the initial impact against the skull.[54] The contrecoup contusion is usually larger than the coup contusion. Of the bleeding injuries, subdural hematomas occur more frequently in older adults, because the bridging veins that pass from the brain to dural sinuses are susceptible to tears. Some subdural hematomas may occur from mild trauma, especially if the victim is taking anticoagulants. Blood flows into the intracranial free space, which is larger in older adults because of physiologic brain atrophy, and so the bleeding may occur for days to weeks before symptoms result, causing a delay in diagnosis.[55] Symptoms may be absent or include headaches, light-headedness, slowness in thinking, apathy and drowsiness, unsteady gait, and occasionally, seizures.[56]

Falls and Fractures

Falls result in multiple injuries, including bruising, abrasions, and head and face injuries as well as fractures. Older adults are prone to falls because of difficulties with balance, coordination, strength, reaction time, and judgment, as in the case of cognitive impairment. Medical conditions that affect bone integrity and increase the potential for fractures include osteoporosis, Paget disease, metastases caused by cancer, and

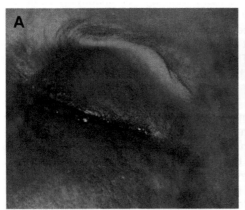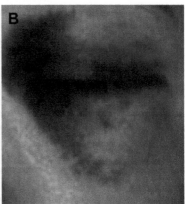

Fig. 27. Black eyes. (*Courtesy of* the Center of Excellence on Elder Abuse and Neglect, University of California, Irvine, CA; with permission.)

malignancies affecting bone, such as multiple myeloma. Spontaneous fractures can occur, but are rare, and the presence of a condition such as osteoporosis increases the vulnerability to a fracture but does not explain how the fracture occurred.

Falls are the cause of significant morbidity caused by fractures and TBI.[49] Only a few studies have described the patterns of injury attributable to falls from any cause, and even fewer describe fall-related injuries from elder abuse. Separating accidental falls from those caused by assault requires consideration of the patient's medical and functional history as well as the story of the fall. This investigation is critical in elder abuse cases, because many abusers claim that a victim's intentional injuries were caused by accidental falls, using the victim's medical and functional problems as distractors.

Patterns of injuries from falls have been described in a few studies. One study described injuries compared with the height of a fall. Height of a fall more than 15 m was associated with injuries in 2 or 3 body regions.[57] In 1 study, patterns of craniomaxillofacial injury in older adults involved concomitant injuries, including brain trauma, upper and lower extremity injury, and thoracic injury. Half of the cases studied were caused by falls. The investigators proposed that injuries to upper extremities may be the result of self-protection with outstretched hands, and injuries to lower extremities may be from weaker bones fractured during a fall.[53] Falls on the outstretched hand or elbow are known to increase the incidence of humeral head and surgical neck fractures in elderly patients.[58] Fracture patterns also stem from the direction of the fall. Some medical conditions, such as Parkinson disease, increase the possibility of falling backwards, for instance.

Because falls may be from intentional forces such as pushing, shoving, kicking, or tripping, physical elder abuse must be considered in the evaluation along with causes of accidental falls, such as cardiac dysfunction or dizziness. Overmedication by a caregiver, causing the older adult to be unsafe during ambulation, is a form of physical abuse. Neglect may be the cause of a fall if a caregiver withholds necessary aids such as a cane or walker, or even eyeglasses. Fractures in persons who are nonambulatory are suspicious.

PLACING PHYSICAL EXAMINATION FINDINGS INTO CONTEXT

Health care providers who discover physical injuries during the course of an examination should be mindful of elder abuse as a cause for the finding. Alternatively, providers who have suspicion for any type of elder abuse should look for signs of physical injury. Some findings are unquestionably traumatic, such as a gunshot wound or a stabbing. However, more often, physical findings are those commonly found in older adults, including bruising and hip fractures. The physical finding is just 1 piece of the puzzle. It must be understood in the context of multiple factors, including physiology, pathophysiology, medical history and function, and the mechanism of injury.

Both the mechanism and story should explain the injury. For example, does a fall from a standing position explain the multiple bruises on the chest and the linear eschars on the anterior shin? This was the claim of the alleged abuser and defense attorney in 1 known case of abuse (see **Figs. 4** and **13**). Does a fall explain multiple bruises to the face of an older woman who is demented and unable to transfer out of bed? Again, this was the claim of the alleged abuser. A man with end-stage dementia brought to the emergency room with obtundation and hypotension died from sepsis seeded by a stage 4 sacral ulcer. The caregiver daughter said she did everything the physician recommended, including turning him every 2 to 3 hours, after taking him from a nursing home. Yet she was absent for most of the day, and home health had been unable to see him for a month. Does one believe the victim with a hoarse voice and conjunctival petechiae when she says that "nothing happened?" The patient with dried feces embedded in a sacral decubitus and wrapped in 4 layers of diapers has not been repositioned or cleaned appropriately despite caregiver denials.

An evaluation of patient's functional abilities is often the key to determining whether abuse has occurred. Assessing functional status informs one's capacity for self-care and identifies caregiving needs. Persons with difficulties in instrumental activities of daily living or activities of daily living are dependent on caregivers and at increased risk for abuse. Understanding what patients can and cannot do for themselves is often the key to determining accidental versus intentional injuries. For instance, if someone alleges that a person in their care caught themselves in the bedrails, causing strangulation, but examination and history show that the victim has multiple contractures and is unable to turn, then, the story is deemed unreasonable. Or if the primary physician knows that a patient is unable to walk without a walker, and no ambulation aid was available at the time of the fall, then, neglect is likely.

DOCUMENTATION

Health care providers should document with the knowledge that the medical record may be used in an elder abuse investigation, by social workers, law enforcement, or prosecutors. Records should be legible. They should list all persons present at the patient encounter and state who the primary caregiver is, as well as their responsibilities. Functional capacity should be included in the history. In addition, pertinent history, such as whether discussions regarding care have occurred in the past, should be included.

Photographs of injuries are often critical to the elder abuse investigation. Following basic guidelines ensures that the images are useful. First, injuries should be measured against a ruler. Even if one lacks a ruler, comparing the injury with an object of familiar size, such as a quarter dollar, is helpful (**Fig. 28**). Serial photographs of injuries are often helpful. For instance, photographing pressure sores serially over time helps

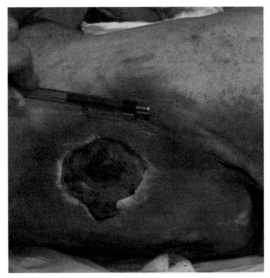

Fig. 28. A standard pen is used in the absence of a ruler. (*Courtesy of* L. Gibbs, MD, Orange, CA.)

the evaluator assess whether the ulcer is healing or worsening. Next, photographs should include the finding from a variety of distances (ie, close-up, regional, and full-body views) to capture detail and place the wound on a specific area of the body. A full-body view leaves no doubt as to which surface or side of the body is affected. Adequate lighting is important for clear images.

SUMMARY

A specific foundation of knowledge is important for evaluating the potential for abuse from physical findings in the older adult. First, the standard physical examination is a foundation for detecting many types of abuse. In addition, an understanding of traumatic injuries, including patterns of injury, in older adults, is important for health care providers. One must have an awareness of elder abuse as ubiquitous and ever present in the differential diagnosis of patient care. One must possess the skills to piece the history, including functional capabilities, and physical findings together, to formulate an educated opinion as to the cause of injury. Armed with this skill set, health care providers will develop the confidence needed to identify and intervene in cases of elder abuse.

REFERENCES

1. Yaar M, Gilchrest BA. Skin aging: postulated mechanisms and consequent changes in structure and function. Clin Geriatr Med 2001;17:617.
2. Gerstein AD. Wound healing and aging. Dermatol Clin 1993;11(4):749–57.
3. Alexandrescu DT, Gallo RL, Alexandrescu DT, et al. The vascular purpuras. Chapter 123. In: Lichtman MA, Kipps TJ, Seligsohn U, et al, editors. Williams hematology. 8th edition. New York: McGraw-Hill; 2010. Available at: http://accessmedicine. mhmedical.com/content.aspx?bookid=358&Sectionid=39835947. Accessed April 27, 2014.
4. Palmer BS, Brodell RT, Mostow EN. Elder abuse: dermatologic clues and critical solutions. J Am Acad Dermatol 2013;68:e37–42.
5. Fowler DR. Forensics. Chapter e263.2. In: Tintinalli JE, Stapczynski J, Ma O, et al, editors. Tintinalli's emergency medicine: a comprehensive study guide. 7th edition. New York: McGraw-Hill; 2011. Available at: http://accessmedicine.mhmedical. com/content.aspx?bookid=348&Sectionid=40381753. Accessed April 26, 2014.
6. Available at: http://www.forensicmed.co.uk/wounds/blunt-force-trauma/bruises/. Accessed April 27, 2014.
7. Child physical abuse. Chapter 8. In: Usatine RP, Smith MA, Chumley HS, et al, editors. The color atlas of family medicine. 2nd edition. New York: McGraw-Hill; 2013. Available at: http://accessmedicine.mhmedical.com/content.aspx? bookid=685&Sectionid=45361042. Accessed April 21, 2014.
8. Mosqueda L, Burnight K, Liao S. The life cycle of bruises in older adults. J Am Geriatr Soc 2005;53(8):1339–43.
9. Wiglesworth A, Austin R, Corona M, et al. Bruising as a marker of physical elder abuse. J Am Geriatr Soc 2009;57(7):1191–6.
10. Friedman LS, Avila S, Tanouye K, et al. A case-control study of severe physical abuse of older adults. J Am Geriatr Soc 2011;59(3):417–22.
11. Murphy K, Waa S, Jaffer H, et al. A literature review of findings in physical elder abuse. Can Assoc Radiol J 2013;64:10–4.
12. Burgess AW, Hanraan NP, Baker T. Forensic makers in elder female sexual abuse cases. Clin Geriatr Med 2005;21:399–412.

13. Available at: https://sites.google.com/site/eforensicmed2/bruises. Accessed April 25, 2014.

14. Fowler DR. Forensics. Chapter e263.2. In: Tintinalli JE, Stapczynski J, Ma O, et al, editors. Tintinalli's emergency medicine: a comprehensive study guide. 7th edition. New York: McGraw-Hill; 2011. Available at: http://accessmedicine.mhmedical.com/content.aspx?bookid=348&Sectionid=40381753. Accessed April 30, 2014.

15. Brown K, Streubert GE, Burgess AW. Effectively detect and manage elder abuse. Nurse Pract 2004;29(8):22–7.

16. Greenbaum AR, Donne J, Wilson D, et al. Intentional burn injury: an evidence-based, clinical and forensic review. Burns 2004;30(7):628–42.

17. Muller MJ, Pegg SP, Rule MR. Determinants of death following burn injury. Br J Surg 2001;88:583.

18. Peck MD. Epidemiology of burns throughout the world. Part II: intentional burns in adults. Burns 2012;38:630–7.

19. Krob MJ, Johnson A, Jordan MH. Burned and battered adults. J Burn Care Rehabil 1986;7:529–31.

20. Bird PE, Harrington DT, Barillo DJ, et al. Elder abuse: a call to action. J Burn Care Rehabil 1998;19:522–7.

21. National Burn Repository, Report of data between 2002–2011, American Burn Association, 2012. Available at: http://www.ameriburn.org/2012NBRAnnualReport.pdf. Accessed May 3, 2014.

22. Demling RH, Demling RH. Burns & other thermal injuries. Chapter 14. In: Doherty GM, Doherty GM, editors. Current diagnosis & treatment: surgery. 13th edition. New York: McGraw-Hill; 2010. Available at: http://accessmedicine.mhmedical.com/content.aspx?bookid=343&Sectionid=39702801. Accessed May 2, 2014.

23. Harper RD, Dickson WA. Reducing the burn risk to elderly persons living in residential care. Burns 1995;21(3):205–8.

24. Chatham N, Carls C. How to manage incontinence associated dermatitis. Wound Care Advisor 2012;1:1. Available at: http://woundcareadvisor.com/wp-content/uploads/2012/05/WCA_M-J-2012_Dermatitis.pdf.

25. Janniger CK, Schwartz RA, Szepietowski JC, et al. Intertrigo and common secondary skin infections. Am Fam Physician 2005;72(5):833–8.

26. Brown KL, Phillips T, Brown KL, et al. Venous ulcers. Chapter 146. In: McKean SC, Ross JJ, Dressler DD, et al, editors. Principles and practice of hospital medicine. New York: McGraw-Hill; 2012. Available at: http://accessmedicine.mhmedical.com/content.aspx?bookid=496&Sectionid=41304127. Accessed May 3, 2014.

27. Section 17. Skin signs of vascular insufficiency. In: Wolff K, Johnson R, Saavedra AP, et al, editors. Fitzpatrick's color atlas and synopsis of clinical dermatology. 7th edition. New York: McGraw-Hill; 2013. Available at: http://accessmedicine.mhmedical.com/content.aspx?bookid=682&Sectionid=45130149. Accessed May 4, 2014.

28. Burkhart CN, Morrell DS, Burkhart CN, et al. Disorders of the hands, feet, and extremities. Chapter 247. In: Tintinalli JE, Stapczynski J, Ma O, et al, editors. Tintinalli's emergency medicine: a comprehensive study guide. 7th edition. New York: McGraw-Hill; 2011. Available at: http://accessmedicine.mhmedical.com/content.aspx?bookid=348&Sectionid=40381734. Accessed May 4, 2014.

29. Collins KA, Presnell SE. Elder neglect and the pathophysiology of aging. Am J Forensic Med Pathol 2007;28(2):157–62.

30. Bliss MR. Lypeaemia. J Tissue Viability 1998;8:4–14.

31. Lyder CH. Pressure ulcer prevention and management. JAMA 2003;289:2.

32. Bates-Jensen BM, Bates-Jensen BM. Pressure ulcers. Chapter 58. In: Halter JB, Ouslander JG, Tinetti ME, et al, editors. Hazzard's geriatric medicine and gerontology. 6th edition. New York: McGraw-Hill; 2009. Available at: http://accessmedicine. mhmedical.com/content.aspx?bookid=371&Sectionid=41587670. Accessed May 4, 2014.

33. The National Pressure Ulcer Advisory Panel (NPUAP); NPUAP Pressure ulcer stages/Categories. Available at: http://www.npuap.org/. Accessed May 4, 2014.

34. Knox DM, Anderson TM, Anderson PS. Effects of different turn intervals on skin of healthy older adults. Adv Wound Care 1994;7:48–52, 54–6.

35. Malvern (PA): Association for the Advancement of Wound Care guideline of pressure ulcer guidelines. Association for the Advancement of Wound Care (AAWC), 2010. Available at: www.guideline.gov/content. Accessed May 4, 2014.

36. Redd M, Gill S, Rochon P. Preventing pressure ulcers: a systematic review. JAMA 2006;296(8):974–84.

37. Brandeis GH, Berlowitz DR, Katz P. Are pressure ulcers preventable? A survey of experts. Adv Skin Wound Care 2001;14(5):244, 245–8.

38. Ziminski CE, Wiglesworth A, Aurstin R, et al. Injury patterns and causal mechanisms of bruising in physical elder abuse. Journal of Forensic Nurs 2013;9(2): 84–91.

39. Wilbur L, Higley M, Hatfield J, et al. Survey results of women who have been strangled while in an abusive relationship. J Emerg Med 2001;21(3):297–302.

40. Plattner T, Bolliger S, Zollinger U. Forensic assessment of survived strangulation. Forensic Sci Int 2005;153:202–7.

41. Karch D, Nunn KC. Characteristics of elderly and other vulnerable adult victims of homicide by a caregiver: national violent death reporting system-17 US States, 2003-2007. J Interpers Violence 2011;26(137):137–57.

42. 1993 National Mortality Followback Survey (NMFS), CDC/National Center for Health Statistics. Available at: http://www.cdc.gov/nchs/nvss/nmfs.htm. Accessed May 6, 2014.

43. Stapczynski JS. Strangulation injuries. Emerg Med Rep 2010;31(17):193–203.

44. Faugno D, Waszak D, Strack GB, et al. Strangulation forensic examination: best practice for health care providers. Adv Emerg Nurs J 2013;3(4): 314–27.

45. Hawley DA, McClane GE, Strack GB. A review of 300 attempted strangulation cases, Part III: injuries in fatal cases. J Emerg Med 2001;21(3):317–22.

46. Holbrook DS, Jackson MC. Use of an alternative light source to assess strangulation victims. J Forensic Nurs 2013;9(3):140–5.

47. Iserson KV. Strangulation. A review of ligature, manual, and postural neck compression in juries. Ann Emerg Med 1984;13:179–85.

48. Smith DJ, Mills T, Taliaferro EH. Frequency and relationship of reported symptomology in victims of intimate partner violence: the effect of multiple attempted strangulation attacks. J Emerg Med 2001;21:323–9.

49. Papa L, Mendes ME, Braga CF. Mild traumatic brain injury among the geriatric population. Curr Transl Geriatr Exp Gerontol Rep 2012;1(3):135–42.

50. Li J, Brown J, Levine M. Mild head injury, anticoagulants, and risk of intracranial injury. Lancet 2001;357:771.

51. Valera E, Berenbaum H. Brain injury in battered women. J Consult Clin Psychol 2003;71:797–804.

52. Munter DW, McGuirk TD, Munter DW, et al. Head and facial trauma. Chapter 1. In: Knoop KJ, Stack LB, Storrow AB, et al, editors. The atlas of emergency medicine. 3rd edition. New York: McGraw-Hill; 2010. Available at: http://accessmedicine.

mhmedical.com/content.aspx?bookid=351&Sectionid=39619700.   Accessed May 10, 2014.

53. Zelken JA, Khalifian S, Mundinger GS, et al. Defining predictable patterns of craniomaxillofacial injury in the elderly: analysis of 1,047 patients. Oral Maxillofac Surg 2014;72(2):352–61.

54. Johnson SC, Johnson SC. Traumatic brain injury. Chapter 68. In: Halter JB, Ouslander JG, Tinetti ME, et al, editors. Hazzard's geriatric medicine and gerontology. 6th edition. New York: McGraw-Hill; 2009. Available at: http://accessmedicine. mhmedical.com/content.aspx?bookid=371&Sectionid=41587682. Accessed May 12, 2014.

55. Ma O, Edwards JH, Meldon SW, et al. Geriatric trauma. Chapter 252. In: Tintinalli JE, Stapczynski J, Ma O, et al, editors. Tintinalli's emergency medicine: a comprehensive study guide. 7th edition. New York: McGraw-Hill; 2011. Available at: http:// accessmedicine.mhmedical.com/content.aspx?bookid=348&Sectionid=40381740. Accessed May 11, 2014.

56. Ropper AH, Samuels MA. Craniocerebral trauma. Chapter 35. In: Ropper AH, Samuels MA, Ropper AH, et al, editors. Adams & Victor's Principles of Neurology. 10th edition. New York, NY: McGraw-Hill; 2014. Available at: http://accessmedicine. mhmedical.com/content.aspx?bookid=690&Sectionid=50910886.   Accessed September 08, 2014.

57. Atanasijevic TC, Savic SN, Nikolic SD, et al. Frequency and severity of injuries in correlation with the height of fall. J Forensic Sci 2005;50(3):608–12.

58. Sartoretti C, Sartoretti-Schefer S, Ruckert R, et al. Comorbid conditions in old patients with femur fractures. J Trauma 1997;43:570.

Medical and Laboratory Indicators of Elder Abuse and Neglect

Veronica M. LoFaso, MS, MD, Tony Rosen, MD, MPH

KEYWORDS

- Elder abuse • Elder neglect • Malnutrition • Dehydration

KEY POINTS

- Elder abuse and neglect are highly prevalent but woefully underdetected and underreported.
- The presentation is rarely clear and requires the piecing together of clues that create a mosaic of the full picture.
- More research needed to better characterize findings that, when identified, can contribute to certainty in cases of suspected abuse.
- Medical and laboratory data can be helpful in the successful determination of abuse and neglect.

INTRODUCTION AND OVERVIEW

As many as 10% of older adults in the United States experience elder abuse each year.[1–3] This maltreatment may include physical abuse, sexual abuse, neglect, psychological abuse, or financial exploitation, and many victims suffer from multiple types of abuse.[1–4] Elder abuse is associated with adverse health outcomes, including emergency department usage,[5,6] hospitalization,[7] depression,[8] nursing home placement,[9,10] and dramatically increased mortality.[11,12] The annual direct medical costs associated with violent injuries to older adults in the United States are estimated at $5.3 billion.[13] This large disease burden and cost are likely to increase significantly because of the anticipated growth of the geriatric population.[14–16]

Despite its frequency, many older adults who suffer from abuse or neglect endure it for years before it is discovered. Studies suggest that as few as 1 in 14 cases of elder abuse is reported to the authorities,[1,17] and much of the associated morbidity and mortality is likely due to this delay in identification and intervention.[18] Victims may be unable to report abuse because of isolation, severe illness, or dementia, or may

Disclosures: None.
New York Presbyterian Hospital, Weill Cornell Medical College, Box 39, 525 East 68th Street, New York, NY 10065, USA
E-mail address: vel2001@med.cornell.edu

be reluctant to report because of fear of reprisal, guilt, desire to protect the abuser, cultural beliefs, or fear of institutionalization. Therefore, recognition and reporting by others is critical for identifying victims and intervening.

Evaluation by health care providers represents an important, underutilized opportunity to identify elder abuse. For many older adults, assessment by health care providers may represent their only contact outside the family. Clinicians, therefore, have a unique opportunity to diagnose suspected elder abuse and initiate further evaluation by Adult Protective Services (APS) and elder abuse teams.[5,6,19–23] Despite this, only 1.4% of cases reported to APS come from physicians,[24] and in a survey of APS workers, of 17 occupational groups physicians were among the least helpful in reporting abuse.[25] Several reasons exist for this missed opportunity, including lack of awareness,[26] inadequate training,[26] insufficient information about available resources, lack of time to conduct a thorough evaluation for abuse, concern about involvement in the legal system, and desire to protect physician-patient confidentiality. Among the most important reasons for underreporting by physicians and health care providers is the difficulty in identifying elder abuse and neglect, and distinguishing between it and the sequelae of accidental trauma and acute or chronic illness. This identification is also made more challenging by the normal physiologic changes that occur with aging.[18,27–30]

Although extreme cases of elder abuse and neglect may be apparent to the provider with a cursory assessment, most are subtle, and require the clinician to maintain a high index of suspicion and to identify clues during the patient evaluation.[31] These clues, often called forensic markers,[31] may include physical findings, injury patterns, and medical or laboratory signs. Potential forensic markers for elder abuse and neglect have been described in the literature for geriatricians, emergency physicians,[5,6,19–23] family physicians,[32,33] nursing home medical directors,[34] burn surgeons,[35] dermatologists,[36] orthopedic surgeons,[37] radiologists,[18] and dentists.[38–40] Most of this existing literature focuses on physical injury patterns suspicious for mistreatment, including bruising, lacerations, fractures, and burns.

In addition to physical injury patterns, however, there are also medical and laboratory markers that should increase suspicion of elder abuse or neglect. Such markers include indicators of malnutrition, dehydration, alterations in status of chronic illness, hypothermia/hyperthermia, rhabdomyolysis, toxicologic findings, and postmortem biochemical values. In many cases, these markers may be the only clue that abuse or neglect has occurred. Though little systematic research exists on the prevalence of these findings in mistreatment, the current literature for each is described herein.

MEDICAL AND LABORATORY INDICATORS OF ELDER ABUSE AND NEGLECT
Malnutrition

Malnutrition and weight loss in the older adult are commonly encountered in geriatric practice (**Table 1**). Malnutrition is a risk for functional decline and vulnerability to many life-threatening diseases, particularly infection.[31] Even in the absence of neglect, older adults have multiple risk factors for malnutrition and weight loss.

Normal aging results in a decrease in taste sensation, and less production of saliva and a dry mouth, making the eating experience less pleasurable. Almost 50% of older adults have a decreased sense of smell, further diminishing their enjoyment of eating and leading to decreased caloric intake.[41] Changes in gastrointestinal tract secretions, such as decrease in prostaglandins, leads to increases in acid that may cause discomfort and lead to avoidance of eating. Decreased

Table 1
Clinical and laboratory findings commonly found in cases of abuse and neglect

Medical Condition	Laboratory Data	Physical Findings	Causes
Dehydration:	Hypernatremia (serum Na >145 mmol/L) Elevated BUN/creatinine ratio >20 Elevated uric acid Elevated Hgb/Hct	Tenting of skin Fecal impaction Dry mucous membranes Sunken eyes Possible orthostatic changes Tachycardia	Withholding fluids Intent to harm Avoid fluid intake to decrease bedwetting Avoid need to provide personal care
Malnutrition	Low serum albumin (<3.5 g/dL) Low prealbumin Low transferrin (<180 mg/dL) Anemia Low cholesterol Low total lymphocyte count (<1500/mm)	BMI <21 kg/m^2 Triceps skin fold <80% normal Muscle wasting Functional decline	Withholding food Unattended dental issues Poor feeding techniques/dysphagia Inattention to food preferences Inability to purchase food: financial abuse
Hyperthermia or hypothermia	Elevated CK Abnormal TFTs	Elevated body temperature Sepsis Dehydration	Lack of AC or heat Excessive clothing or inadequate clothing NMS (hyperthermia: neuroleptic use)
Rhabdomyolysis	Elevated CK: serum Myoglobin: urine Hypernatremia (dehydration) Hypophosphatemia (malnutrition) Hypokalemia Acute renal insufficiency	Signs of bruising/falls Signs of wrist/ankle restraints Signs of malnutrition or dehydration Hypo/hyperthermia	Trauma: muscle injury Prolonged immobility (restrained) Severe malnutrition or dehydration Hypo-/hyperthermia: lack of AC/heat Overuse/misuse of neuroleptic medications (NMS)
Toxicology	Presence in blood/hair samples of recreational or prescription drugs or toxins not prescribed by a practitioner. ie: ETOH LSD Marijuana Amphetamines Narcotics Sedative/hypnotics	Sedations/somnolence Euphoria Cognitive impairment Depression Cardiovascular events	Inappropriate administration of medication with intent to chemically restrain or sedate Intent to harm
Infection	Recurrent UTI Aspiration pneumonia on CXR Sexually transmitted diseases; +VDRL, GC swab+ Infected pressure ulcers	Urinary frequency/ burning Vaginal discharge Recurrent choking with feeding Advanced-stage or multiple ulcers with signs of infection or poor care	Sexual abuse Force feeding Neglect of personal hygiene/turning in bed/nutrition

The abnormalities of laboratory values can be seen in other disease states and are not pathognomonic to elder abuse. They must be evaluated in the context of the presenting clinical situation.

Abbreviations: AC, air conditioning; BMI, body mass index; BUN, blood urea nitrogen; CK, creatine kinase; CXR, chest radiography; ETOH, ethanol; GC, *Neisseria gonorrhoeae*; Hct, hematocrit; Hgb, hemoglobin; LSD, lysergic acid diethylamide; NMS, neuroleptic malignant syndrome; TFTs, thyroid function tests; UTI, urinary tract infection; VDRL, Venereal Disease Research Laboratory test.

esophageal contractions and lower esophageal sphincter pressure occur with aging, resulting in dysphagia and gastroesophageal reflux disease, potentially increasing food avoidance.

End-stage dementia, highly prevalent in our aging society, can cause increased production of tumor necrosis factors and other cytokines that contribute to weight loss. In addition, patients with dementia and other neurologic conditions (eg, amyotrophic lateral sclerosis, stroke, Parkinson disease) may have dysphagia, contributing to poor oral intake and inadequate nutrition. Malnutrition can also occur in the setting of cancer, intestinal disorders such as celiac disease, and depression. Mechanical problems such as temporomandibular joint syndrome or the absence of teeth can also contribute to decreased caloric intake. Many commonly encountered medical disorders, such as thyroid, cardiovascular, and pulmonary disease, often lead to unintentional weight loss through increased metabolic demand and decreased appetite and caloric intake.[42]

Clinicians have long recognized that changes in weight may reflect change in health or wellness of an individual. A body mass index (BMI) of less than 21 kg/m^2 is concerning for malnutrition,[27] and a loss of 40% of total body weight can result in death.[31] Triceps skinfold, and a mid-arm circumference less than 80% of normal, is also a clinical marker of malnutrition.[43] Significant weight loss should prompt the clinician to evaluate for medical and psychosocial causes. Elder abuse or neglect should be considered in this differential, especially when the individual depends on others for their care or if they suffer from dementia or significant mental illness that impairs judgment.[44]

Medical examiners have identified malnutrition as among the most relevant factors in determining abuse or neglect.[45] A large retrospective 10-year review of elder abuse cases of the State Medical Examiner's Office serving a large metropolitan area revealed that 36.4% of postmortem neglect cases were severely malnourished (BMI <17.5 kg/m^2), 40.9% were underweight (BMI 17.5–20.0 kg/m^2), and only 22.7% had a BMI of greater than 20.0 kg/m^2.[46] These data highlight the importance of clinicians documenting and charting body habitus over time, as cachexia is highly prevalent in neglect cases.

Malnutrition is certainly not unique to inadequate caregiving or neglect in the home setting. Studies have shown that poor nutrition is seen in anywhere from 8% to 27% of nursing home residents.[47] As many as 40% to 60% of nursing home residents have been reported to have dysphagia contributing to inadequate caloric intake.[48] Other studies find the incidence of malnutrition ranges from 12% to 50% among the hospitalized elderly population and from 23% to 60% among institutionalized older adults. Polypharmacy, mood disorders, and staff attentiveness to feeding needs are often the cause of malnutrition in the absence of an underlying disease process. Loneliness, especially when combined with recent bereavement or poor social support, has been shown to be a common and significant risk factor for malnutrition in institutions.[47] Patients' cultural food preferences are often overlooked in the institutional setting. Although most experts agree that there is a great need for institutions to respond to nutritional deficits, there are no clear data to quantify how much of the nutritional deficits are due to systems problems and how much are due to underlying metabolic and disease processes.

Determining if abuse or neglect is a contributing factor when an older adult presents with malnutrition is challenging, given the issues already discussed. No single biochemical marker on its own serves as a satisfactory screening test for malnutrition. When reviewing clinical data, certain constellations of findings raise one's level of suspicion for abuse or neglect. Laboratory data represent a key piece of a more detailed assessment that incorporates many data points.

Laboratory findings suggestive of malnutrition

In addition to history and physical examination findings suggestive of malnutrition, laboratory markers may be helpful. Serum proteins synthesized by the liver, including albumin, transferrin, retinol-binding protein, and thyroxine-binding prealbumin, may serve as markers of nutritional status. Traditionally, low serum albumin (<3.5 g/dL) has been the most widely accepted of these because it has been shown to predict mortality and morbidity.[43,49] Many factors other than undernutrition, such as infection and inflammation, affect these proteins, limiting their usefulness, especially in the acutely ill. In addition, owing to the long half-life of albumin, serum albumin does not respond to short-term changes in caloric or protein consumption. Low serum transferrin (<180 mg/dL)[43] appears to be a more sensitive early indicator of acute protein-energy malnutrition, but is unreliable in conditions including iron deficiency, hypoxemia, chronic infection, and hepatic disease. A low total lymphocyte count (<1500/mm)[43,49] has been postulated as a sign of poor nutrition. Malnutrition may contribute to age-related immune dysregulation, including decreased lymphocyte proliferation.[49] In addition, serum protein levels have been used to evaluate malnutrition, a low total cholesterol level has been correlated with the risk of malnutrition, and some suggest that obtaining values of vitamin and trace elements such as thiamine, riboflavin, pyridoxine, calcium, vitamin D, vitamin B_{12}, folate, and ferritin may also be helpful indicators.[49]

Anemia is common among older adults, with prevalence estimated at 8% to 25% for community-dwelling older adults and 48% to 63% of nursing home residents.[50] Though an important marker of malnutrition, the differential diagnosis for anemia in a geriatric patient is broad, including anemia of chronic disease, iron deficiency, and renal insufficiency, and most cases are multifactorial.[50] Therefore, using anemia to identify malnutrition resulting from elder abuse or neglect is challenging. Nevertheless, because a complete blood count is a laboratory test commonly ordered in a wide variety of clinical scenarios, unexplained anemia may be the only clue of malnutrition, and its presence should encourage the provider to pursue additional evaluation and testing.

Dehydration

Dehydration is a common finding in older adults, and has significant associated morbidity and mortality. There are several factors associated with normal aging that contribute to dehydration in the elderly. Older adults experience decreased thirst sensation and decreased total body water. In the aging kidney, effectiveness of arginine vasopressin is decreased and the ability to concentrate urine is reduced (even in the setting of normal renal function tests). Medications, including diuretics, and comorbid illnesses causing diarrhea and vomiting, may contribute to dehydration.[51]

Neglectful caregivers may withhold hydration from older adults, putting them at risk for serious adverse health effects. Liquids may be withheld because of passive negligence, especially if a care recipient cannot communicate the need for fluids. Alternatively, a caregiver may actively withhold hydration from the older adult with incontinence to reduce the need for clothing and bedding changes. Even worse, hydration may be withheld with the intent to harm the individual. Older adults have less physiologic reserve, and dehydration as a result of abuse or neglect may contribute to their death.[44]

The prevalence of dehydration in nursing home patients is reported to be as high as 35%, given the advanced chronic medical illnesses from which many residents suffer.[52,53] Hypernatremic dehydration in an institutionalized patient should be considered as possible neglect in the absence of clear documentation of attempts made to correct the problem.[19] Deaths in nursing homes attributable to malnutrition or dehydration, though common, are also very seldom investigated.[44] Unfortunately, physicians consistently fail to order autopsies in older adults, even in cases where severe malnutrition or dehydration is noted at the time of death, strongly suggesting that the possibility of abuse or neglect is not being considered. Of note, researchers have found that death certificates with malnutrition or dehydration listed as the primary or secondary cause of death were not subject to postmortem examination or other investigation after the fact.

In the living victim of neglect, dehydration may manifest with tachycardia and orthostatic hypotension, tenting of skin, dryness of mucous membranes, and hard or impacted stool. A study of emergency room patients aged 60 years and older found that the following physical examination characteristics correlated best with the severity of dehydration: tongue dryness, longitudinal tongue furrow, dryness of mucous membranes of the mouth, upper body muscle weakness, confusion, speech difficulty, and sunken eyes.[54] In postmortem evaluations, physical findings included tenting of skin, "stickiness of serosal surfaces," sunken orbits, and fecal impaction.[28]

Laboratory findings suggestive of dehydration

Hypernatremia, defined as serum sodium level greater than 145 mmol/L, is the most commonly noted laboratory finding in dehydration. Hypernatremic dehydration (from fluid deprivation) disproportionately affects the youngest and oldest, but unlike in the pediatric population, elderly patients may be asymptomatic until the sodium level exceeds 160 mmol/L.[55]

Hypernatremic dehydration portends poor outcomes. One study found a 33% mortality rate for patients admitted to a geriatrics ward with serum sodium levels in the range of 151 to 153 mEq/L. Another investigation found that nearly 50% of patients hospitalized with dehydration died within a year, and among those with a sodium level higher than 154 mEq/L, mortality was 71.4%.[56] Researchers studied 116 patients admitted to a large university hospital with hypernatremia (serum sodium >145 mmol/L): 66% expired and 34% survived. Cognitive changes such as delirium, obtundation, and altered speech were more prominent in the group that expired.[57] Many studies reported febrile illness secondary to infection as a common cause of dehydration in the elderly.[58]

Severe dehydration is also an important forensic finding. Collins and colleagues[92] reported the results of forensic evaluation of 8 elder neglect cases (6 postmortem and 2 premortem). In 3 cases (37.5%), dehydration was the cause of death. In those cases vitreous chemistries revealed sodium levels ranging from 164 to 180 mmol/L and urea nitrogen 76 to 310 mg/dL.

Other more subtle clues to dehydration might include elevations in hematocrit, blood urea nitrogen and creatinine ratio, uric acid, and calcium. If present, these laboratory values might prompt the clinician to query further about the cause of the clinical presentation.

Chronic Illness Management

Abuse and neglect often present in a subtle manner, and the first clue may be a change in previously well-controlled chronic illnesses. Older adults who depend on others for their care and who present to clinicians with sudden or unexplained declines in their chronic disease state should have a thorough medical and psychosocial evaluation. Caregiver mistreatment, disruption in delivery of medications, and negligence in bringing the dependent older adult to their appointments can all result in poor medical outcomes. For example, recurrent hospitalizations for cardiac patients, especially for exacerbations in heart failure, should prompt questioning about medication compliance with diuretics and dietary intake of sodium. Many possible abuse or neglect scenarios may lead to acute change in the status of a previously well-controlled chronically ill patient.

More subtle insults to the health of the chronically ill elderly can be environmental. Examples include neglectful caregivers smoking in the vicinity of a patient with chronic obstructive pulmonary disease, having the older adult with ambulatory problems in an upstairs bedroom far from a bathroom or in a cluttered environment, and poor regulation of temperature leading to hyperthermia or hypothermia. In addition, the depression, anxiety, embarrassment, and functional decline which often accompany abuse may contribute to future nonadherence to medical regimens and avoidance of the health care system.

Medication misuse

When an elderly patient presents with an acute decline caused by exacerbation of a chronic illness, laboratory testing can be helpful in identifying the cause and assessing medication adherence. Drug levels of many commonly prescribed medications (eg, digoxin, warfarin, phenytoin) should be followed on a regular basis. Misuse of medications by caregivers can present in the following ways:

1. Overdosing or underdosing of prescription medications prescribed to the patient
2. Administration of over-the-counter or prescribed medications belonging to other persons that were not prescribed by the patient's physician
3. Failing to follow health care instructions for drug-level monitoring for routine maintenance or dosing adjustments

Laboratory findings suggestive of mismanagement of chronic illness

Diabetics should have their hemoglobin A_{1C} levels monitored regularly. Repeated episodes of hypoglycemia or hyperglycemia, or hemoglobin A_{1C} levels markedly elevated above acceptable levels, suggest poor dietary compliance or medication nonadherence. In the dependent patient with dementia, these findings would be concerning for neglect or abuse. Exogenous administration of insulin to do harm can be detected by checking C-peptide and insulin levels in the blood.

Erratic levels of anticoagulants (as measured by international normalized ratio) in previously well-controlled patients might prompt further questioning about administration and diet. An elevated digoxin level can be used to confirm digoxin toxicity in the appropriate clinical setting. Thyroid function tests are used to monitor appropriate dosing of thyroid medication in the hypothyroid patient, with the exception of acute illness when the specificity of sensitive thyroid-stimulating hormone is reduced. Uncontrolled seizure disorders should prompt the clinician to check levels of antiseizure medications (eg, phenytoin, valproic acid, phenobarbital).

Uncontrolled chronic pain or escalating use of pain medications when seemingly adequate doses of medication are being prescribed should raise a red flag to check for medication diversion. Caregivers may be using opiate pain medications themselves or selling them for personal financial gain.[59]

Hypothermia and hyperthermia Alterations in temperature may also be a subtle sign that should trigger providers to consider the possibility of elder abuse or neglect. An older adult presenting to the emergency department with mental status changes may be suffering from hypothermia or hyperthermia. Older adults are particularly susceptible to both hypothermia (body temperature <35 C), hyperthermia (body temperature >37.5 –40 C); and malignant nonexertional heat stroke (>40 C),[28,60–63] which are common, underrecognized, and may lead to significant morbidity and mortality.[61,62] Perception of environmental temperature and acute temperature change is decreased in the elderly,[28,64] as is the body's ability to regulate core temperature.[26,27,60,63] Thus, even slight environmental changes may have a significant effect.[62,65,66]

Hypothermia risk is increased by muscular atrophy and a decrease in adipose tissue, reducing protection and insulation.[27,28,67,68] The basal metabolic rate decreases with age, as does the capacity for shivering thermogenesis.[28] A vasoconstrictive response to manage heat loss is decreased in older adults.[28,60,63] Chronic conditions common among elderly patients may also contribute to hypothermia, including diabetes mellitus, liver disease, cerebrovascular disease, adrenal and pituitary insufficiency, and hypothyroidism.[28]

Hyperthermia risk is increased because older adults also have decreased vasodilation, often because of peripheral vascular disease.[28] In addition, reduced cardiac output[28,60,63] and impaired sweat response decreases the body's capacity to lose excess heat.

Polypharmacy, common among geriatric patients, can precipitate hypothermia or hyperthermia, as medications such as benzodiazepines and narcotics can impair thermoregulatory ability[28,69] and antipsychotic medications can cause hyperthermia associated with neuroleptic malignant syndrome.[70,71] Alcohol consumption can cause vasodilation, which accelerates hypothermia,[28,69] and use of stimulants such as cocaine[72] may lead to hyperthermia.

Environmental circumstances of older adults may increase the risk of hypothermia and hyperthermia. Many live in older, less well insulated homes, leading to a greater loss of heat during cold weather and increased difficulty keeping rooms cool during warm weather.[73] In addition, many elders living on a modest fixed income may limit their use of heat and electricity in an attempt to save money.[73]

Temperature is routinely assessed orally, temporally, or aurally in adults in most clinical settings, but these have been shown to be inaccurate,[74] particularly in older adults. Therefore, providers should consider checking a rectal temperature in patients with significant concern for hypothermia or hyperthermia.

Although temperature is not commonly reported as a marker of elder abuse or neglect, hypothermia has been described in cases[73,75] and identified as a cause of death in victims.[75] It is also recognized as a potential indicator of child abuse.[76] Many elder abuse and neglect scenarios may lead to dangerous hypothermia or hyperthermia. Most commonly, caregivers fail to protect an older adult from environmental temperatures, which may be due to the lack of appropriate heat or cooling. Heat and air conditioning may be turned off for reasons of nonpayment. Caregivers may leave windows open or closed inappropriately, leading to dangerous indoor temperatures.[77,78] Moreover, use of inadequate or excessive clothing and bed coverings may contribute to hypothermia or hyperthermia.[77,78] Even in skilled nursing facilities this can be a problem,[62] with extreme cases often reported in the media.[79,80]

In addition to environmental exposure, hypothermia and hyperthermia may occur with other types of elder abuse and neglect. Hypothermia is a frequent complication in patients with traumatic injury, and contributes to morbidity and mortality.[81,82] Hypothermia may also complicate sepsis[61,62] and other severe medical illnesses. Hypothermia, and particularly hyperthermia, may occur because of inappropriate medication dosing,[28,77,78] as in the case of benzodiazepines and narcotic pain medications already noted.

Rhabdomyolysis Rhabdomyolysis is the breakdown of skeletal muscle and release of intracellular contents, including creatine phosphokinase and the heme-containing protein myoglobin, into the blood.[50,60] Rhabdomyolysis may have a mild, asymptomatic course or may lead to severe electrolyte imbalances and acute renal failure.[50,60] Providers may check for rhabdomyolysis by measuring serum creatine phosphokinase and checking urine for the presence of heme protein (present in myoglobin), and the absence of red blood cells.[60]

Severe rhabdomyolysis in geriatric patients is typically caused by prolonged immobility after falls[50,61–64] or acute illness.[50] Geriatric patients may be particularly susceptible to rhabdomyolysis because aging muscle is more vulnerable to hypoxic injury.[50]

Though infrequently mentioned as a sign of elder abuse,[65] rhabdomyolysis has been well recognized as a potential complication in child abuse[66–73] and as a potential clue in cases when abuse is not otherwise suspected.[68] Rhabdomyolysis is also documented in younger adult victims of intentional blunt trauma and physical torture.[74,75] Therefore, the presence of rhabdomyolysis in an elderly patient with other evidence of traumatic injury should raise concern for elder abuse.

In addition to blunt physical trauma, rhabdomyolysis may occur after prolonged struggling against physical restraints.[76] These restraints, including Posey vests, and wrist and ankle restraints made of leather, plastic, or cloth, have historically been used in skilled nursing facilities to control unsafe or challenging behaviors in older adults. Use of physical restraint has been shown to increase the chance of serious injury or death, and may cause additional significant complications including loss of mobility, pressure ulcers, incontinence, and delirium.[77–80,83] Therefore, many commentators advocate avoidance of physical restraints in nursing home practice,[81] and some suggest that use of physical restraint in a noncritical situation may represent both physical abuse and neglect.[31] Unfortunately, though controversial,[77,83] the use of physical restraint is still common in nursing home practice[81] with no evidence of a decreasing prevalence. Rhabdomyolysis, in the appropriate clinical scenario, should trigger concern for prolonged, inappropriate use of restraint by caregivers.

Rhabdomyolysis may also be present in specific elder abuse syndromes in conjunction with other medical and laboratory markers (see earlier discussion). Hypernatremia may cause rhabdomyolysis,[82,84] as may hypokalemia or hypophosphatemia from malnutrition. An adverse drug-related or toxicologic event, particularly neuroleptic malignant syndrome associated with antipsychotics,[85] may lead to rhabdomyolysis. Moreover, rhabdomyolysis may occur in severe cases of hyperthermia and heat stroke[86,87] or hypothermia[88–90] because of exposure.

Infection

Serious, life-threatening infections are highly prevalent in the older population, and it would be unrealistic to consider abuse or neglect in every patient who presented with infection. However, infections are often the final common pathway by which older adults, and especially neglected or abused older adults, die. Precursors to infection may include dehydration or malnutrition states. Dysphagia and force feeding can lead to aspiration pneumonia. Inappropriate care of pressure ulcers can lead to infection, osteomyelitis, and sepsis. Delayed care for patients with nonspecific symptoms, such as altered mental status or lack of appetite, leads to worse infections at presentation, such as urosepsis instead of an uncomplicated urinary tract infection. Identifying patterns of recurrent or suspicious infections can help add to an overall picture of neglect or abuse.

Microbial cultures of blood, urine, lung, and wounds can be helpful in piecing together the cause of death. Collins and Presnell[91] reviewed 8 cases of fatal neglect in victims 74 to 94 years old. Causes of death were sepsis caused by severe pressure ulcers or dehydration. Five of the 8 cases had positive blood cultures. Organisms identified were *Staphylococcus aureus*, Enterococcus, *Proteus penneri*, *Proteus mirabilis*, and *Pseudomonas aeruginosa*. In 3 of the cases the cultures from pressure ulcers correlated with blood culture results (*P penneri*, *P aeruginosa*, *P mirabilis*, and/or *S aureus*). In these types of cases, an investigation should ensue to determine whether a delay in medical care for ulcers placed the patient at risk for sepsis.

Elderly patients who present with recurrent urinary tract infections or new vaginal infections should be screened for sexual abuse. Cervical, rectal, and oral swabs may show evidence of sexually transmitted infections that would be atypical in the older adult. Evidence of spermatozoa, prostatic acid phosphatase, p30 glycoprotein, and DNA can help corroborate suspicion of sexual abuse. Hair and nail clippings and fibers from clothing may also be helpful.[27,92]

Toxicology

Polypharmacy is a common problem in the older population. Older patients presenting to the emergency department take an average of 4.2 medications per day, with 91% taking at least 1, 13% taking 8 or more, and some taking as many as 17. Of these patients, 31% have been prescribed a combination of medications that may lead to at least 1 potentially adverse drug interaction.[93]

Abusive or neglectful caregivers can either withhold or overadminister these medications, resulting in serious adverse health outcomes for the patient. Medications may be given in excess to pharmacologically restrain an older adult to avoid nighttime waking or to render communication with the outside world impossible. Financial abuse can render older adults unable to afford their chronic medications. Reviewing medication bottles and tracking prescription patterns is necessary for determining abuse related to medications. Communication with community pharmacists can be a very helpful practice if medication mismanagement is suspected.

Caregivers may force or deceive patients into taking medications. Common agents include benzodiazepines (eg, flunitrazepam, lorazepam), hypnotics (eg, zopiclone, zolpidem), sedatives (neuroleptics; some anti-H1 receptors), or anesthetics (eg, γ-hydroxybutyrate, ketamine). Cannabis, ecstasy, LSD, ethanol, and other drugs of abuse may also be used by abusers to chemically sedate or harm older adults. In a large review of elder homicides reviewed by researchers, 17% of elders had detectable levels of ethyl alcohol in their system.[91]

Serum drug levels may not be detected because of several factors such as rapid clearance from the body, a short half-life, or unstable chemical properties. Hair samples may be used as a helpful adjunct to serum and urine samples to detect toxic substances, especially when there is delay in presentation to the medical team and the window of opportunity to detect these substances in the blood has passed.[94]

Pain medication and psychotropic medications are commonly stolen by caregivers and diverted for their own use or sold to others. Drug levels of medications can determine whether the medication is present in the patient's system as it should be if taken correctly. The absence of a chronically prescribed medication in the blood should raise suspicion for mismanagement and possible neglect or abuse, as should the presence of a medication that is not prescribed.

The use of toxicology screening during autopsy of older adults varied greatly among medical examiners, but most at least checked medication levels.[45] Unfortunately, the medical examiner does not often have the complete list of prescription medications, and therefore cannot thoroughly evaluate the contribution of substances to the demise of the victim. In addition, postmortem drug levels cannot be correlated with serum normative values in living subjects,[95] but can be helpful when interpreted using formulas that account for known postmortem changes.[96]

POSTMORTEM BIOCHEMISTRY

Unfortunately, many cases of elder abuse and neglect are not discovered during the older adult's life. Therefore, medical examiners play a significant role in the assessment and identification of elder mistreatment. In addition to traditional autopsy, medical examiners may use postmortem biochemical markers to complement their investigation of the cause of death. Questions still exist about the reliability of the science, and robust databases do not exist to assist with interpretation of results.[97] Despite this, biochemical tests do exist, and others are in development, which may complement traditional autopsy evaluation and shed light on the cause of death.[98] Given the likelihood that many abuse and neglect cases are not identified even during postmortem examination, the availability of these biochemical markers and their potential application to assessment of elder mistreatment is encouraging.

Some of the more reliable and conventional markers such as blood urea nitrogen and creatinine, both in blood and other body fluids such as pericardial fluid, can be helpful in evaluating postmortem azotemia and dehydration. For example, although serum creatinine may be elevated by significant skeletal muscle injury caused by trauma or physical abuse, pericardial creatinine levels remain unaffected. This fact can help distinguish creatinine elevations caused by dehydration from creatinine elevations attributable to abuse.

Abnormalities in antemortem serum sodium concentrations are considered equivalent to postmortem vitreous humor levels, allowing for diagnosis of hyponatremia or hypernatremia at the time of death.

Myocardial markers, including cardiac troponin 1 (cTN1) and creatine kinase MB (CK-MB), have recently come into common use for the postmortem investigation of the cause of death. Some researchers have found that elevations of cTN1 and CK-MB in blood and pericardial fluids are related to ischemic, hypoxic, and cytologic myocardial damage, and can be characteristic of the cause of death (myocardial infarction, stroke, hyperthermia, methamphetamine abuse, asphyxia, and carbon monoxide poisoning).[99] Cardiac troponin levels should be interpreted in context of other clinical findings and pathologic findings, and with consideration of the postmortem period.[98] Myoglobin levels (present in more abundance in skeletal muscle) are elevated in pericardial and cerebrospinal fluids in cases of fatal hyperthermia and methamphetamine abuse.[100] High postmortem urinary myoglobin levels may be suggestive of significant skeletal muscle trauma or muscle hyperactivity, such as seizures.[99] Although these postmortem biochemical techniques remain somewhat new, they may help to identify muscle trauma in physical abuse, attempts to harm through inappropriate drug use, or the time and cause of death for purposes of prosecution in legal cases.

SUMMARY

Elder abuse and neglect are highly prevalent but woefully underdetected and underreported. The presentation is rarely clear, and requires the piecing together of clues that create a mosaic of the full picture. More research is needed to better characterize findings that, when identified, can contribute to certainty in cases of suspected abuse.

However, even with the current state of knowledge, medical and laboratory data can be helpful in the successful determination of abuse and neglect.

REFERENCES

1. Acierno R, Hernandez MA, Amstadter AB, et al. Prevalence and correlates of emotional, physical, sexual, and financial abuse and potential neglect in the United States: the National Elder Mistreatment Study. Am J Public Health 2010;100:292–7.
2. Lachs MS, Pillemer K. Elder abuse. Lancet 2004;364:1263–72.
3. Berman J, Lachs MS. Under the Radar: New York State Elder Abuse Prevalence Study: self-reported prevalence and documented case surveys. Report prepared by Lifespan of Greater Rochester, Inc., Weill Cornell Medical Center of Cornell University, New York City Department for the Aging; 2011.
4. Council NR. Elder mistreatment: abuse, neglect and exploitation in an aging America. Washington, DC: The National Academies Press; 2003.
5. Dong X, Simon MA. Association between elder abuse and use of ED: findings from the Chicago Health and Aging Project. Am J Emerg Med 2013;31:693–8.
6. Lachs MS, Williams CS, O'Brien S, et al. ED use by older victims of family violence. Ann Emerg Med 1997;30:448–54.
7. Dong X, Simon MA. Elder abuse as a risk factor for hospitalization in older persons. JAMA Intern Med 2013;173:911–7.
8. Dyer CB, Pavlik VN, Murphy KP, et al. The high prevalence of depression and dementia in elder abuse or neglect. J Am Geriatr Soc 2000;48:205–8.
9. Lachs MS, Williams CS, O'Brien S, et al. Adult protective service use and nursing home placement. Gerontology 2002;42:734–9.
10. Dong X, Simon MA. Association between reported elder abuse and rates of admission to skilled nursing facilities: findings from a longitudinal population-based cohort study. Gerontology 2013;59:464–72.
11. Lachs MS, Williams CS, O'Brien S, et al. The mortality of elder mistreatment. JAMA 1998;280:428–32.
12. Dong XQ, Simon MA, Beck TT, et al. Elder abuse and mortality: the role of psychological and social wellbeing. Gerontology 2011;57:549–58.
13. Mouton CP, Rodabough RJ, Rovi SL, et al. Prevalence and 3-year incidence of abuse among postmenopausal women. Am J Public Health 2004;94:605–12.
14. Report on: the future of geriatric care in our nation's emergency departments: impact and implications. 2008. Available at: http://www.acep.org/WorkArea/DownloadAsset.aspx?id=43376.http://www.acep.org/WorkArea/DownloadAsset.aspx?id=43376. Accessed June 23, 2011.
15. Roskos ER, Wilber ST. 210: the effect of future demographic changes on emergency medicine. Ann Emerg Med 2006;48:65.
16. Wilber ST, Gerson LW, Terrell KM, et al. Geriatric emergency medicine and the 2006 institute of medicine reports from the committee on the future of emergency care in the U.S. Health System. Acad Emerg Med 2006;13:1345–51.
17. Pillemer K, Finkelhor D. The prevalence of elder abuse: a random sample survey. Gerontology 1988;28:51–7.
18. Murphy K, Waa S, Jaffer H, et al. A literature review of findings in physical elder abuse. Can Assoc Radiol J 2013;64:10–4.
19. Bond MC, Butler KH. Elder abuse and neglect: definitions, epidemiology, and approaches to emergency department screening. Clin Geriatr Med 2013;29:257–73.

20. Geroff AJ, Olshaker JS. Elder abuse. Emerg Med Clin North Am 2006;24: 491–505.
21. Friedman LS, Avila S, Tanouye K, et al. A case-control study of severe physical abuse of older adults. J Am Geriatr Soc 2011;59:417–22.
22. Heyborne RD. Elder abuse: keeping the unthinkable in the differential. Academic Emergency Medicine 2007;14:566–7.
23. Chan KL, Choi WM, Fong DY, et al. Characteristics of family violence victims presenting to Emergency Departments in Hong Kong. J Emerg Med 2013;44: 249–58.
24. Teaster PB, Dugar TA, Mendiondo MS, et al. The 2004 survey of state adult protective services: abuse of adults 60 years and older. Report prepared by The National Committee for the Prevention of Elder Abuse and The National Adult Protective Services Association. Washington, DC: National Center on Elder Abuse; 2007.
25. Blakely BE, Dolon R. Another look at the helpfulness of occupational groups in the discovery of elder abuse and neglect. J Elder Abuse Negl 2003;13:1–23.
26. Jones JS, Veenstra TR, Seamon JP, et al. Elder mistreatment: National Survey of Emergency Physicians. Ann Emerg Med 1997;30:473–9.
27. Collins KA. Elder maltreatment: a review. Arch Pathol Lab Med 2006;130: 1290–6.
28. Collins KA, Presnell SE. Elder neglect and the pathophysiology of aging. Am J Forensic Med Pathol 2007;28:157–62.
29. Collins KA, Sellars K. Vertebral artery laceration mimicking elder abuse. Am J Forensic Med Pathol 2005;26:150–4.
30. Rosenblatt DE, Cho KH, Durance PW. Reporting mistreatment of older adults: the role of physicians. J Am Geriatr Soc 1996;44:65–70.
31. Dyer CB, Connelly MT, McFeeley P. The clinical and medical forensics of elder abuse and neglect. In: Bonnie RJ, National Research Council (US) Panel to Review Risk and Prevalence of Elder Abuse and Neglect, editors. Elder mistreatment: abuse, neglect, and exploitation in an aging America. Washington, DC: National Academies Press; 2003.
32. Kurrle S. Elder abuse. Aust Fam Physician 2004;33:807–12.
33. Yaffe MJ, Tazkarji B. Understanding elder abuse in family practice. Can Fam Physician 2012;58:1336–40.
34. Liao S, Mosqueda L. Physical abuse of the elderly: the medical director's response. J Am Med Dir Assoc 2006;7:242–5.
35. Bird PE, Harrington DT, Barillo DJ, et al. Elder abuse: a call to action. J Burn Care Rehabil 1998;19:522–7.
36. Palmer M, Brodell RT, Mostow EN. Elder abuse: dermatologic clues and critical solutions. J Am Acad Dermatol 2013;68:e37–42.
37. Chen AL, Koval KJ. Elder abuse: the role of the orthopaedic surgeon in diagnosis and management. J Am Acad Orthop Surg 2002;10:25–31.
38. Senn DR, McDowell JD, Alder ME. Dentistry's role in the recognition and reporting of domestic violence, abuse, and neglect. Dent Clin North Am 2001;45: 343–63, ix.
39. Golden GS. Forensic odontology and elder abuse–a case study. J Calif Dent Assoc 2004;32:336–40.
40. Cowen HJ, Cowen PS. Elder mistreatment: dental assessment and intervention. Spec Care Dentist 2002;22:23–32.
41. Duthie EH, Katz P, editors. Practice of geriatrics. 3rd edition. Philadelphia: WB Saunders; 1998.

42. Bouras EP, Lange SM, Scolapio JS. Rational approach to patients with unintentional weight loss. Mayo Clin Proc 2001;76(9):923–9.
43. Tomaiolo P, et al. Preventing and treating malnutrition in the elderly. JPEN J Parenter Enteral Nutr 1981;5(1):46–8.
44. Lachs MS, Otto J. Elder abuse roundtable: detection and diagnosis; what are the forensic markers for identifying physical and psychological signs of elder abuse and neglect? National Institute of Justice; 2000.
45. Kim L, Mitchell S, Dyer C. Do medical examiners determine elder mistreatment as a cause of death? Forensic Sci Med Pathol 2007;3:9–13.
46. Shields L, et al. Abuse and neglect: a ten-year review of mortality and morbidity in our elders in a large metropolitan area. J Forensic Sci 2004;49:122–7.
47. Wallace JI. Malnutrition and enteral/parenteral alimentation. In: Hazzard WR, Blass JP, Ettinger WH Jr, et al, editors. Principles of geriatric medicine and gerontology. 4th edition. New York: McGraw-Hill; 1999. p. 1455–69.
48. Shanley C, O'Loughlin G. Dysphagia among nursing home residents; an assessment and management protocol. J Gerontol Nurs 2000;26:243–56.
49. Harris D. Malnutrition screening in the elderly population. J R Soc Med 2005; 98(9):411–4.
50. Marcus EL, Rudensky B, Sonnenblick M. Occult elevation of CK as a manifestation of rhabdomyolysis in the elderly. J Am Geriatr Soc 1992;40:454–6.
51. Ayus JC, et al. Abnormalities of water metabolism in the elderly. Semin Nephrol 1996;16:277–88.
52. Silver A. Aging and risks for dehydration. Cleve Clin J Med 1990;57:341–4.
53. Himmelstein D, et al. Hypernatremic dehydration in nursing home patients: an indicator of neglect. J Am Geriatr Soc 1983;31:466–71.
54. Gross C, et al. Clinical indicators of dehydration severity in elderly patients. J Emerg Med 1992;10:267–74.
55. Adrogue H, et al. Hypernatremia. N Engl J Med 2000;342:1493–9.
56. Warren L, et al. The burden and outcomes associated with dehydration in the elderly, 1991. Am J Public Health 1994;84:1265–9.
57. Mandal AK, Saklayen MG, Hillman NM, et al. Predictive factors for high mortality in hypernatremic patients. Am J Emerg Med 1997;15:130–2.
58. Borra SI, et al. Hypernatremia in the aging: causes, manifestations, and outcomes. J Natl Med Assoc 1995;87(3):220–4.
59. Baumrucker SJ, Carter GT, VandeKieft G, et al. Diversion of opioid pain medications at end-of-life. Am J Hosp Palliat Care 2009;26(3):214–8.
60. Marx J, Hockberger R, Walls RJ. Rhabdomyolysis. Rosen's emergency medicine - concepts and clinical practice. 8th edition. Philadelphia: Elsevier, Saunders; 2013. p. 1667–75.
61. Ratcliffe PJ, Ledingham JG, Berman P, et al. Rhabdomyolysis in elderly people after collapse. Br Med J 1984;288:1877–8.
62. Mallinson WJ, Green MF. Covert muscle injury in aged patients admitted to hospital following falls. Age Ageing 1985;14:174–8.
63. Swain DG, Nightingale PG, Gama R, et al. Cardiac enzyme changes in elderly fallers. Age Ageing 1990;19:207–11.
64. Ratcliffe PJ, Berman P, Griffiths RA. Pressure induced rhabdomyolysis complicating an undiscovered fall. Age Ageing 1983;12:245–8.
65. Yamazaki M, Nakatome M, Takikita S, et al. A fatal case of elder abuse with rhabdomyolysis. Japanese Journal of Legal Medicine 52:43.
66. Roy D, Al Saleem BM, Al Ibrahim A, et al. Rhabdomyolysis and acute renal failure in a case of child abuse. Ann Saudi Med 1999;19:248–50.

67. Peebles J, Losek JD. Child physical abuse and rhabdomyolysis: case report and literature review. Pediatr Emerg Care 2007;23:474–7.
68. DiGiacomo JC, Frankel H, Haskell RM, et al. Unsuspected child abuse revealed by delayed presentation of periportal tracking and myoglobinuria. J Trauma 2000;49:348–50.
69. Schwengel D, Ludwig S. Rhabdomyolysis and myoglobinuria as manifestations of child abuse. Pediatr Emerg Care 1985;1:194–7.
70. Rimer RL, Roy S 3rd. Child abuse and hemoglobinuria. JAMA 1977;238:2034–5.
71. Leung A, Robson L. Myoglobinuria from child abuse. J Urol 1987;29:45–6.
72. Mukherji SK, Siegel MJ. Rhabdomyolysis and renal failure in child abuse. Am J Roentgenol 1987;148:1203–4.
73. Rosenberg HK, Gefter WB, Lebowitz RL, et al. Prolonged dense nephrograms in battered children. suspect rhabdomyolysis and myoglobinuria. J Urol 1983;21: 325–30.
74. Malik GH, Sirwal IA, Reshi AR, et al. Acute renal failure following physical torture. Nephron 1993;63:434–7.
75. Naqvi R, Ahmed E, Akhtar F, et al. Acute renal failure due to traumatic rhabdomyolysis. Ren Fail 1996;18:677–9.
76. Mohr WK, Petti TA, Mohr BD. Adverse effects associated with physical restraint. Can J Psychiatry 2003;48:330–7.
77. Evans LK, Cotter VT. Avoiding restraints in patients with dementia: understanding, prevention, and management are the keys. Am J Nurs 2008;108:40–9.
78. Miles SA. Case of death by physical restraint: new lessons from a photograph. J Am Geriatr Soc 1996;44:291–2.
79. Miles SH. Restraints and sudden death. J Am Geriatr Soc 1993;41:1013.
80. Mohr WK, Mohr BD. Mechanisms of injury and death proximal to restraint use. Arch Psychiatr Nurs 2000;14:285–95.
81. Feng Z, Hirdes JP, Smith TF, et al. Use of physical restraints and antipsychotic medications in nursing homes: a cross-national study. Int J Geriatr Psychiatry 2009;24:1110–8.
82. Abramovici MI, Singhal PC, Trachtman H. Hypernatremia and rhabdomyolysis. J Med 1992;23:17–28.
83. Cotter VT. Restraint free care in older adults with dementia. Keio J Med 2005;54: 80–4.
84. Acquarone N, Garibotto G, Pontremoli R, et al. Hypernatremia associated with severe rhabdomyolysis. Nephron 1989;51:441–2.
85. Becker BN, Ismail N. The neuroleptic malignant syndrome and acute renal failure. J Am Soc Nephrol 1994;4:1406–12.
86. Yeo TP. Heat stroke: a comprehensive review. AACN Clin Issues 2004;15: 280–93.
87. Semenza JC. Acute renal failure during heat waves. Am J Prev Med 1999;17:97.
88. Borel Y, Kilham L, Hyslop N, et al. Isologous IgG-induced tolerance to benzyl penicilloyl. Nature 1976;261:49–50.
89. Shoji S, Karasawa K, Miyagi K, et al. Serum creatine kinase in primary hypothermia. Clin Chem 1989;35:2254–5.
90. Bosker G. Elderly abuse: patterns, detection and management. Resident Staff Physician Magazine 1990;30:39–44.
91. Collins K, Presnell S. Elder homicide a 20 yr review. Am J Forensic Med Pathol 2006;27:183–7.
92. Collins K. The laboratory's role in detecting sexual assault. Lab Med 1998;29: 361–5.

93. Hohl CM, Dankoff J, Colacone A, et al. Polypharmacy, adverse drug-related events, and potential adverse drug interactions in elderly patients presenting to an Emergency Department. Ann Emerg Med 2001;38:666–71.

94. Kintz P. Chemical abuse in the elderly: evidence from hair analysis. Ther Drug Monit 2008;30:207–11.

95. Ferrer R. Post-mortem clinical pharmacology. Br J Clin Pharmacol 2008;66: 430–43.

96. Launiainen T, Ojanpera I. Drug concentrations in post-mortem femoral blood compared to therapeutic concentrations in plasma. Drug Test Anal 2013. http://dx.doi.org/10.1002/dta.1507.

97. Luna J. Is postmortem biochemistry really useful? Why is it not widely used in forensic pathology? Leg Med 2009;11(Suppl 1):S27–30.

98. Maeda H. Significance of postmortem biochemistry in determining the cause of death. Leg Med 2009;11:46–9.

99. Zhu BL, et al. Postmortem urinary myoglobin levels with reference to the causes of death. Forensic Sci Int 2001;115:183–8.

100. Wang Q, et al. Combined analysis of creatine kinase MB, cardiac troponin 1 and myoglobin in pericardial and cerebrospinal fluids to investigate myocardial and skeletal muscle injury in medicolegal autopsy cases. Leg Med 2011;5: 226–32.

Common Presentations of Elder Abuse in Health Care Settings

James S. Powers, MD[a,b],*

KEYWORDS

- Elder abuse • Health care setting • Risk factors • Caregivers

KEY POINTS

- Health care professionals encounter elder abuse in the community and in medical offices, emergency rooms, hospitals, and long-term care facilities.
- Keen awareness of elder abuse risk factors and the variety of presentations in different health settings helps promote detection, treatment, and prevention of elder abuse.

INTRODUCTION

Respect for seniors and their caregivers is at the heart of patient-centered care. Orientation of services to achieve positive outcomes as viewed from the patient's perspective is the ultimate goal. These principles can be adapted to elder abuse and its prevention in all health care settings and levels of care.

The White House Conference on Aging promoted a patient Bill of Basic Human Rights for Older Americans (**Box 1**). These principles are important and set the benchmark in promoting dignity for elder care in all locations of care.

Every older person deserves our respect. Caregivers also need assistance, and there is a need to support the caregiver to best help vulnerable elders. Seventy-five percent of caregivers are family members, and 70% are female, who function with little assistance, many with unmet physical and emotional needs of their own.[1–4]

Patients flow across a continuum of care, from ambulatory to custodial nursing home care, to access resources according to their needs. Each level of care (**Box 2**) has its own unique characteristics with patients at different stages of disease, function, and vulnerabilities. In general, more functional individuals reside in the community where financial abuse, scams, and isolation are more prevalent. As some age,

[a] Tennessee Valley Health System Geriatric Research, Education and Clinical Center, 1310 24th Avenue, South Nashville, TN 37212, USA; [b] The Center on Aging, Vanderbilt University School of Medicine, 7159 Vanderbilt Medical Center East, Nashville, TN 37232, USA
* Corresponding author. Tennessee Valley Health System Geriatric Research, Education and Clinical Center, 1310 24th Avenue, South Nashville, TN 37212.
E-mail address: james.powers@vanderbilt.edu

Clin Geriatr Med 30 (2014) 729–741
http://dx.doi.org/10.1016/j.cger.2014.08.004
0749-0690/14/$ – see front matter Published by Elsevier Inc.

geriatric.theclinics.com

Box 1
Basic human rights for older Americans

1. The right to freedom, independence and the free exercise of individual initiative. This should encompass not only opportunities and resources for personal planning and managing one's lifestyle but support systems for maximum growth and contributions by older persons to their community.

2. The right to an income retirement which would provide an adequate standard of living. Such income must be sufficiently adequate to assure maintenance of mental and physical activities which delay deterioration and maximize individual potential for self-help and support. This right should be assured regardless of employment capability.

3. The right for opportunity for employment free from discriminatory practices because of age. Such employment when desired should not exploit individuals because of age and should permit utilization of talents, skills, and experience of older persons for the good of self and community. Compensation should be based on the prevailing wage scales of the community for comparable work.

4. The right for an opportunity to participate in the widest range of meaningful civic, educational, recreational, and cultural activities. The varying interests and needs of older Americans require programs and activities sensitive to their rich and diverse heritage. There should be opportunities for involvement with persons of all ages in programs which are affordable and accessible.

5. The right to suitable housing. The widest choices of living arrangements should be available, designed, and located with reference to special needs at costs which the older person can afford.

6. The right to the best level of physical and mental health services needed. Such services should include the latest knowledge and techniques science can make available without regard to economic status.

7. The right to ready access to effective social services. These services should enhance independence and well-being, yet provide protection and care as needed.

8. The right to appropriate institutional care when required. Care should provide full restorative services in a safe environment. This care should also promote and protect the dignity and rights of the individual along with family and community ties.

9. The right to a life and death with dignity. Regardless of age, society must assure individual citizens of the protection of their constitutional rights and opportunities for self-respect, respect and acceptance from others, a sense of enrichment and contribution, and freedom from dependency. Dignity in dying includes the right of the individual to permit or deny the use of extraordinary life support systems.

We pledge the resources of this nation to the ensuring of these rights for all older Americans regardless of race, color, creed, age, sex, or national origin, with the caution that the complexities of our society be monitored to assure that the fulfillment of one right does not nullify the benefits received as a result of another entitlement. We further dedicate the technology and human skill of this nation so that later life will be marked in liberty with the realization of the pursuit of happiness.

From the White House Conference on Aging, Administration on Aging, Department of Health, Education, and Welfare, AOA Pub. No. 148. Washington, DC: 1971.

---

they may be susceptible to isolation, injuries and conditions such as falls, malnutrition, or dehydration if caregiving and health care needs are not met. More physically dependent individuals require higher levels of care and, because of their dependence, are more prone to trauma and decubiti during lapses of caregiving. For those who live alone in the community, dementia or depression can lead to self-neglect.

Box 2
Glossary of levels of care

Adult Day Care

Structured day programs for older adults and disabled individuals permitting family caregivers time to pursue personal and employment opportunities while still maintaining affected individuals in the home setting.

Respite Care

Temporary in-home assistance or placement (foster home, nursing home, or hospital) of a disabled individual (often several days to weeks) to allow a rest period for family caregivers. This frequently permits resumed acceptance of caregiving functions and long-term maintenance in the home setting.

Assisted Living

Residence that provides a variety of services designated to facilitate continued residence in the community for older adults and disabled persons. Assistance may include: meals, administration of medication, homemaker services, transportation, health reminders, and personal care.

Board and Care

Residence for infirm individuals who are able to ambulate, or self-propel in a wheelchair. Meals, personal care, medicine administration, and group living environment are provided.

Nursing Home Level I (Intermediate Care)

Institutional care for individuals whose functional disability prevents assistance at a lower level of care. Many seniors with stroke, cancer, and cardiovascular disease reside in long-term care facilities.

Nursing Home Level II (Skilled Care)

Institutional care for individuals with skilled nursing needs. This includes frail elderly with feeding tubes, postoperative care, wound care, and rehabilitation.

When caring for elders, health care providers not only see patients in clinics, emergency rooms, and hospitals but also care for them by working in their sites of living. In doing so, providers interface with the various sites of care, including adult day health care, adult day care, assisted living facilities, board and care homes, respite care homes, and nursing homes. Each time older persons interface with the health care system, there are invaluable opportunities for health care providers to detect and intervene in abusive situations.

PRESENTATIONS OF ELDER ABUSE IN COMMUNITY LIVING
Home Environment

Identification of abuse in the home requires a high level of suspicion, whereas in health care facilities incidents are more likely to be directly observable and quickly discovered. The home environment reveals clues to abuse that office or hospital visits may not. Patients presenting in the office may not be able to reveal all concerns, especially if accompanied by the caregiver. Telltale signs of fear, silence, or inability to interview the patient alone are warning signs to the provider of possible abuse. The abuse can take many forms and is often not directly observable. Community occurrences related to caregiving deficits often go unreported by the patient. The affected individual fears abandonment or institutionalization and so tolerates continued abuse.

Health care professionals oversee the care of persons living at home through home health services, home hospice care, adult day care, adult day health care, and PACE

(Program for the All-inclusive Care of the Elderly) programs. Acting as agents of the provider, staff reports of abuse need to be taken seriously by the provider. Home care nurses may be the first and only professionals to notice signs of multiple types of abuse in the home. Neglect may be apparent from lack of food and proper hygiene, or developing decubiti ulcers despite active treatment. Home care staff may uncover evidence of restraints or bruising in suspicious places. Hospice nurses may observe that pain medications are being refilled too quickly, even though the hospice patient remains in pain, leading to the realization that the caregiver is using it for themselves. Patients in assisted living facilities (ALFs) are eligible for home health services as are persons in their own homes, and, in addition, have an ALF staff, which provides another level of oversight. Health care providers, therefore, have the benefit of information provided by ALF staff and in-home care. ALFs are often licensed by states and must meet fire and building safety standards; however, they are not reimbursed by Medicare and Medicaid, and therefore are not inspected by state agencies. Residents of ALFs may be less prone to financial abuse and neglect of hygiene or nutritional needs in comparison with community-dwelling elders[5]; however, a survey of ALF administrators suggests that abuse is indeed prevalent, although there has been little study of this in comparison with nursing homes.[6]

Nursing Homes

Nursing homes provide a very high level of oversight and care because residents have an average of 3 or more functional deficits. Nursing homes are licensed to provide skilled or nonskilled services (**Box 3**), or both. Residents of nursing homes have professional staff availability round the clock. Long-term care staff members, however, are prone to overwork and stress. Low staff-to-patient ratios, high staff turnover, and urban environments where staff does not have long-term knowledge of the resident all contribute to increased risk of abuse. Neglect is the most common type of elder abuse in facilities. In addition to high levels of care, nursing homes are licensed by state agencies, and are subject to state surveys and statutory regulations.[7] These surveys include yearly unannounced state inspections with deficiencies graded on a scope and severity grid. Major quality indicators are also posted for public inspection on Nursing Home Compare (http://www.medicare.gov/nursinghomecompare/?AspxAutoDetectCookieSupport=1).

Focusing on caregivers, whether in the home or facility, is crucial to understanding and intervening in elder abuse. Although caregivers may inflict all forms of abuse, neglect is the most prevalent form of abuse in the frail elderly (**Box 4**).[8] Caregiver fatigue, burnout, and failure to provide care occurs more often with certain patient factors, including dependency, mental health, and dementia, and caregiver factors, including illness, lack of control, mental health needs, and lack of financial and support services. The failure of the caregiver relationship often results in institutionalization.[9,10]

Box 3
Nursing home services

Skilled	Nonskilled
Acute rehabilitation	Dementia
Wound care	Functional dependency
Intravenous antibiotics	Incontinence
Changing oxygen, insulin requirements	Lack of caregiver

Box 4
Risk factors for inadequate or abusive caregiving

Cognitive impairment in the patient, caregiver, or both

Dependency of the caregiver on the patient, or vice-versa

Family conflict

Family history of abusive behavior, alcohol or drug misuse or abuse, mental illness, or mental retardation

Financial distress or lack of funds to meet caregiver health demands

Isolation of the patient, caregiver, or both

Living arrangements inadequate to the needs of the ill person

Stressful events in the family such as death of a loved one or loss of employment

From Fulmer T. Mistreatment of older adults. In: Durso SC, Sullivan GM, editors. Geriatrics review syllabus: a core curriculum in geriatric medicine. 8th edition. New York: American Geriatrics Society; 2013. p. 105; with permission.

FINDINGS ASSOCIATED WITH ELDER ABUSE

Elder abuse is notoriously underreported but appears to be more common in the community, and is estimated to occur in 1% to 2% of the elderly population. In a national survey of adult protective service agencies conducted in 2000, less than 8.3% of abuse occurred in institutional settings and 60.7% of cases were domestic. Substantiated reports in institutional settings represented 8.5%, and domestic settings 42.5%. Of institutional complaints filed, nursing home staff made 2.6% and long-term care ombudsmen made 0.5%.[5]

There are 6 major categories of elder abuse (**Box 5**). Financial abuse relates to the exploitation or misappropriation of an elderly person's assets for personal or monetary gains. Physical abuse consists of willful acts carried out with the intent of causing pain or injury. Sexual abuse includes nonconsensual sexual activity with a nonconsenting or incompetent older person. Emotional abuse includes willful acts or threats intended to cause emotional anguish or pain. Caregiver neglect is the most common form of abuse, and consists of intentional or unintentional failure of the designated caregiver to meet the needs necessary for the elderly person's physical and mental well-being. Self-neglect is present among individuals living alone who, by choice or because of

---

Box 5
Classification of elder abuse

Financial

Physical

Sexual

Emotional

Caregiver neglect

Self-neglect

Data from Lachs MS, Pillemer K. Abuse and neglect of elderly persons. N Engl J Med 1995;332:437–43; and Kruger RM, Moon CH. Can you spot the signs of elder mistreatment? Postgrad Med 1999;106:169–83.

---

dementia or mental health concerns, fail to act in their own self-interest with subsequent deterioration in health and functional status.

Each of these different forms of abuse is associated with hallmark findings (**Table 1**). Financial abuse occurs when the affected individual is a victim of fraud or scams, or family exploitation. If the abuse is perpetrated by a caregiver, the victim may feel helpless because of dependency on the abuser and fear of placement into an institution. Caregivers may use resources for personal gain and neglect patient needs. The presence of dementia or extreme dependency needs may limit the victim's ability to obtain help or comprehend the seriousness of the abuse. In the office setting, the patient may

Table 1 Screening for mistreatment of older adults	
Assessment Domain	**Key Indicators**
General	Clothing: inappropriate dress, soil, or disrepair Hygiene (including appearance of hair and nails) Nutritional status Skin integrity
Abuse	Anxiety, nervousness, especially toward caregiver Bruising, in various healing stages, especially bilateral or on inner arms or thighs Fractures, especially in various healing stages Lacerations Repeated emergency department visits Repeated falls Signs of sexual abuse Statements about abuse by the patient
Neglect	Contractures Dehydration Depression Diarrhea Failure to respond to warning of obvious disease Fecal impaction Malnutrition Medication underuse or overuse or otherwise inappropriate use Poor hygiene Pressure ulcers Repeated falls Repeated hospital admissions Urine burns Statements about neglect by the patient
Exploitation	Evidence of misuse of patient's assets Inability of patient to account for money and property or to pay for essential care Reports of demands for money or goods in exchange for caregiving or services Unexplained loss of Social Security, pension checks Statements about exploitation by the patient
Abandonment	Evidence that patient is left alone unsafely Evidence of sudden withdrawal of care by caregiver Statements about abandonment by the patient

Data from Fulmer T. Elder mistreatment assessment. Try this: best practices in nursing care to older adults. 2008;15. Available at: www.consultgerirn.org/. Accessed March 17, 2014; and Fulmer T. Mistreatment of older adults. In: Durso SC, Sullivan GM, editors. Geriatrics review syllabus: a core curriculum in geriatric medicine. 8th edition. New York: American Geriatrics Society. 2013. p. 105.

only reveal information when directly questioned. Clues for health care providers may include inability to obtain prescriptions, medication diversion, statements of the patient regarding exploitation, or repeated requests from family members for money.

Physical abuse may occur in the home or institutional setting. Signs may include bruises, skin tears, fractures, burns, and other injuries. Patients may present to the emergency room immediately after the event or after a delay. Clues to physical abuse may be found after inspection of the injuries, which commonly involve skin, the head, and bone. Most often, the physical injury must be evaluated in the context of the history for a determination of abuse to be made. Certain locations of bruising are considered suspicious, with large bruises, facial and lateral arm bruises, and posterior torso bruises suggestive of abuse.[11] Band- and belt-like markings or patterns suggest restraints.

Sexual abuse occurs in the setting of incompetent or frail and dependent patients. Signs include depression, fear, dysuria, tender genitalia, and venereal diseases. The victim may express fear in the presence of the perpetrator. Sexual abuse occurs primarily in the home setting, with 70% occurring in the home compared with 30% in facilities according to a 2006 report to the US Department of Justice, which surveyed an expert working group regarding cases reported to Adult Protective Services or the criminal justice system.[12] Occurrences in facilities signify sentinel events that may lead to grave sanctions.

Emotional abuse may be suspected when the interaction between patient and caregiver seems tense and strained. Silence, depression, and an ever-present or controlling caregiver are also signs. In general, emotional abuse occurs in all settings between caregivers and recipients, and is often detected in health care settings. It may be suspected if the caregiver refuses to leave the patient or speaks for the patient, or if the victim expresses fear in the presence of the caregiver or makes statements regarding fear or exploitation.

Caregiver neglect may present as weight loss, dehydration, falls, fears, and poor hygiene. Such signs occur primarily in patients living in the home setting and board and care residences, or in nursing home patients with severe dementia or acute illnesses. The caregivers may be overwhelmed. If it occurs in long-term care facilities, neglect suggests low staffing levels, poor staff training, and lack of leadership.

Self-neglect occurs among persons living alone. Often depression or dementia are present. Malnutrition, repeated falls, decubitus ulcers, contractures, medication nonadherence, missed appointments, and poor hygiene can be clues. Fear of loss of home or possessions, and inability to access services and assistance, are often present.[13]

FACTORS ASSOCIATED WITH ELDER ABUSE IN DIFFERENT SETTINGS

The home setting, board and care, and foster home encompass care by family or nonrelated individuals. Awareness of financial resources is crucial in understanding caregiver needs, especially when the caregiver depends on the finances of the care recipient. Patient-directed benefits sponsored by the state, or the Veterans Administration (VA), permit individuals to purchase caregiving services. Although background checks reduce the potential for abuse, the possibility for abuse and neglect remains. Oversight by state agencies and the VA helps to promote safe patient-centered care and helps patients remain in their homes.

Caregivers are subject to stress, illness, competing roles with other family concerns, and loss of employment when caregiving results in work absences. Often caregivers assume their roles with little preparation and no training for the skills required of them. Some 70% of family caregivers work out of a sense of duty, often without relief and benefit of respite.[14] Other family members may avoid sharing responsibilities, further burdening the designated caregiver. A VA State of the Art Conference on Geriatric Care in 2008 reported a listing of caregiver needs (**Box 6**).[15]

The presence of dementia in the patient increases the caregiving burden. The requisite constant supervision is difficult to maintain. Incontinence is a major contributor to caregiver burden. Behavioral problems including safety concerns can be sudden and unexpected. Training in communication and management strategies for persons with dementia, such as acknowledgment and redirecting, takes time to develop.

Other factors include social and geographic isolation, which produces loneliness and lack of oversight. Residence in remote areas may include lack of readily available assistance and fewer support services for caregivers. In the community, scams involving the elderly are common, especially those who live alone or have cognitive impairment. Unscrupulous and unsolicited marketing for home repairs, investment, and sweepstakes traps many elderly each year. Transportation needs are universal requirements for frail elders. Lack of accessible transportation or difficulty in scheduling transportation contributes to increased isolation. Caregiver assistance and provision of information is required for transportation to be a functional service.

Cultural issues and low education contribute to the caregiver profile. Lower social status and lack of experience or training all affect caregiver function. The female caregiving role is predominant, although 30% to 40% of caregivers are men.[14] Training and expectations of informal family caregivers differ considerably from the expectations of licensed health care professionals.

HEALTH CARE SETTINGS

In ambulatory care practices, routine office visits offer the opportunity to screen for abuse. Clues include missed visits, lack of routine screenings and immunizations, poor attainment of disease management targets, and medication nonadherence. Diversion of medications, poor hygiene, and a poor relationship between patient and caregiver may be other clues (see **Table 1**).

Elder abuse presents in the emergency department (ED) in the setting of acute medical conditions and trauma, which may be directly related to abuse and neglect. Careful observation for signs of medication nonadherence, multiple injuries, and fears and concerns expressed by the patient often lead to the detection of elder abuse. Hospitalization, involvement of social work, and reporting to Adult Protective Services and law enforcement may be indicated, especially if there are concerns about the safety of

---

Box 6
Caregiver needs

Information, education (illness specific), eligibility and availability of community resources

Home-based and community-based resources

Emergency contact information

Group support

Transportation

Help with personal caregiver needs, medical and mental health

the victim on returning to the home environment. Unfortunately, although health care providers are mandated reporters, they continually underreport. A study of ED nurses in Florida found that 83% reported seeing evidence of elder abuse but only 36% had reported abuse.[16] In another survey, ED nurses reported seeing severe injuries such as skull fractures, sexual assault, bites, and severe bruising although only 36% reported abuse, despite medical personnel reporting requirements.[17]

Institutional abuse and neglect in nursing homes includes the most vulnerable and frail of all elders. Some 7% of all complaints regarding institutional facilities reported to long-term care ombudsmen were complaints of abuse, neglect, or exploitation.[18] A 2000 study involving 2000 nursing home residents reported that 44% claimed to have been abused, and 95% said they were personally neglected or saw another resident neglected.[19,20] Abuse may involve restraints, poor skin care evidenced by bad hygiene or soiled clothing, or even decubiti. Falls, injuries during transfers, lack of equipment, low staffing levels, and poorly trained staff with high turnover may be present. Clues include falls during lapses in observation, inappropriate medication, lack of activity, dehydration, and use of restraints.

A 1987 survey of 577 nursing home staff members from 31 facilities found that 36% witnessed at least 1 incident of physical abuse during the preceding 12 months, including excessive use of restraints, pushing, shoving, grabbing, or biting. Ten percent reported they had committed such acts themselves.[20] National data from the Centers for Medicare and Medicaid Services (CMS 2010) delineate a prevalence of verbal abuse, physical abuse, or socially inappropriate behavior in 19% of long-term residents with psychiatric illnesses, and 7% among residents without psychiatric illness.[21] Resident-on-resident assaults are more common in the setting of dementia, psychiatric illness, dignity violations, disordered sleep, and staff isolation.[22] To reduce the prevalence of patterns of neglect, nursing homes are required to perform reviews of quality indicators and quarterly submission of minimum dataset (MDS) reports, which track many conditions potentially related to abuse and neglect.

Hospitalized patients are more physically dependent, and the potential for neglect is present. Because of the short length of stay in acute care settings and the high level of training of most personnel, abuse is less likely. Safety during transfers, management of delirium and behavioral disturbances, lapses in supervision, and inattention to comfort are potential contributors to falls, unwarranted use of restraints and urinary catheters, and development of pressure sores.

ADDRESSING ELDER ABUSE IN DIFFERENT SETTINGS

Home-based and community-based resources must be accessed and individualized to address specific patient needs. Deciding on whether it is safe to return to the home setting, and which resources need to be added, requires detailed information about the patient and family circumstances in addition to clinical skill and knowledge of available resources. The more complex patients may benefit from interdisciplinary team input to achieve optimum results.

The United States lags behind many other developed countries with respect to caregiver support services in proportion to its investment in acute care services.[23] Medicare home services traditionally offer only acute skilled rehabilitation services, and do not cover maintenance or restorative care visits. However, there is an increasing realization of the need for these services and a corresponding increase in availability of support services. Resources for caregivers include Web sites, support groups, individual counseling by social workers, and nursing personnel from hospital or home agencies. Community agencies and churches are also helpful in supporting caregivers.

Support groups for caregivers are sponsored by organizations including local affiliates of the Alzheimer's Association, Mental Health Association, specific disease-oriented foundations, and the VA. These groups offer education about specific disease processes, management and coping strategies, and even respite care programs. Addressing competing caregiver roles and responsibilities, managing unrealistic expectations, stress management, and emotional and social support serve as invaluable assistance to many caregivers.

Home care team meetings provide the opportunity to discuss particular patients with the involvement of nursing, social work, and physician and occupational therapy These meetings, which may include involvement of the primary care provider and additional community resources, can complete wellness checks, identify gaps in care, and address needs for both caregiver and patient.

For patients, victim empowerment support groups discuss problems, strengths, solutions, and resources to safely maintain independence and protection from unwanted influence and abuse. Buddy systems are also promoted, providing nonprofessional help, listening, and support to promote appropriate responses, improve self-esteem, and maintain personal control.[24] For individuals living alone, medic alert systems can add protection. Some senior residences may offer regular wellness checks to add another margin of safety to independent living. Community education regarding scams is often provided by community nonprofit agencies and is publicized in the media to educate elderly consumers.

In instances of immediate concern for the safety of the patient resulting from caregiver neglect or self-neglect, immediate removal to a safe environment may be necessary. It is the duty of the health care professional to involve the local department of Adult Protective Services to determine the extent of the situation, including personal and family resources. This approach provides the legal recourse to determine the capacity of the affected individuals to make decisions on their own behalf, and to appoint a guardian. The individual may also be removed to a safe residence.

Institutional needs and resources vary greatly. In long-term care facilities, recruitment and retention of experienced staff is a challenge. The average tenure of nursing aids, the largest pool of nursing home staff, is 6 months. Long-term care facilities are constantly training new staff to care for our most vulnerable citizens. Leadership and professionalism, in addition to providing a career ladder, is crucial in addressing this important workforce issue. Staffing levels in long-term care average 3.57 (0.8) hours per resident day according to a review of the 2004 online screening certification and reporting system (OSCAR).[25]

Hospitals also are challenged to provide attentive staff for frail elders and additional sitters for unstable or delirious patients. Periodic in-house services on geriatric topics and training designed to address management strategies for difficult patients, especially nonpharmacologic management of agitation and other special needs of frail elderly, are important ways to address this need (**Box 7**).[26–28]

Both hospital and nursing home care planning meetings can focus on patients and families with caregiving challenges, permitting an interdisciplinary approach to difficult issues. Quality improvement metrics such as falls, injuries, use of restraint, use of psychotropic medication, and MDS quarterly reports in the case of long-term care facilities can permit focus on areas of concern using a PDSA (plan-do-study-act) process improvement, or, in the case of unusually concerning problems, a root cause analysis process.

Box 7
Nonpharmacologic management of agitation in dementia

Attention to patient comfort (ie, toileting, bathing, temperature, dietary preferences)

Therapeutic environment of care

Maintain normal sleep-wake cycle

Assess for pain

Assess for sensory deprivation (hearing and vision)

Removal of restraints

Behavioral therapy (ie, stimulus control, differential reinforcement of desirable behaviors, redirection)

Structured activities such as exercise and outdoor walks

Staff training (ie, empathy, skills, focused nurturing care)

Pet therapy, companion animals

Massage, music therapy, aromatherapy

Video or audio recordings of family members

Individual and group reminiscence therapy

Activities of daily living skills retraining

Cognitive retraining, reality orientation

Reduced stimulation unit

Patient assaults, including patient-on-patient, patient-on-staff, and staff-on-patient assaults, are particularly difficult problems.[22] The presence of dementia, psychiatric diagnoses, anger, and history of assaults are particularly important antecedents. Individualized care planning to provide patient-centered care, a therapeutic environment of care, enhanced staff communication, and a change of shift communication protocol are helpful strategies in addressing this important problem.

REFERENCES

1. Drinka TJ, Smith JC, Drinks PJ. Correlates of depression and burden for informal caregivers of patients in a geriatrics referral clinic. J Am Geriatr Soc 1987;35: 522–5.
2. Conlin MM, Caranosos GJ, Davidson RA. Reduction of caregiver stress by respite care: a pilot study. South Med J 1992;85:1096–100.
3. Colerick EJ, George LK. Predictors of institutionalization among caregivers of patients with Alzheimer's disease. J Am Geriatr Soc 1986;34:493–8.
4. Zarit SH, Reever KE, Bach-Peterson J. Relatives of the impaired elderly: correlates of feelings of burden. Gerontologist 1980;20:649–55.
5. National Center on Elder Abuse. A response to the abuse of vulnerable adults: the 2000 survey of state adult protective services. In: Teaster PB, editor. Washington, DC: 2003. Available at: http://www.elderabusecenter.org/pdf/research/apsreport030703.pdf. Accessed March 17, 2014.
6. Castle N. An examination of resident abuse in assisted living facilities. Available at: https://www.ncjrs.gov/pdffiles1/nij/grants/241611.pdf. Accessed March 17, 2014.
7. Levenson S. Medical direction in long term care: a guidebook to the future. Durham (NC): Carolina Academic Press; 1993.

8. Teaster PB, editor. The 2004 survey of state adult protective services: abuse of adults 60 years of age and older. Washington, DC: The National Committee for the Prevention of Elder Abuse and t\ The National Adult Protective Services Association; 2006. Prepared for The National Center on Elder Abuse. Available at: http://www.napsa-now.org/wp-content/uploads/2012/09/2-14-06-FINAL-60+REPORT.pdf.

9. Shulz R, Beach SR. Caregiving as a risk factor for mortality, the caregiver health effects study. JAMA 1999;282:2215–9.

10. Elder abuse and neglect. Council on Scientific Affairs. JAMA 1987;257:966–71.

11. Ziminski CE, Wiglesworth A, Austin R, et al. Injury patterns and causal mechanisms of bruising in physical elder abuse. J Forensic Nurs 2013;9:84–91.

12. Burgess AW. Elderly victims of sexual abuse and their offenders. Report to the US Department of Justice. 2006. Available at: https://www.ncjrs.gov/pdffiles1/nij/grants/216550.13. Accessed March 17, 2014.

13. Gurley RJ, Lum N, Sande M, et al. Persons found in their home helpless or dead. N Engl J Med 1996;334:1710–39.

14. A NAC, 2004: National Alliance for Caregiving/AARP, Caregiving in the U.S, 2004. Available at: http://assets.aarp.org/rgcenter/il/us_caregiving_1.pdf. Accessed March 17, 2014.

15. Shay K, Burris JF, State of the Art Planning Committee. Setting the stage for a new strategic plan for geriatrics and extended care in the Veterans Health Administration: summary of the 2008 VA State of the Art Conference, "The changing faces of geriatrics and extended care: meeting the needs of veterans in the next decade". J Am Geriatr Soc 2008;56:2330–9.

16. Reynolds E, Stanton S. Elder abuse: a nursing perspective. In: Kosberg JI, editor. Abuse and maltreatment of the elderly: causes and interventions. Boston (MA): John Wright; 1983. p. 391–403.

17. Pettee EJ. Elder abuse: implications for staff development. J Nurs Staff Dev 1997; 13:7–12.

18. Department of Health and Human Services, Administration on Aging. 2010 National ombudsman reporting system data tables. Washington, DC: US Department of Health and Human Services, Administration on Aging; 2010.

19. Broyles K. The silenced voice speaks out: a study of abuse and neglect of nursing home residents. A report from the Atlanta long term care ombudsman program and Atlanta Legal Aid Society to the National Citizen's Coalition for Nursing Home Reform. Atlanta (GA): National Citizen's Coalition for Nursing Home Reform; 2000.

20. Pillemer K, Moore DW. Abuse of patients in nursing homes: findings from a survey of staff. Gerontologist 1989;29:314–20.

21. Centers for Medicare & Medicaid Services. MDS quality indicator report. 2010. Available at: http://www.cms.gov/Research-Statistics-Data-and-Systems/Computer-Data-and-Systems/MDSPubQIandResRep/qmreport.html. Accessed March 17, 2014.

22. Powers J, Gwirtsman H, Erwin S. Psychiatric illness and resident assaults among veterans in long-term care facilities. J Gerontol Nurs 2014;40(4):25–30. http://dx.doi.org/10.3928/00989134-20131028-05.

23. Murray CJ, Frenk J. Ranking 37th – measuring the performance of the US health care system. N Engl J Med 2010;362:98–9.

24. Reis M, Nahmiash D. When seniors are abused: an intervention model. Gerontologist 1995;35:666–71.

25. Mueller C, Arling G, Kane R, et al. Nursing home staffing standards: their relationship to nurse staffing levels. Gerontologist 2006;46:74–80.

26. Cohen-Mansfield J. Non-pharmacologic interventions for inappropriate behaviors in dementia, a review, summary and critique. Am J Geriatr Psychiatry 2001;9: 361–81.

27. Wolff JC, Rand-Giovannette E, Palmer S, et al. Caregiving and chronic care: the guided care program for families and friends. J Gerontol A Biol Sci Med Sci 2009; 64:785–91.

28. Burns R, Nichols LO, Martindale-Adams J, et al. Primary care interventions for dementia caregivers: 2-year outcomes from the REACH study. Gerontologist 2003; 43:547–52.

Prevention and Early Identification of Elder Abuse

Jason Burnett, PhD[a,b,*], W. Andrew Achenbaum, PhD[a,b,c],
Kathleen Pace Murphy, PhD[a,b]

KEYWORDS

- Elder abuse • Screening • Ageism • Adult protective services • Mistreatment

KEY POINTS

- Early identification and prevention of elder abuse requires challenging ageist perceptions.
- Increasing public awareness and health professional training is needed to differentiate abuse in older adults from "normal" aging.
- More research is needed to identify characteristics that increase the risk of elder abuse and subsequent studies to inform best practices for reducing harmful outcomes.
- Concise assessments can be used effectively during brief clinical visits with older adults to identify risk factors and indicators of abuse.

INTRODUCTION

The United States is undergoing an aging boom. Every day, 8000 Baby Boomers reach the retirement age of 65. Currently, adults 65 years and older represent 14% of the US population; by 2050, this number is expected to reach 25%.[1] This upsurge in societal aging will most likely be accompanied by a sharp increase in callous acts of abuse for many older adults, causing horrific suffering regardless of social class, gender, or ethnic and cultural background. Elder abuse escalates the burden on limited public health resources.[2] We need both effective prevention strategies to protect an aging population at risk for elder abuse as well as early detection of warning signs and symptoms.

[a] Division of Geriatric and Palliative Medicine, Department of Internal Medicine, Harris Health System, Texas Elder Abuse and Mistreatment Institute (TEAM), UT Health, 3601 North MacGregor Way, Houston, TX 77004, USA; [b] Consortium on Aging, Texas Elder Abuse and Mistreatment Institute (TEAM), UT Health, 3601 North MacGregor Way, Houston, TX 77004, USA; [c] Graduate School of Social Work, The University of Houston, 110 HA Social Work Building, Houston, TX 77204, USA
* Corresponding author. Division of Geriatric and Palliative Care, Department of Internal Medicine, UT Health, 3601 North MacGregor Way, Houston, TX 77004.
E-mail address: Jason.Burnett@uth.tmc.edu

Clin Geriatr Med 30 (2014) 743–759
http://dx.doi.org/10.1016/j.cger.2014.08.013   geriatric.theclinics.com

DEFINITION

Over the past 30 years, elder abuse has received greater and greater attention from health and social service professions and law enforcement agencies. The US Centers for Disease Control and Prevention,[3] the US Administration on Aging (now known as the US Administration on Community-Living),[4] and the World Health Organization have made it a priority.[5] Although there is no universally accepted definition of elder abuse, existing ones are consonant with the (1985) Elder Abuse Prevention, Identification and Treatment Act, which defines abuse as "the willful infliction of injury, unreasonable confinement, intimidation or cruel punishment with resulting physical harm or pain or mental anguish or the willful deprivation by a caretaker of goods or services which are necessary to avoid physical harm, mental anguish or mental illness."[6] The World Health Organization further describes elder abuse as an act of violence and a human rights violation.[7] Given the latitude of interpretations under this definition, it is not surprising that public officials and interprofessional researchers broaden their understanding of the scope of elder abuse. Identifying and addressing the causes and consequences of elder abuse, broadly understood, speaks to many comorbidities and environmental hazards associated with late-life vulnerabilities.

TYPES OF ELDER ABUSE

The US National Center on Elder Abuse identifies 7 unique types of elder abuse and provides definitions for each: Physical abuse, sexual abuse, financial exploitation, caregiver neglect, psychological and emotional abuse, abandonment, and self-neglect.[8] **Table 1** lists definitions for each type of abuse along with their most recent US population-based prevalence estimates.[8,9] These estimates represent self-reported abuse by cognitively intact community-dwelling older adults.

Table 1
Abuse types, definitions and 1-year US population-based incidence estimates for community-dwelling cognitively intact adults 65 years of age and older

Type	Definition	Prevalence (%)
Physical abuse	Bodily injury, physical pain or impairment owing to use of physical force	1.6
Sexual abuse	Any kind of non-consensual sexual contact	0.6
Psychological/emotional abuse	Verbal or non-verbal acts that cause emotional and/or psychological anguish, pain, or distress	3.2
Financial exploitation	Improper or illegal use of an older adult's money, property or assets	5.2
Caregiver neglect[a]	Failure or refusal to fulfill one's caregiver obligation or duties to an older adult	5.1
Self-neglect[a]	Older adult self-behaviors that threatens the individual's own health and safety	5.1
Abandonment	Desertion of an older adult by a person who assumed responsibility for their care	—

Note: The incidence estimates represent the findings of the most recent US population-based study of elder abuse in cognitively intact community-dwelling older adults. These rates are estimated to be higher among the cognitively impaired.
[a] Self-Neglect and caregiver neglect were combined in this study for a prevalence of 5.1%.

INCIDENCE AND PREVALENCE

That the full extent of elder abuse, both in the US and worldwide, remains unclear reflects difficulties in detecting the problem; there are variations in mandatory reporting standards and substantiation criteria, as well as in the methods used to obtain prevalence estimates.[10,11] The elder abuse literature suggests approximately 80% of true elder abuse cases are not reported to authorities.[12] For these reasons, estimates probably are greatly underestimated. Several US population-based studies provide annual elder abuse incidence estimates ranging from 1% to 10%.[13,14] The most recent US population-based prevalence study found that 11% of cognitively intact community-dwelling older adults 65 years of age and older experienced at least 1 form of abuse in the 12 months before the study. As shown in **Table 1**, financial exploitation was the most commonly reported type of abuse, closely followed by neglect.[9] Given that overall estimates of older adults constitute 14% of the US population, anywhere from at least 400,000 to 4,000,000 older adults are currently mistreated. Worldwide, the World Health Organization estimates that anywhere from 1% to 35% of older adults have been victimized or will experience elder abuse.[15] With a rapidly aging population around the globe, the problem of elder abuse will grow exponentially worse in the coming years unless preventive measures are set in place.

MORBIDITY AND MORTALITY

The elderly are the most heterogeneous segment of the population. Many older adults are healthy. Many older adults suffer from multiple chronic health conditions, including those who have lower physiologic and psychological reserves limiting their ability to cope with stressful situations. They experience 2- to 3-fold increases in all-cause mortality compared with older adults that are not abused.[16,17] Alarmingly, what emerges from the data is that elder abuse significantly predicts mortality in older adults independent of a broad range of other social, functional, physical, medical, mental health, and demographic qualities. Elder abuse is such an adverse and burdensome event that mistreated older adults with little or no disease symptomatology seem to be at risk for early mortality.

RISK FACTORS

Every older person is at risk. Elder abuse occurs across many different socioeconomic statuses and cultures. There are certain characteristics that place older adults at greater risk for being victimized. Although older persons who lend money to children owing to a hardship may not be at high risk for abuse, evidence suggests that the risk increases significantly, although not ubiquitously, if co-residency or substance abuse are preconditions. Because elder abuse is enmeshed with many factors, we must explore characteristics of both the victim and the perpetrator that increase the likelihood of abuse. So, although the risk factors are fairly well established, there is a compelling need for evidence-based studies that determine whether certain social, environmental, and individual risk factor combinations pose differential risks of subsequent victimization. **Table 2** provides a list of common victim and perpetrator risk factors.[18–20]

EARLY IDENTIFICATION AND PREVENTION: STATE OF THE LITERATURE

Much more research needs to be completed in the field of elder abuse to improve effective prevention and early identification. Despite substantial work to date, this is a relatively new field; we need better prevention and early identification strategies.

Table 2
Elder abuse victim and perpetrator characteristics

Victim/Perpetrator	Characteristics
Victim	Female, advanced age, cognitive impairment, co-habitation with others (especially family members), social isolation and poor social support networks, mental health problems, substance abuse, dependency on perpetrator for care, frailty
Perpetrator	Cognitive impairment, family history of abusive behavior, male, mental illness or mentally challenged, $\geq$40 y of age, financial or substance abuse dependency, adult child

This requires (1) addressing ageism, (2) expanding knowledge about subjective and objective abuse indicators, (3) increasing elder abuse screening in clinical settings, and (4) establishing elder abuse detection and prevention as routine medical care.

Ageism

In 1969, a pioneer in the field of aging, Dr Robert Butler coined the term "ageism" to capture discrimination against older adults simply based on their age and the aging process.[21] Ageist assumptions can lead to inattention toward older adult health problems or equating aging with poor health. The blindness that results shadows health care professionals, patients, and society as a whole. Researchers have linked negative views of aging to functional decline, depression, isolation, despair, and disability, thereby increasing the risk for abuse and early mortality.[22] Ageism has unexpected consequences; it impedes progress toward enhancing the prevention and early identification of elder abuse.

Ascribing serious medical problems to the vicissitudes of "normal" aging may divert true attention from the circumstances surrounding a health problem. For instance, decubitus ulcers, which have been linked to elder abuse, could result from severe end-stage diseases affecting mobility and malnutrition, but they may also indicate caregiver neglect.[23] Similarly, depression is a common mental health problem among abused elders.[24] Abuse may either lead to depression or contribute to a patient's vulnerability. If health problems such as ulcers and depression are categorized as natural consequences of aging, rather than signs suggestive of abuse, vulnerable older adults may be left to endure and suffer ongoing abuse, a condition often occurring for years before it is detected.[25]

Disparities in preventive care and medical treatment disparities also exist owing to age. Older adults are less likely than younger individuals to receive preventive care and, thus, may experience an increased likelihood of becoming dependent.[22] Conversely, older people can positively or adversely contribute to their overall well-being by the relative degree to which they eat and drink in moderation, exercise regularly, and monitor their sleeping habits. The same goes for aggressive medical treatments, which providers may not deem appropriate for adults advancing in years. Foregoing treatment typically accorded people in their prime may reduce an elder's ability to perform activities of daily living and engage in social activities, thus increasing isolation or dependency and subsequent abuse. For instance, a frail elder patient may be offered a wheelchair rather than physical therapy, further diminishing her musculoskeletal system and accelerating functional decline in several activities of daily living, which increases the likelihood of dependence.

There is a national shortage of geriatric trained medical professionals. Even now, only 10% of US medical schools require students to participate in geriatric coursework or rotations.[22] Because many health care professionals may not be able to detect the signs of elder abuse, much less how to screen for it, we must enhance training in geriatric medicine nationwide if we are going to improve prevention and early detection of elder abuse.

Increasing Awareness and Elder Abuse Indicators

Detecting elder abuse is rarely an easy task, even for individuals trained to identify it.[26] Aspects of abuse complicate detection. Roughly 95% of older adults live in their homes, the site of the abuse. By the time the targeted older adult is seen by a physician, family member, or a neighbor, the elder's injuries or psychological abuse may have dissipated to a subclinical level undetected by a brief physical examination or clinical visit. Likewise, in many cases the signs of abuse are subtle, masked by the aging process.[27] As noted, not knowing what overt and subtle signs to look for diminishes early identification. However, there are indicators and markers of elder abuse. Using them in a thorough patient assessment is important for an accurate diagnosis. The older adult patient should be examined alone and away from the caregiver. A complete physical examination in a patient gown is warranted in suspected abuse. Physicians should pay particular attention to areas often hidden by clothing, socks, and shoes. This approach allows the physician to ask direct and nonthreatening questions to ascertain the history behind the clinical picture. **Table 3** provides a list of indicators for the different types of abuse.[28]

Table 3
Elder abuse types and indicators of abuse

Abuse Type	Indicators
Physical abuse	Fractures, welts, lacerations, bite marks, burns, bruises, untreated injuries, internal injuries, repeated history of falls, repeated emergency department visits, traumatic alopecia
Sexual abuse	Difficulty walking or sitting, pain or itching in the genital area, unexplained sexually transmitted diseases, vaginal or anal bleeding, torn, stained or bloody underclothing, bruising around genital or breast regions
Psychological/emotional abuse	Emotional upset, agitation, depression, suicidal ideation, hyper vigilance toward abuser, withdrawn, unusual behavior such as sucking, biting, rocking, crying, self-mutilation
Financial exploitation	Sudden changes in bank accounts, inability to afford medications, unexplained disappearance of possessions, unexplained asset transfer(s), unexplained loss of pension or social security checks
Caregiver neglect	Dehydration, malnutrition, decubitus ulcers, unexplained deterioration in health, failure to thrive, lack of routine medical care or medications, urine burns, multiple hospital and emergency department admissions, repeated falls, poor hygiene, unexplained weight loss
Abandonment	Cognitively-impaired older adult left in emergency department, victim place on public transportation with a 1-way ticket, older adult is left alone unsafely for periods of time
Self-neglect	Unkempt appearance, withdrawn, depressed, isolated, hazardous or unsafe living conditions, unexpected to unexplained deterioration in health, untreated health conditions, weight loss, dehydration, poor hygiene

Adapted from Brandl B, Dyer CB, Heisler CJ, et al. Elder abuse detection and intervention-a collaborative approach. Springer Series on Ethics, Law and Aging. New York: Springer Publishing Company; 2007. p. 79–100.

Bruising and Fall-Related Injuries

Physical indicators provide evidence used to determine whether an elder's injury occurred as a result of an accident or an intentional act of abuse. In 2007, unintentional injury in adults 65 years of age and older was the ninth leading cause of death. In 2009, falls were both the most common type of unintentional injury in older adults as well as the seventh leading cause of violence-related injury in older adults.[29] Research focused on types of injury to distinguish accidental causes from trauma is helpful.

In 2005, Mosqueda and colleagues[30] studied the association between bruising and physical abuse in older adults. The placement of bruises, the study found, differentiate accidental bruising from nonaccidental bruising. In fact, an estimated 90% of accidental bruises presented on the extremities of the older adults, not on the head or neck region, buttocks, genitalia, or soles of the feet. This study also examined the color and duration of bruising only to find that these indicators were not reliable evidence regarding the intentionality of the injuries.

In 2009, Wiglesworth and colleagues[31] extended the earlier bruising study to examine location and size of bruising associated with physical abuse. This project relied on 67 older adults reported to Adult Protective Services (APS) for physical abuse. After an expert panel reviewed the case history and determined, by consensus, whether physical abuse occurred, the investigators compared bruise size and location between the groups. Their findings that bruises associated with elder abuse are commonly large (>5 cm), and are present on the face, lateral right arm, and posterior torso, support the Mosqueda (2005) study.[30]

There is evidence that traumatic injuries of patients presenting to health care providers may be missed. For example, approximately 23% of emergency department visits occur in older adults with injuries.[29] In 2011, Friedman and co-wrokers[32] investigated the injuries of traumatic elder abuse victims treated in an emergency department. This study found that wounds in the forms of fractures, internal injuries, and open and penetrating wounds were more common in elder abuse victims than unabused older adults.

In 2012, Ziminski and colleagues[29] conducted a 2-year retrospective study of emergency department visits by older adults. They assessed the relation between emergency department visits and injuries in cognitively challenged older adults. Cognitive impairment was not significantly related to falls, but the data indicate that individuals with cognitive impairment suffered more injuries in the head, neck, and face region; lower limb; upper limb; and trunk. In contrast, those whose injuries were not related to falls were far more likely to suffer open wounds. These open wounds could be the result of trauma related to physical abuse by caregivers or self-neglect. A recent case-control study by Burnett and colleagues (2013),[23] investigating the forensic markers of elder abuse in older decedents found that a history of decubitus ulcers were predictive of prior elder abuse substantiation by APS.

Burns and Lacerations

Burns and lacerations are common injuries seen in health care settings. Burns often are indicative of abuse in older adults. Studies estimate that approximately 40% to 70% of burns in older adults are linked to elder abuse.[33] Clinical and forensic investigations of burn patterns in older adults resemble those found in child abuse[34] and, thus, should increase suspicion of abuse rather than assuming these injuries occurred by accident.

Lacerations are equally difficult to attribute to elder abuse because skin integrity is reduced as part of aging. Lacerations are more likely to occur in older adults as a result of blunt force trauma, restraints, and friction, but leave less evidence regarding the type of abuse. Nonetheless, abrasions retain the form of the device used to create the trauma.[27]

SCREENING AND MONITORING FOR ELDER ABUSE RISK FACTORS

Systematic screening for risk factors and indicators of abuse are critical for early detection and prevention. Multiple studies show that declines in physical and mental health as well as limited social networks, cohabitation, and isolation lead to higher risks for increased dependency and subsequent elder abuse.[18,19,28] Unfortunately, very little systematic screening of elder abuse and its risk factors occurs in clinic settings.[35] Physicians are in a position to oversee screening and prevention of elder abuse. They often see their elderly patients 5 or more times per year.[36] Thus, physicians develop trusting relationships with the patients and have multiple opportunities to observe and discuss changes in cognition, function, mental health, social, living, and financial statuses.

Comprehensive Geriatric Assessments

Comprehensive geriatric assessments (CGA) are the gold standard for assessing the health and well-being of older adults. CGAs often incorporate the physical health, mental health, and social and cognitive domains important for quality of life and protection from elder abuse.[35] Although this approach has been shown to be helpful in identifying problem areas, CGAs are cumbersome and time consuming, and may require additional training, making them impractical for brief clinical visits with older adults. Therefore, family physician practices, nongeriatric specialists, and emergency departments are not likely to perform CGAs, suggesting the need for alternative approaches.

Referrals for Comprehensive Geriatric Assessments

Geriatric medical teams are trained in CGA and accustomed to completing some combination of these assessments on a routine basis. Such teams can be a resource for non–geriatrics-trained health care professionals. Referrals to geriatric medicine teams for an annual CGA would afford a baseline evaluation of the different risk factors for elder abuse. Alternatively, the primary care provider might choose to perform a CGA to monitor changes over the year that may warrant further investigation into the possibility of elder abuse. For emergency department personnel, consultations with geriatric medicine teams might facilitate determining the presence of abuse or whether older adults upon discharge are at risk for abuse.

Periodic Assessment of Elder Abuse Risk Factors

Clearly not every clinical visit can include a lengthy battery of elder abuse risk factor measures. Nonetheless, it would be beneficial to assess executive functioning, memory, depression, and activities of daily living at routine intervals. Several standardized tests, which are relatively quick and efficient for these subtle domains, could be performed once or twice a year and supported by vigilant monitoring of changes in status in subsequent visits. Depression may undergo more rapid development, but these other domains are not likely to change significantly in short periods of time. Should changes be noticed, further investigation should ensue to rule out elder abuse as a potential contributing cause for the change in health status. Likewise, health care professionals should be skeptical of repeated "accidental injuries" in older adults; a significant portion of these injuries may be related to abuse.

Social history and qualitative interviews

An older adult may choose not to reveal being abused out of shame, fear of further abuse, protection of a loved one, or simply because they are unable to communicate these incidents owing to cognitive impairment.[19] This does not mean that questions regarding elder abuse should not be routinely asked. Patients and caregivers should be questioned separately. Health care providers should at the very least ask open-ended questions regarding the older adult's social engagement, financial decision making, and fear of being unsafe or injured. Questions even as neutral as "Is there anything going on at home that you would like to talk about?" might reveal information indicative of potential elder abuse. This may lead to a confession of being injured or to other vague complaints that may be coded communication regarding ongoing abuse. Other questions to consider include: "Has anyone touched you without your permission?"; "Has anyone hurt, hit or treated you roughly?"; "Has anyone taken your personal possessions such as your money, car, or valuables without your permission?"; "Has anyone yelled or sworn at you?"; and "Has anyone made fun of you or hurt your feelings?"

The verbal information gained from these exchanges may be diminished when victims of abuse exhibit behaviors such as withdrawal, anxiety, missed appointments, depression, stress, or trauma. In these cases, it may be helpful to assess the cause of these behaviors to rule out the suspicion of elder abuse. In addition, if the caregiver insists on answering for the patient, downplays the patient's complaints, acts overly compassionate, refuses to allow the interview with the patient to take place without the caregiver present, or cancels the patient's appointments, the clinicians' suspicion for abuse should be elevated.

ELDER ABUSE CLINICAL ASSESSMENTS

The American Medical Association recommends that all geriatric patients receive elder abuse screening.[37] In cases where injuries are not extensive or do not require emergency care, an older adult may not present to a physician until after the salient indicators are gone. Thus, relying on physical signs may not be informative. Since 1975, when Burston first reported on "granny battering" in the British Medical Journal, there have been considerable efforts to develop elder abuse assessments despite the lack of available criteria.[38] Because the burden of identification is falling on the shoulders of health care professionals, most of the assessments were designed to identify suspicion of elder abuse during brief clinical visits, such as emergency departments and outpatient settings.

Some of the measures such as the CGAs and conflict tactics scale[39] provide an indirect assessment of elder abuse. Other measures such as the Elder Abuse Assessment Instrument,[40] Brief Abuse Screen for the Elderly,[35] Indicators of Abuse,[41] Hwalek-Sengstock Elder Abuse Screening Test,[42] Elder Abuse Suspicion Index,[43] American Medical Association Screening of Abuse,[19] the Vulnerability to Abuse Screening Survey,[44] and the Geriatric Mistreatment Scale[45] were specifically designed to detect possible elder abuse. These assessments vary in length, elder abuse types assessed, and psychometric appraisal. Although most elder abuse assessments have internal reliability testing, many have not undergone more rigorous construct validation or measurement invariance testing to determine whether these assessments are equally useful across different genders and ethnic/cultural contexts. Despite these limitations, these assessments can still be used to screen older adults to provide potential early identification and prevention. After all, a positive screen does not ubiquitously mean that elder abuse is occurring, but rather that further information should be gathered. **Table 4** provides a list of elder abuse assessments that may be suitable for clinical settings.

Table 4
Elder abuse assessments and clinical suitability

Assessment	Items	Administration	Psychometrics	Clinical Suitability
Elder Assessment Instrument (EAI)	42	Completed by a professional to assess physical, social, medical, independence in older adults. Also provides a summary	Content and construct validity; good inter-rater agreement; sensitivity = 0.71 specificity = 0.93; item-reliability = 0.84; test-retest = 0.83	Good psychometrics, but lengthy
Brief Abuse Screen for the Elderly (BASE)	5	Training required to assess physical, psychological, financial mistreatment and neglect; takes 1 min to complete	Face validity and inter-rater agreement	Brief, but requires specialized training
Hwalek-Sengstock Elder Abuse Screening Test (HS-EAST)	6	Self-report or interview by a professional	Construct and predictive validity, weak item reliability, but good cross-cultural adaptation	Brief, but primarily assesses domestic violence
Elder Abuse Suspicion Index (EASI)	6	Completed by health care professional to assess risk, neglect, verbal, psychological, emotional, financial, physical and sexual abuse over a 12-mo period; 2 min to complete	Sensitivity = 0.77; specificity = 0.44	Brief with adequate ability to detect true cases of abuse, but may result in higher numbers of false positive findings of abuse
American Medical Association Abuse Screen (AMAAS)	9	Brief assessment by health care professional to assess for social isolation, financial exploitation, sexual abuse, caregiver neglect, and emotional/verbal abuse	None reported	Brief, but no psychometric performance assessment
Vulnerability to Abuse Screening Scale (VASS)	12	Self-report of dependency, dejection, coercion, and vulnerability	Moderate ranges of reliability and moderate to good construct validity	Brief, but not unreliable in assessing coercion by others
Geriatric Mistreatment Scale (GMS)	22	Assesses physical, psychological and sexual abuse, caregiver neglect and financial exploitation	Internal reliability ranging from 0.55 (financial abuse) to 0.87 (sexual abuse)	Good psychometrics, but lengthy and need for training

Elder Assessment Instrument

The Elder Assessment Instrument is a 41-item instrument containing 7 sections. The instrument's first 5 sections assess clinical manifestations and subjective patient responses related to general assessment and, more specifically, elder abuse, neglect, exploitation, and abandonment indicators. The Elder Assessment Instrument uses a Likert scale, resulting in a quantitative value for each elder abuse domain. The sixth section is a summary section where the assessor provides an overall likelihood of the presence of elder abuse for the individual patient. The last section invites comment and prompts development of a follow-up plan. This tool has been shown to have acceptable construct validity, interrater agreement, and good sensitivity and specificity. Unfortunately, its length diminishes its appropriateness in busy clinical settings.[40]

Brief Abuse Screen for the Elderly

The Brief Abuse Screen for the Elderly contains only 5 items. It has good interrater agreement, but no other psychometric evaluations have been conducted. Despite only taking 1 minute to complete, deploying the Brief Abuse Screen for the Elderly requires training. The Brief Abuse Screen for the Elderly discriminates between abusive and nonabusive caregivers, but it does not include a question on self-neglect.[41]

Hwalek-Sengestock Elder Abuse Screening Test

The Hwalek-Sengestock Elder Abuse Screening Test (HS-EAST)[42] has been reduced to a 6-item risk assessment of domestic violence in older adults and vulnerability to physical harm. This scale could certainly serve clinicians as a brief elder abuse screening tool. Recent psychometric evaluation has shown that the HS-EAST can be cross-culturally adapted to assess for elder abuse and vulnerability in Portuguese populations.

Elder Abuse Suspicion Index

The Elder Abuse Suspicion Index is a 6-item assessment designed to identify older adults who may be being abused. It takes approximately 2 minutes to administer. The Elder Abuse Suspicion Index was validated in family practices and ambulatory care settings. Its sensitivity and specificity are recorded as 0.47 and 0.75, respectively. These values suggest that, although the Elder Abuse Suspicion Index may not always identify abuse when it is occurring, it performs fairly well at identifying those that have not been abused. An additional strength is that it was validated against a detailed elder abuse Social Work Evaluation. The first 5 questions are asked directly to the patient. These questions cover basic and instrumental activities of daily living dependency, neglect, emotional abuse, financial exploitation, and sexual abuse. The last question directs the treating physician(s) to assess for various patient behaviors and characteristics uncommon for the older adult and associated with elder abuse. These cues include withdrawn nature, poor eye contact, malnutrition, medication noncompliance, cuts, bruises, poor hygiene, and inappropriate clothing. Yes to any of these questions indicates potential abuse.[43]

American Medical Association Abuse Screen

The American Medical Association Abuse Screen is a brief assessment with only 9 questions. The questions listed in this assessment evaluate the domains of social isolation, financial exploitation, sexual abuse, caregiver neglect, and emotional and psychological abuse. Although very brief, the questions in this assessment could be quite informative. Questions include: "Are you alone a lot?", "Are you afraid of anyone at home?", and "Has anyone ever touched you without your consent?" Affirmative answers should, at the very least, raise suspicion and prompt further discussion.[19]

Vulnerability to Abuse Screening Scale

The Vulnerability to Abuse Screening Scale is a 12-item scale with 4 domains that cover vulnerability, dependence, dejection, and coercion. This scale is specifically designed to assess for elder abuse, and combines 10 questions from the original HS-EAST screening test with 2 additional items, including threatening behavior from others and whether or not the older adult is afraid of anyone in their family. Its vulnerability and coercion scales demonstrate moderate to good construct validity. Overall, the reliability of the different domains on the Vulnerability to Abuse Screening Scale ranges from 0.31 (coercion) to 0.74 (dependency), which are indicated to be adequate for brief screening.[44]

Geriatric Mistreatment Scale

The Geriatric Mistreatment Scale is a 22-item assessment designed to assess 5 domains of elder abuse. Each question refers to the 12 months before the interview. The domains include physical and psychological abuse, caregiver neglect, financial exploitation, and sexual abuse. The Geriatric Mistreatment Scale also asks who is responsible for the abuse. The overall internal reliability of the scale is reported to be good with a Cronbach's alpha of 0.83. The reliabilities for the domains were psychological abuse (0.82), physical abuse (0.72), financial abuse (0.55), caregiver neglect (0.80), and sexual abuse (0.87). All domains except for financial abuse have adequate to good item reliabilities, indicating the ability for the items to all measure their targeted type of abuse.[45]

In-Home Assessments

Like most behaviors punishable by law, attempts are often made to conceal elder abuse and occurrences often happen in privacy. In fact, acts of elder abuse occur mostly in the privacy of the older adult's home.[28] As mentioned, perpetrators and victims often try to hide these abuses from physicians, neighbors, and social services. Therefore, treating older adults in clinical settings provides only a partial picture of the dynamic sociocultural context wherein most elder abuse occurs. To gain a more complete picture of potential abuse, it may be important to complete an in-home assessment and determine if proper care of the older adult is being provided. Because home visits are time intensive, it may be prudent to perform home visits for patients when suspicion for potential abuse is high. Also, this may be the only effective way to detect self-neglect in older adults.

FEASIBILITY OF CLINICAL SCREENING

Within the United States, the Joint Commissions that accredits hospitals requires emergency departments to screen every patient for potential abuse or neglect regardless of age. Bond and Butler[19] (2013) recommend use of the EASI or the American Medical Association Abuse Screen to identify elder abuse in emergency departments.

A recent study by Russell and colleagues[46] (2012) reported on the feasibility of elder abuse screening in dental clinics. Older adult patients were approached in the waiting rooms and asked to answer sensitive questions for the HS-EAST regarding elder abuse. One third of the older adult patients refused to participate. Of those who participated, an alarming 28% scored high enough to indicate a high likelihood of current elder abuse. This feasibility study is especially important because it demonstrates that older adults, while waiting to be seen by a health care provider, are willing to undergo elder abuse screening. It is worth noting that the screening does not have to be completed by the physician in most cases. When using the EASI, however, the physician or treating clinician must provide an answer to the last question regarding changes in the patients status over time.

REPORTING AND RESPONDING TO ELDER ABUSE

In 1975, the US federal government mandated states to establish social service agencies across the country.[47] In 2004, the federal government spent approximately one half of a billion dollars on state APS agencies across the country.[48] These monies were used by APS to investigate, substantiate, and provide services to adults with disabilities and older adults. Currently, 44 states have mandatory reporting laws for its citizens. Even in these states, many cases are unreported for multiple reasons including ageism, lack of public awareness regarding the identification of elder abuse, and lack of knowledge about where to report cases.

In 2004, Kennedy and colleagues[49] surveyed 250 family physicians and 250 general internists to assess the perceived magnitude of elder abuse and to determine their sense of responsibility for detecting, reporting, and intervening. Unanimously, physicians agreed that identifying and treating elder abuse is important. The vast majority (75%) reported that physicians could intervene effectively in elder abuse cases and 78% believed that primary care physicians were in the best position to detect elder abuse. These statistics are surprising; physician-initiated elder abuse reports to social service agencies account for less than 2% of the reported cases.[50]

The same study provided evidence that 63% of the physicians polled never asked about elder abuse and only 31% reported encountering elder abuse in the 12 months before the survey. For those physicians who did encounter elder abuse, an alarming 94% stated that they were unable to prove elder abuse had occurred or decided not to report their cases to APS. Equally discouraging is the finding that 98% of those surveyed reported the perception of being inadequately trained to effectively detect, treat, and manage elder abuse cases.[49]

In 2010, a separate study by Almogue and colleagues[51] echoed these findings by showing that medical and nursing staff had low levels of knowledge regarding elder abuse issues and that they were unaware of laws and protocols for detection and reporting. Almogue and colleagues also reported that physicians wanted to be absolutely certain that abuse was occurring before reporting their patients to social services. Likewise, 75% of home health care providers stated that they would need conclusive evidence, such as eye witness to abuse, before proceeding.

Although some cases of elder abuse are obvious, many may be subtle and require further investigation for supportive evidence. Accordingly, it is important for health care providers to report potential elder abuse cases to APS even when definitive evidence is not available. A high suspicion of abuse by a health care professional warrants further investigation. In clinical settings, elder abuse should be treated like any other disease state. If there are symptoms, then further steps should be taken to confirm the diagnosis. Capezuti and colleagues[52] (2011) provide a 3-pronged approach for health care providers to follow to improve the early identification and prevention of elder abuse:

- Recognition of real or potential abuse;
- Referral to proper source(s) for intervention; and
- Ongoing follow-up and evaluation.

These steps indicate both the need to screen for elder abuse and seek conclusive evidence, as well as the necessity to report potential cases of abuse to the proper authorities and investigative agencies. This approach presupposes continual ongoing care and management of the older adults to improve early detection and prevent recurrent cases of elder abuse in the future.

A CLINICIAN'S POCKET GUIDE TO EARLY DETECTION AND PREVENTION OF ELDER ABUSE

As mentioned, physicians and health care providers woefully underreport elder abuse. **Fig. 1** presents a familiar reporting structure to help with the early identification of and

Subjective

The following statements may be a red flag indicating further investigation:

Abandonment: I am all alone. I have no one who cares for me.

Physical Abuse: They hurt me. Please don't tell anyone about the injury. Stories that do not correlate to the type of injury and/or physical signs and symptoms.

Exploitation: I don't know what happened to my money. I can no longer afford ...I have misplaced my jewelry or my money. I don't understand what happened.

Neglect: My caregiver is so busy, it is not their fault that they don't have time to feed me, get my medications, or change my diaper.

Psychological Abuse: I don't want to complain, my son/daughter yell if I complain. Please don't make fun of me.

Self-Neglect: I'm fine, I don't feel like taking my medications or taking care of myself. I'd don't need to bathe much, I'm clean enough as I am.

Objective

Physical Manifestation	Psychological Manifestation	Sociological/Environmental Manifestation
– Bruising in various stages of healing	Assess for Caregiver and Patient	
– Contractures	– Anxiety	– Recent Inability to pay bills
– Falls	– Anxiety toward CG*	– Left alone in Emergency Room
– Dehydration	– Anger by patient toward CG*	– Nonadherence to medication
– Fractures in various stages of healing	– Depression	– Repeated ER admissions
– Lacerations	– Fearfulness	– Repeated hospital admissions
– Diarrhea	– Impatience toward CG	
– Fecal Impaction	– Irritability toward CG	
– Malnutrition	– Nervousness	
– Inappropriate use of medications	– Nervousness toward CG	
– Poor hygiene	– CG impatience toward patient	
– Sexual abuse signs	– CG irritability toward patient	
– Pressure ulcers		
– Urine burns		
– Delirium		

*CG=caregiver

See Table II for Additional Risk Factors

Assessment

Patient in immediate danger from abuse or neglect

Unexplained or inconsistent explanations for physical findings, suspicious for mistreatment

Diminished decision-making ability (risk of self-neglect)

Not suspicious of elder abuse or neglect

Plan

• Refer to emergency services and Adult Protective Services (APS)

• Refer to APS and emergency services if recent sexual abuse to gather forensic evidence

• Utilize health care proxy, durable power of attorney if available
• Refer to APS if no family or friend available
• Contact primary care provider or referral to evaluate cognitive impairment

• Complete routine medical exam
• Refer to other health care providers if needed

Assessment and Plan reprinted with permission of from Elsevier.

Fig. 1. Subjective, objective, assessment, and plan (SOAP) process for identifying, reporting and preventing elder abuse. (*Adapted from* Chang AL, Wong JW, Endo JO, et al. Geriatric dermatology part II. Risk factors and cutaneous signs of elder mistreatment for the dermatologist. J Am Acad Dermatol 2013;68(4):533.e1–10; with permission.)

response to patients who may be experiencing the various types of elder abuse. The SOAP note has been taught in medical schools throughout the country for years. SOAP is an acronym for Subjective, Objective, Assessment, and Plan. Subjective data are the statements made by the patient or the caregiver. Subjective data include the reason for the visit (patient's chief complaint) and other pertinent historical information, such as the history of the present illness, review of body systems, medical and surgical history, and family and social history, medical review and the patient's allergies. Objective data are the signs the health care provider observes throughout the physical examination. These observations include the interactions between the older adult and the caregiver. Assessment is the health care provider's critical thinking, which formulates the differential diagnoses. The plan consists of interventions prescribed to address the patient's chief concern and the diagnoses identified.

In elder abuse, vague statements may often be a call for help. Further investigation of these comments may open the door for the elder person to expound on their particular situation. It is important to interview the older adult alone and away from the caregiver to allow the patient to speak freely and openly. They may directly state they have been hit and plead with you not to mention this anyone. It is also common for older adults to defend the caregiver's behaviors by reasoning that the caregiver was busy or overly stressed in response to caring for the older adult. For these reasons, it is also important to talk to with caregiver and understand their view of the situation. In **Fig. 1**, the different types of elder abuse are listed with potential "red flag" comments by older adults that may indicate abuse. For example, in abandonment, older adults may state: "I am all alone"; "I have no one to take me to the grocery store or pharmacy since my child has left"; or "I haven't seen my kids in months – they're so busy." In physical abuse, the physical examination often is the primary source of objective data. In the current health care structure, patients are often seen in their clothes rather than a patient gown and physical signs may be missed. Based on the older adult's chief complaint and further inquiry, the clinician may be able to ascertain that the history and the nature of the injury do not correlate as described. Home visits are often more revealing. The older adult's response to questions regarding lack of cleanliness in the home, lack of food and medication, and overall safety of the environment provide substantial information for further investigation. Older adults experiencing psychological abuse may be the least verbal. Thus, asking direct questions about incidents of psychological abuse (ie, yelling, ridicule) may be the best approach to detection.

Objective observations and clinical training can provide a lifeline to older adults experiencing any one of these type of abuse. We have divided the objective data into the physical, psychological, and sociologic/environmental manifestations. This biopsychosocial and environmental model will be helpful in any health care setting. Clinical manifestations of physical abuse have been discussed previously. It is important to complete a thorough skin examination. Psychological manifestations include evaluating the behaviors of both the older adult as well as the caregiver (if present). Do you observe impatience, anger, irritability, or "bullying" behaviors by the caregiver toward the older adult? Does the older adult patient seem to be more anxious, fearful, impatient, or nervous when the caregiver is in the room? These types of behaviors must be explored further through separate interviews with both the older adult and the caregiver. The sociologic and environmental manifestations may be red flagged in your electronic medical review. Is there a history of repeated emergency department or hospital admissions? Are electronic prescriptions filled? During geriatric home visits or interprofessional rounds, evidence should be documented regarding conditions such as disconnected utilities, financial strain, and level of concern regarding available social services that may be affecting the older adults health maintenance and personal safety. This is especially important for older adults who depend on another for their care.

Remembering the elder abuse risk factors outlined in **Table 2** in conjunction with the older adult's subjective data and your objective biopsychosocial, physical, and environmental examination will lead to your assessment of this person's current health situation. In **Fig. 1**, we provide a limited assessment and plan of care depending on whether the patient is in immediate danger from abuse or neglect, has unexplained or inconsistent explanations for physical findings, has diminished decision making capacity or is not suspicious of elder abuse or neglect. This SOAP format provides a framework for daily clinical practice. It is easily incorporated into clinical practice so that increasing numbers of elder abuse can be detected and addressed.

SUMMARY

Elder abuse is often undetected, but nonetheless emerges as a critical medicosocial problem in an aging society. These cruelties are detrimental to the overall health, well-being, and survival of older adults. Despite advances over the last 20 years, society continues to face challenges that impede the protection of older adults from abuse. Factors such as ageism and the lack of health care professional training on elder abuse, uniform reporting standards, and clinical screening all diminish the chances for early detection and prevention. Protecting older adults from abuse requires finding ways to overcome these barriers in hopes of creating a society where aging is revered and those in the golden years can live safely without fear.

REFERENCES

1. AARP. Boomers @65: celebrating a milestone birthday. Available at: http://www.aarp.org/personal-growth/transitions/boomers_65/. Accessed January 15, 2014.
2. Teaster PB, Otto JM, Dugar TA, et al. The 2004 survey of state adult protective services: abuse of adults 60 yrs and older. Available at: http://vtdigger.org/vtdNewsMachine/wp-ontent/uploads/2011/08/20110807_surveyStateAPS.pdf. Accessed January 29, 2014.
3. US Centers for Disease Control and Prevention. Preventing elder abuse. Available at: http://www.cdc.gov/features/elderabuse/. Accessed January 15, 2014.
4. National Center for Elder Abuse, Administration on Aging. Statistics/data. Available at: http://www.ncea.aoa.gov/Library/Data/index.aspx. Accessed January 15, 2014.
5. World Health Organization. Elder abuse. Available at: http://www.who.int/ageing/projects/elder_abuse/en/. Accessed January 15, 2014.
6. Gorbien MJ, Eisenstein AR. Elder abuse and neglect: an overview. Clin Geriatr Med 2005;21(2):279–92.
7. World Health Organization. Abuse of the elderly. Available at: http://www.who.int/violence_injury_prevention/violence/world_report/factsheets/en/elderabusefacts.pdf. Accessed January 15, 2014.
8. National Center for Elder Abuse, Administration on Aging. Types of abuse. Available at: http://ncea.aoa.gov/FAQ/Type_Abuse/. Accessed January 15, 2014.
9. Acierno R, Hernandez MA, Amstadter AB, et al. Prevalence and correlates of emotional, physical, sexual, and financial abuse and potential neglect in the united states: the national elder mistreatment study. Am J Public Health 2010;100(2):292–7.

10. Mysyuk Y, Westendorp RG, Lindendberg J. Added value of elder abuse definitions: a review. Ageing Res Rev 2013;12:50–7.
11. Abbey L. Elder abuse and neglect: when home is not safe. Clin Geriatr Med 2009;25:47–60.
12. National Center for Elder Abuse, Administration on Aging. Fact sheet: elder abuse prevalence and incidence. Available at: http://www.ncea.aoa.gov/Resources/Publication/docs/FinalStatistics050331.pdf. Accessed January 15, 2014.
13. Laumann EO, Leitsch SA, Waite LJ. Elder mistreatment in the United States: prevalence estimates from a nationally representative study. J Gerontol B Psychol Sci Soc Sci 2008;63(4):S248–54.
14. Lachs MS, Pillemer K. Elder abuse. Lancet 2004;364(9441):1263–72.
15. World Health Organization. A global response to elder abuse and neglect: building primary health care capacity to deal with the problem worldwide: main report. Available at: http://www.who.int/ageing/publications/ELDER_DocAugust08.pdf. Accessed January 15, 2014.
16. Lachs MS, Williams CS, O'Brien S, et al. The mortality of elder mistreatment. JAMA 1998;280(5):428–32.
17. Dong X, Simon M, Mendes de Leon C, et al. Elder self-neglect and abuse and mortality risk in a community-dwelling population. JAMA 2009;302(5):517–26.
18. Lachs MS, Pillemer K. Abuse and neglect of elderly persons. N Engl J Med 1995;332:437–43.
19. Bond MC, Butler KH. Elder abuse and neglect: definitions, epidemiology, and approaches to emergency department screening. Clin Geriatr Med 2013;29:257–73.
20. Bonnie RJ, Wallace RB. Elder mistreatment: abuse, neglect and exploitation in an aging America. Washington, DC: National Academies Press; 2003.
21. Butler RN. Ageism: a foreword. J Soc Sci 1980;36(2):8–11.
22. Alliance for Aging Research. Available at: http://www.agingresearch.org/newsletters/view/156. Accessed August 25, 2014.
23. Burnett J, Mitchell RA Jr, Cloyd EA, et al. Forensic markers associated with elder mistreatment and self-neglect: a case-control study. Acad Forensic Pathol 2013;3(4):458–67.
24. Dyer CB, Pavlik VN, Murphy KP, et al. The high prevalence of depression and dementia in elder abuse or neglect. J Am Geriatr Soc 2000;48(2):205–8.
25. Jackson SL, Hafemeister TL. Pure financial exploitation vs. hybrid financial exploitation co-occurring with physical abuse and/or neglect of elderly persons. Psychol Violence 2012;2(3):285–96.
26. Taylor K, Dodd K. Knowledge and attitudes of staff towards adult protection. J Adult Protect 2003;5:26–32.
27. Dyer CB, Connolly MT, McFreely P. The clinical and medical forensics of elder abuse and neglect. In: Bonnie RJ, Wallace RB, editors. Elder mistreatment: abuse, neglect and exploitation in an aging America. Washington, DC: National Academies Press; 2003. p. 339–81.
28. Brandl B, Dyer CB, Heisler CJ, et al. Elder abuse detection and intervention-a collaborative approach. Springer series on ethics, law and aging. New York: Springer; 2007. p. 79–100.
29. Ziminski CE, Phillips LR, Woods DL. Raising the index of suspicion for elder abuse: cognitive impairment, falls and injury patterns in the emergency department. Geriatr Nurs 2012;33(2):105–12.
30. Mosqueda L, Burnight K, Liao S. The life cycle of bruises in older adults. J Am Geriatr Soc 2005;53(8):1339–43.

31. Wiglesworth A, Austin R, Corona M, et al. Bruising as a marker of physical elder abuse. J Am Geriatr Soc 2009;57:1191–6.
32. Friedman LS, Avila S, Tanouye K, et al. A case-control study of severe physical abuse of older adults. J Am Geriatr Soc 2011;59:417–22.
33. Bowden ML, Grant ST, Vogel B, et al. The elderly, disabled and handicapped adult burned through abuse and neglect. Burns Incl Therm Inj 1988;14(6): 447–50.
34. Greenbaum AR, Horton JB, Williams CJ, et al. Burn injuries inflicted on children or the elderly: a framework for clinical and forensic assessment. Plast Reconstr Surg 2006;118:46–8.
35. Fulmer T, Guadagno L, Dyer CB, et al. Progress in elder abuse screening and assessment instruments. J Am Geriatr Soc 2004;52:1–8.
36. Yaffee MJ, Bachir T. Understanding elder abuse in family practice. Can Fam Physician 2012;58:1336–40.
37. American Medical Association. Available at: http://www.ama-assn.org//resources/doc/csaph/a08-csaph7-ft.pdf. Accessed January 15, 2014.
38. Burston GR. Granny battering. Br Med J 1975;3(5983):592.
39. Straus MA. Measuring intrafamily conflict and violence: the conflict tactics (CT) scale-form A. J Marriage Fam 1979;41:75–88.
40. Fulmer T, Paveza G, Abraham I, et al. Elder neglect assessment in the emergency department. J Emerg Nurs 2000;26:436–43.
41. Reis M, Nahmiash D, Shrier R, et al. When seniors are abused: an intervention model. Gerontologist 1995;35:666–71.
42. Neale A, Hwalek M, Scott R, et al. Validation of the Hwalek-Sengstock elder abuse screening test. J Appl Gerontol 1991;10:406–18.
43. Yaffe MJ, Weiss D, Wolfson C, et al. Detection and prevalence of abuse of older males: perspectives from family practice. J Elder Abuse Negl 2007;19(1–2): 47–60.
44. Schofield MJ, Mishra GD. Validity of self-report screening scale for elder abuse: Women's Health Australia Study. Gerontologist 2003;43(1):110–20.
45. Giraldo-Rodriguez L, Rosas C. Development and psychometric properties of the geriatric mistreatment scale. Geriatr Gerontol Int 2013;13:466–74.
46. Russell SL, Fulmer T, Singh G, et al. Screening for elder mistreatment in a dental clinic population. J Elder Abuse Negl 2012;24(4):326–39.
47. Dyer CB, Pickens S, Burnett J. Vulnerable elders: when it is no longer safe to live alone. JAMA 2007;298(12):1448–50.
48. Naik AD, Burnett J, Pickens-Pace S, et al. Impairment in instrumental activities of daily living and the geriatric syndrome of self-neglect. Gerontologist 2008;48(3): 388–93.
49. Kennedy RD. Elder abuse and neglect: the experience, knowledge, and attitudes of primary care physicians. Fam Med 2005;37(7):481–5.
50. Stark SW. Blind, deaf and dumb: why elder abuse goes unidentified. Nurs Clin North Am 2011;46:431–6.
51. Almogue A, Weiss A, Marcus EL, et al. Attitudes and knowledge of medical and nursing staff toward elder abuse. Arch Gerontol Geriatr 2009;51:86–91.
52. Capezuti E, Kagan SH, Happ MB, et al. Recognizing and referring suspected elder mistreatment. Geriatr Nurs 2011;32(3):209–11.

Elder Physical Abuse

Lisa M. Young, MD, MBA

KEYWORDS

- Elder abuse • Physical abuse • Injury • Assault • Restraint
- Adult protective services • Ombudsman

KEY POINTS

- Physical abuse of the elderly is a significant public health concern. The true prevalence of all types, including trauma, restraints, and misuse of medications, is unknown, and underreporting is known to be significant.
- The geriatric population is projected to increase dramatically over the next 10 years, and the number of abused individuals is projected to increase as well.
- It is critical that health care providers feel competent in addressing physical elder abuse.
- The cases presented illustrate the variety of presenting symptoms that may be attributed to physical elder abuse.
- Recognition of abuse by clinicians and reporting suspicion of abuse to the proper authorities will improve the care of older adults and prevent serious morbidity and mortality.

INTRODUCTION

Elder physical abuse consists of injury, assault, or restraint of an older person. Abuse is most often perpetrated by a family member who is acting as a caregiver. The true prevalence of elder abuse, including physical abuse, is unknown, because of underreporting. However, over half a million older adults are estimated to be subject to abuse yearly in the United States. Clinician awareness and recognition of physical elder abuse are important to ensure the safety of patients. Signs, symptoms, and patterns of injuries may indicate that a patient is the victim of abuse. In many cases, these can be distinguished from normal signs of aging. Certain characteristics of the caregiver and care recipient are correlated with an increased risk of abuse. Once a health care provider has a suspicion of abuse, it should be reported to Adult Protective Services, or the ombudsman, if the victim lives in a facility. Many states require mandatory reporting of the suspicion of elder abuse to the appropriate authorities. In addition, law enforcement should be notified in most cases of physical abuse. The victim must be assured of his or her safety, as well as appropriate medical care.

Disclosures: None.
HealthCare Partners, 3330 West Lomita Boulevard, Torrance, CA 90505, USA
E-mail address: liyoung@healthcarepartners.com

Clin Geriatr Med 30 (2014) 761–768
http://dx.doi.org/10.1016/j.cger.2014.08.005   geriatric.theclinics.com

DEFINITION AND PREVALENCE

Physical abuse of an elder is defined by the Centers for Disease Control and Prevention (CDC) as an injury, assault or threat with a weapon, or inappropriate restraint of a person aged 60 and older by a caregiver or other person in a position of trust.[1]

A 2013 report by the CDC states that an estimated 500,000 older adults are subject to elder maltreatment yearly in the United States.[2] The extent of the problem is thought to be underestimated due to lack of reporting by abuse victims to authorities. The National Institute of Justice sponsored a study to determine the prevalence of elder maltreatment in community-dwelling older adults completed in 2009. The study was performed via telephone survey and consisted of over 5000 participants aged 60 years or older. The study found the prevalence of physical mistreatment among the surveyed population to be 1.6%. Of the survey participants alleging abuse, only 31% reported the abuse to law enforcement.[3] A prevalence study of elder abuse in New York published in May 2011 found that the number of elders reporting physical abuse in the study was 20 times greater than the number of physical abuse cases reported to authorities.[4]

RISK FACTORS ASSOCIATED WITH ELDER ABUSE

Many studies have identified characteristics of the abusers and victims. A diagnosis of dementia and living with the abuser are the risk factors most strongly correlated with abuse of an elder.[5] Problematic behaviors associated with dementia and psychiatric illness further increase the risk of physical abuse.[6] Social isolation, an inadequate social support system, and history of conflicts with family members also increase the risk of an elder being abused.[7] Disability of an elder person has not been found to be an independent risk factor for abuse, but may increase their vulnerability if other risk factors are present.[5] For instance, impaired vision, gait, and balance place one at an increased risk of falls from force. Pavlik and colleagues[8] found in a study of abuse cases reported in Texas that female gender and older age are correlated with risk of abuse. With each 10-year increase in age, the risk of an Adult Protective Services report being filed for abuse doubled.[8]

An epidemiologic study of elder abuse in Boston published in 2012 revealed that two-thirds of the abusers were spouses, and one-third were the adult children of the abuse victim.[5] Substance abuse by the caregiver increases the risk of abuse, as does caregiver mental illness, such as depression.[5,9] Caregivers who are dependent on the elder person for housing or financial assistance are at high risk for perpetrating abuse.[5] Other factors increasing the risk of abuse include inadequate social support and insufficient caregiver training.[3] Exposure to abuse in early life, a history of violence, and antisocial behavior increase risk for a family member or caregiver to become abusive.[5]

TYPES OF PHYSICAL ABUSE

Several types of physical abuse have been identified. The most common acts of abuse are hitting, slapping, or striking the elder with an object.[5] Restraints may be considered a form of physical abuse.[10,11] Restraints can be physical, using bindings, or chemical, using medications.[10] Examples include overmedication with psychoactive medications administered to keep a patient sedated in bed. Undermedication may include withholding neurologic or psychoactive medications. For example, withholding dopamine agonist medication may cause increased muscle rigidity in a person with Parkinson disease, resulting in gait difficulty. Force-feeding is another form of abuse.[10] A patient with dementia may refuse to eat or eat very slowly. Force-feeding a person with dementia can result in increasing oral stasis and aspiration. Aspiration pneumonitis and pneumonia are serious sequelae resulting from force-feeding.

SIGNS AND SYMPTOMS OF ELDER PHYSICAL ABUSE

The most common injuries of physical abuse are unexplained bruises, skeletal fractures, abrasions, and head injury.[5] These types of injuries may occur as secondary effects from medications, chronic disease, or accident, making the distinction from physical abuse difficult. However, in these cases, the history is critical to understanding the context of the injury. Patterns of injuries may support a diagnosis of abuse. Multiple injuries in different stages of healing should raise the clinician's suspicion of elder abuse. A bruising study of older adults, published in 2005, evaluated accidental bruising in the elderly. The results showed that approximately 90% of accidental bruises occurred on the extremities, with no accidental bruising on the genitalia, plantar surface of the feet, ears or neck.[12] The color of bruising was not found to be a good indicator of the age of the bruise.[12] Other factors such as anticoagulant medications did increase the number of bruises, but did not lead to prolonged resolution of bruises.[12] However, the location of the bruises was more suggestive of abuse than any of the other factors. A subsequent study of geriatric patients with bruises as a result of physical abuse, found that unlike accidental bruising, bruises as a result of physical abuse are greater than 5 cm, and more often occur on the face, back, and lateral aspect of the right arm.[13] Fractures in the elderly that result from bone disease such as osteoporosis, or injury, such as an accidental fall, commonly occur in the vertebrae and hips for women over age 75 and wrists for women under age 75.[14] Fractures of the head, cervical spine, and trunk are more likely to result from physical assault than limb fractures. However, spiral fractures of the large bones of the limbs and fractures with a rotational component are more diagnostic of physical abuse.[14] Signs of elder abuse also include fear of a caregiver or family member, a decline in maintenance of the elder person's hygiene, and social withdrawal.[7,15,16]

REPORTING ELDER ABUSE

Once elder abuse is suspected, clinicians have a duty to ensure the safety of their elderly patients. Mandated reporting laws for suspected elder abuse exist in 42 states.[5] Many of the states that require reporting provide immunity to physicians who report in good faith.[5] The threshold for reporting is a suspicion of abuse, not absolute proof, much like in the case of suspected child abuse. Reports of suspected abuse are made to Adult Protective Services for community-dwelling elders. Once a suspected abuse report is filed, an evaluation by social services is initiated to determine if there is evidence to support an investigation and legal action. In cases of imminent danger to the elderly patient, law enforcement should be contacted immediately to intervene and investigate the suspected abuse. In addition, law enforcement should be contacted with signs of physical injury thought to be the result of assault.

If the patient who is suspected of being abused resides in a long-term care or board-and-care facility, a report is made to the ombudsman associated with the facility. The Nursing Home Ombudsman program was established by the Older Americans Act of 1976 to provide an advocate for residents of long-term care facilities in cases of abuse and neglect. Facilities are required to post contact information for the ombudsman in plain view.

CASE STUDIES
Case 1

L.J. was a right hand-dominant 90-year-old woman with mild-to-moderate Alzheimer dementia who presented to her primary care physician's office for a routine visit. She sat in her wheelchair, accompanied by her adult grandson, with whom she lived. The patient appeared well groomed. Her vital signs and weight were stable from the previous visit. She had no complaints. On examination, she was noted to have pain in her left shoulder with range of motion. The shoulder joint was slightly deformed and tender. She and her grandson denied trauma to her shoulder. A radiograph of the left shoulder revealed an anterior dislocation. Discussion was held with the patient in private, who denied a fall or injury in the home. The patient's grandson was interviewed in private and complained of his grandmother exhibiting increasing debility and behaviors. She required assistance with transfers, dressing, toileting, and bathing. She refused to comply with his requests at times. He admitted to increasing frustration and difficulty with caring for her. He had no other family to assist him with caring for the patient. Questioning further, he related that his grandmother had an episode of incontinence the prior day while transferring to the toilet from her wheelchair. He grabbed her left arm and pulled her up and out of the wheelchair in an attempt to quickly transfer her to the toilet. He admitted she complained of pain in her left shoulder after the transfer.

Case 1 discussion

The patient has suffered abuse at the hand of her grandson, albeit unintentional per his report. A shoulder dislocation, particularly of the nondominant arm, would not be expected to occur accidentally. Characteristics that put the patient at risk for abuse include her advanced age, female gender, living with her grandson, and her diagnosis of Alzheimer dementia. Risk factors associated with her grandson that point to risk of abusing the patient include increasing caregiver burden and inadequate support, as there is no other family to provide assistance with care of the patient. An Adult Protective Services report was filed in this case. Legal action was not undertaken, but resources and oversight were provided to ensure no further abuse.

Case 2

E.W was a 75 year old functionally independent man with a history of atrial fibrillation, on warfarin for anticoagulation, and with an automatic implantable cardiac defibrillator (AICD). He was brought to the emergency department by his daughter for increasing confusion and weakness. He was found to have an acute on chronic subdural hematoma on computed tomography (CT) scan of the brain. The patient's daughter, who did not live with the patient, reported that the patient's wife stated he fell in his home. He was admitted to the intensive care unit (ICU). Neurosurgery was consulted, and serial monitoring with CT scans was recommended without surgical intervention. Serial CT scans of the brain were performed with no extension of the subdural hematoma. The patient was transferred to a telemetry bed for continued care. While ambulating to the bathroom with a nurse, the patient experienced a syncopal episode. His AICD was found to have fired due to rapid atrial fibrillation on interrogation. The AICD had not fired at the time that the fall reportedly occurred in the home. The patient's medications are adjusted with rate control of the atrial fibrillation. A discussion was held with the patient's daughter to arrange discharge from the hospital. She reported that the patient lives with his second wife and her son, who is 45 years old and unemployed. The daughter reported that the patient's stepson is "hot headed" and argues with the patient and his mother frequently. The daughter related her concern of possible abuse, as she found her father with a "black eye" in the recent past. She stated the stepson does not allow anyone in the home, including family members. On review of the patient's electronic medical record, his primary care physician evaluated the patient 2 months prior following an emergency room visit for a syncopal fall that occurred when he came between his wife and stepson during an altercation. The patient suffered a large hematoma to the occipital scalp. The evaluation in the emergency room at that visit was negative for a cause of the syncope.

Case 2 discussion
There was suspicion of intentional physical abuse of the patient by the patient's stepson. The patient suffered a potentially life-threatening injury resulting in an ICU stay. His daughter had previously noted the patient with a bruise to his face, which is a location suggestive of abuse. He has had a prior injury documented by his primary physician that may have resulted from the patient being pushed by his stepson when he attempted to come to the aid of his wife during an altercation with her son. Again, the resulting head injury was suggestive of abuse. Risk factors for abuse of the patient by his stepson include cohabitation and financial dependence on the patient, as the stepson is unemployed. Commonly, more than 1 type of abuse is present at one time; in this case, aside from possible physical and financial abuse, the son is also isolating the patient from family and friends. The stepson reportedly does not allow anyone other than the patient and his mother into the home, leading to social isolation and possible antisocial behavior. An Adult Protective Services report was filed, leading to police investigation of the case.

Case 3

H.P. was a 91-year-old woman with history of Parkinson disease and dementia who was admitted to the hospital for increasing weakness, declining oral intake, and lethargy. The patient was cared for in her home by her adult daughter. The patient was found to be dehydrated. Decubitus ulcers were noted over the coccyx and right ischium. She had no evidence of infection. Brain imaging was negative for an acute cerebral vascular event. The patient's advanced Parkinson disease and dementia were determined to be the cause of her presenting symptoms. A nasogastric tube was placed for feeding, as the patient was found to have dysphagia on evaluation of her swallow function. After a 3-day hospital stay, her condition was stable for transfer to a rehabilitation facility. Her daughter was at the bedside when the attending physician at the rehabilitation facility evaluated the patient. The patient was noted to have rigidity of the muscles of the extremities. She was nonverbal but moaned when repositioned by staff. She did not follow commands. The decubitus ulcers over the coccyx, right ischium, and bilateral heels were unstageable, with discoloration of the skin around the ulcerations. The attending physician discussed the patient's medical condition and the home situation with the patient's daughter. Even though the electronic medical records noted Parkinson disease, the patient's daughter denied that the patient has this and stated that her dementia was mild. She reported that the patient was walking and talking in the home just prior to the hospitalization. Medications in the home setting were reported to be a variety of supplements with no medications for Parkinson disease or dementia. The patient's daughter reported that the bedsores occurred in the emergency department and worsened during her hospitalization. The physician noted the daughter was middle-aged, cachectic, and disheveled. She was restless throughout the conversation, slurring her words when she spoke.

Case 3 discussion

This case is an example of physical abuse and neglect. The decubitus ulcers were noted to be on pressure points consistent with lying in bed for extended periods without being repositioned, consistent with neglect. The patient's muscle rigidity resulted from withholding dopamine agonists. Withholding the dopamine agonist has resulted in pain with repositioning due to muscle stiffness as evidenced by the patient moaning with movement. Risk factors for the patient to be abused include advanced dementia, advanced age, female gender, and residing with her abuser. Factors associated with caregiver abuse include caregiver burden and possible substance abuse versus mental illness. An Adult Protective Services report was filed by the emergency department physician on presentation to the hospital. It was found that a previous Adult Protective Services report had been filed by the patient's primary physician due to the decubitus ulcers. The case remains under investigation.

Case 4

C.M. was an 82-year-old woman with dementia who suffered a mechanical fall in her home, fracturing her hip. She underwent surgical repair and was sent to a skilled nursing facility for rehabilitation postoperatively. She was reported by family members to be "worse off" with regards to her cognition after the surgery. The patient had episodes of crying out and attempting to exit her bed without assistance at the nursing facility. The patient was evaluated by the attending physician after the facility staff expressed concern for the patient's safety. The facility requested medications to calm the patient as she exhibited anxiety. After speaking to the patient's family member and medical decision maker, consent was obtained for use of a low dose of lorazepam ordered every 12 hours as needed for anxiety. The patient tolerated the lorazepam without adverse effects. She was reported by staff to be less anxious and did not attempt to exit her bed. Her attending physician went out of town for 3 days to a medical conference. A hospital physician agreed to take call for the attending physician's patients during the day. Nursing staff reported to the covering physician that the patient continued to cry out frequently. Nursing requested adjustment of the lorazepam dose as the patient's behaviors were disruptive to other patients. The attending physician returned to the nursing facility to see the patient following the conference. The patient was lethargic and more confused than during the previous visit. On review of the medication administration record, it was found that lorazepam had been ordered every 8 hours as needed. The nursing staff had been administering the lorazepam every 8 hours around the clock, documenting anxiety and behaviors as the reason for administration. Discussion with the nursing staff revealed that nonpharmacologic measures, such as staff members sitting with the patient, to calm the patient were not used prior to lorazepam administration. Diagnostic studies were performed to ensure that there was no cause for the change of condition other than the medication change with a negative evaluation. The patient was weaned from the lorazepam with improvement of the lethargy and delirium. She was noted to have increased muscle weakness despite improvement in her alertness following discontinuation of lorazepam.

Case 4 discussion

This case illustrates physical abuse through overmedication. The ombudsman was contacted, as the abuse occurred in a rehabilitation facility. Risk factors predisposing the patient to abuse include female gender, advanced age, and dementia, with behaviors of attempting to exit her bed without assistance and frequent crying out. The patient's debility following her hip fracture contributed to her risk of abuse, as she placed an increased burden on facility staff for her care. The facility staff members were found to have difficulty dealing with the patient's behaviors due to lack of training in nonpharmacologic interventions and lack of staff to implement such interventions when interviewed by the ombudsman. The staff utilized a medication ordered by the physician with the intention of intermittent use on a scheduled basis to chemically restrain the patient, preventing behaviors from occurring. The facility was required to develop protocols to intervene using nonpharmacologic measures in cases of patients with dementia exhibiting unsafe or disruptive behaviors. Staff members underwent mandatory training in utilization of these alternative measures as part of a corrective action plan.

SUMMARY

Physical abuse of the elderly is a significant public health concern. The true prevalence of all types, including trauma, restraints, and misuse of medications is unknown, and under-reporting is known to be significant. The geriatric population is projected to increase dramatically over the next 10 years, and the number of abused individuals is projected to increase also. It is critical that health care providers feel competent in addressing physical elder abuse. The cases presented illustrate the variety of presenting symptoms that may be attributed to physical elder abuse. Recognition of abuse by clinicians and reporting suspicion of abuse to the proper authorities will improve care of older adults and prevent serious morbidity and mortality.

REFERENCES

1. Available at: www.cdc.gov/ViolencePrevention/eldermaltreatment/definitions. Accessed January 12, 2014.
2. Available at: www.cdc.gov/features/elderabuse. Accessed January 12, 2014.
3. Acierno R, Hernandez-Tejada M, Muzzy W, et al. The national elder mistreatment study. Washington, DC: National Institute of Justice; 2009. Document No. 226456.
4. Lachs M, Irene F, Psaty IR, et al. Under the radar: New York state elder abuse prevalence study. Final report. Rochester (NY): Lifespan of Greater Rochester, Inc; 2011.
5. Lachs M, Pillemer K. Abuse and neglect of elderly persons. N Engl J Med 1995; 332:437–43.
6. Johannesen M, LoGiudice D. Elder abuse: a systematic review of risk factors in community-dwelling elders. Age Ageing 2013;42(3):292–8.
7. Shugarman L, Fries B, Wolf R, et al. Identifying older people at risk of abuse during routine screening practices. J Am Geriatr Soc 2003;51:24–31.
8. Pavlik V, Hyman D, Festa N, et al. Quantifying the problem of abuse and neglect in adults—analysis of a statewide database. J Am Geriatr Soc 2001;49:45–8.
9. Wiglesworth A, Mosqueda L, Mulnard R, et al. Screening for abuse and neglect of people with dementia. J Am Geriatr Soc 2010;58:493–500.
10. Available at: www.ncea.aoa.gov/FAQ/Type_Abuse/index.aspx. Accessed February 15, 2014.
11. Friedman L, Avila S, Tanouye K, et al. A case–control study of severe physical abuse of older adults. J Am Geriatr Soc 2011;59:417–22.
12. Mosqueda L, Burnight K, Liao S. The life cycle of bruises in older adults. J Am Geriatr Soc 2005;53:1339–43.
13. Wiglesworth A, Austin R, Corona M, et al. Bruising as a marker of physical elder abuse. J Am Geriatr Soc 2009;57:1191–6.

14. Dyer C, Connolly M, McFeeley P. The clinical and medical forensics of elder abuse and neglect. In: Bonnie RJ, Wallace RB, editors. Elder mistreatment: abuse, neglect, and exploitation in an aging America. Washington, DC: National Academies Press; 2003. p. 339–81.

15. Schofield M, Powers J, Loxton D. Mortality and disability outcomes of self-reported elder abuse: a 12-year prospective investigation. J Am Geriatr Soc 2013;61:679–85.

16. Dong X. Advancing the field of elder abuse: future directions and policy implications. J Am Geriatr Soc 2012;60:2151–6.

Elder Neglect

Tessa del Carmen, MD*, Veronica M. LoFaso, MS, MD

KEYWORDS

- Elder mistreatment • Elder abuse • Elder maltreatment • Elder neglect
- Adult protective services

KEY POINTS

- Elder neglect is the most common form of elder abuse. Identifying patients who are vulnerable to neglect allows clinicians to intervene early and potentially prevent situations that can escalate and lead to harm or even death.
- Health care workers have a unique opportunity to uncover these unfortunate situations and in many cases may be the only other contact isolated vulnerable patients have with the outside world.
- Responding appropriately and quickly when neglect is suspected and using a team approach can improve the health and well-being of older victims of neglect.

INTRODUCTION

Elder neglect is the most commonly reported form of elder mistreatment[1,2] and has the potential for serious and often fatal consequences for the victims.

Elder neglect and mistreatment remain under-reported.[3] Barriers for health care providers to reporting neglect to proper authorities include lack of provider knowledge, time constraints, or fear of retaliation of the abuser to the victim.[4] Victims are often frail and reticent to report a family member or caregiver because of shame or fear. In many neglect cases, the victims may not have the ability or be willing to testify against the abuser, making attempts at prosecution difficult.

Clinicians are frequently challenged to make a definitive diagnosis of neglect. Unlike other forms of elder mistreatment where injuries are more obvious (fractures, burns, contusions, and lacerations), neglect may present with more subtle findings. Awareness of red herrings and maintaining a high index of clinical suspicion are necessary to detect and assess neglect. Failure to identify neglect and mistreatment can lead to a detrimental effect on an older person, because there is a 3-fold increase in mortality in elder mistreatment and neglect victims compared to non-abused older adults.[5]

Division of Geriatrics and Palliative Medicine, New York Presbyterian Hospital, Weill Cornell Medical College, Baker 14, 525 East 68th Street, New York, NY 10065, USA
* Corresponding author.
E-mail address: tmd9004@med.cornell.edu

Clin Geriatr Med 30 (2014) 769–777
http://dx.doi.org/10.1016/j.cger.2014.08.006
0749-0690/14/$ – see front matter © 2014 Elsevier Inc. All rights reserved.
geriatric.theclinics.com

DEFINITION AND PREVALENCE

According to the National Center on Elder Abuse, neglect is defined as failure to provide basic care and necessities to a person for whom one has accepted caregiving responsibilities. These responsibilities include, but are not limited to, providing the basic necessities of daily living, such as food and hydration, and the ability to provide a safe physical environment, administer medications, attend to a person's hygiene, and maintain a comfortable and stable living environment.

Neglect can be passive or active, intentional or unintentional.[6] Intentional neglect is the act of knowingly failing to provide the necessary care for an elder person. Unintentional neglect can be the lack of ability to provide proper care or unknowingly placing an elder person in harm through their actions or lack of actions.

The prevalence of neglect is staggering. In a study by Acierno and colleagues,[7] 1 in 10 community-residing elders of 5777 respondents reported being mistreated in the past year, with more than 5% of the participants reporting potential neglect. The incidence of elder abuse in nursing homes ranges from 20% to 30%.[8,9] Neglect was reported in nursing homes at 9.8% and in assisted living facilities, neglect is reported to be 9.8%.[8,9] Although research in assisted living facilities is limited, long-term care ombudsman notes frequent reports of neglect in assisted living facilities.[10]

According to a US House of Representatives report in 2001,[11] 1 of 10 nursing homes had violations that caused residents harm. In another study of nursing home residents, 95% said they had been neglected or witnessed another resident being neglected[2,12] and in a separate study of nursing homes staff, more than 50% admitted to mistreating older patients, and two-thirds of this mistreatment was neglect.[13]

A majority of abusers are family members[2] of victims who live in the community, but for others who suffer neglect in nursing homes or assisted living facilities, abusers may be staff members, visitors or other residents.[6]

SIGNS AND SYMPTOMS

Common physical signs of neglect include malnutrition, dehydration, poor hygiene, and inadequate or inappropriate clothing. Malnutrition and poor hygiene can lead to pressure ulcers. Nutritional deficiencies are a risk factor for pressure ulcers.[14] Pressure ulcers can also be caused by a lack of proper repositioning of immobile patients or placing a person on bed restraints for prolonged periods of time.[5] Although there are other medical conditions that can lead to poor wound healing and increased risk for pressure ulcers, such as diabetes mellitus, vascular diseases, and wounds that occur at the end of life, also known as Kennedy Terminal Ulcers, most clean pressure ulcers with adequate blood supply should show signs of healing in 2 to 4 weeks if treated properly.[15] Victims of neglect may be missing necessary assistive devices, such as walkers, hearing aides, glasses, or dentures. These assistive devices are necessary to keep patients aware of their surroundings. Without these, patients are susceptible to dangers that can increase their morbidity and mortality, like falls, which can lead to fractures and decreased functional status.

Other clues to neglect include an unexpected deterioration in a person's health. This may indicate lack of access to the health care system or neglectful withholding of the proper medications and treatments required to manage their health problems.

Factors that place patients at risk for neglect/abuse include[4]

- Interdependence between the patient and potential abuser
- Social isolation
- Shared living environment

Common characteristics of neglectful/abusive caregivers include[4]

- Mental illness
- Drug abuse/alcohol abuse
- Developmentally delay
- Dementia
- Physical impairment
- Financial dependence on the victim
- Lack of knowledge or experience in caregiving

APPROACHES TO SCREENING

There are multiple screening and assessment tools for elder mistreatment and elder neglect. To date, there is no widely accepted screening tool or method. A high level of suspicion and clinical judgment by a health care professional are critical for detection.

The American Medical Association recommends that all physicians routinely inquire about the physical, sexual, and psychological abuse of an elder patient as part of the medical history analysis. Patients and caregivers should be interviewed separately.

Suggested questions for patients when screening for neglect or abuse include[16]

- Do you feel safe?
- Do you feel your needs are being met?
- Has someone hurt you or is hurting you?
- Are your needs being met?
- Has your caregiver ignored you or left you alone for some time?
- Does your caregiver depend on you financially?
- Does your caregiver have any history of alcohol or drug abuse or mental disorder?

Suggested questions for an alleged abuser when screening for neglect or abuse include[16]

- What kind of help does the person you care for need?
- What is the person you care for able to do for him/herself?
- What are the expectations from you by the person you care for and are you able to meet those expectations?
- Do you feel frustrated caring for this person?
- Is there anything you need to help you better care of the person?

CLINICAL EVALUATION

An evaluation for neglect should include a complete history and physical examination with special attention to function and psychosocial stressors. An interdisciplinary approach to the assessment and plan if available is preferable.

The history should be conducted in a private space with the patient separated from the caregiver. Any assisted devices needed for communication should be provided (ie, hearing devices, amplifiers, glasses, and dentures). The health care professional should conduct the interview in a culturally sensitive manner cognizant of the fact that different cultures may disagree on what constitutes elder neglect. Reluctance on the part of the caregiver to leave the patient alone may be an indicator of mistreatment. The cognitive status and level of capacity of the patient must always be ascertained and, if further clarification is needed, neurologic or psychiatric consultations may be warranted. A complete medical examination is crucial to differentiate possible signs and symptoms of abuse and neglect from conditions that might occur as part of normal aging. The physical examination should be comprehensive. It should begin with a general observation of the patient's interaction with the examiner, including appearance, possible signs of dehydration, weight loss, and personal hygiene. The examination should pay special attention to the skin for any evidence of possible physical abuse, skin rashes, or pressure ulcers. Functional status evaluation, including activities of daily living (ADLs) and instrumental ADLs (IADLs), allows practitioners to formulate a plan specifically tailored to patients' needs and abilities.

INTERVENTION

If a patient needs assistance in the home, it is essential to find out if the patient has access to assistance as well as the knowledge of who is to provide it. Any medical aides required, such as hearing devices, glasses, and walking devices, should be supplied for the patient. Living arrangements are vital to understand because patients and the alleged neglectors may live within the same household. Determining who manages patients' finances and the resources they have can help determine if a patient is dependent on others or if a patient has dependents for living and personal expenses. Social support should be determined because victims are often socially isolated by abusers.

Once neglect is suspected, the health care provider must determine whether the patient is safe or in immediate danger. If there is an immediate threat, local authorities may need to be called or the patient may need hospitalization.

If a patient it is able to return home safely, a home visit and safety evaluation are appropriate. The situation should be discussed with the patient if he or she has decision-making capacity. Consulting with social work may be necessary to arrange other services, such as counseling, arranging alternate living arrangements, and referring to local agencies. A person who has capacity has a right to refuse intervention. Guardianship, conservatorship, or special court proceedings may be necessary if a victim lacks capacity. Medical intervention should include any needs that have been unmet, such as pain control, blood pressure control, and wound care.

REPORTING

Legal interventions differ from state to state, but knowing a state's reporting system is important. The laws differ from state to state but all health care providers are mandated in 42 states to report suspected elder abuse to Adult Protective Services (APS).[17–30] In some states, health care providers can be found negligent if they do not report suspected mistreatment.

Reporting of potential abuse occurring in nursing homes or assisted living facilities should be reported to the local long-term care ombudsman and APS.

Case 1

A 64-year-old woman with a history of systolic heart failure, diabetes mellitus, osteoarthritis, and severe spinal stenosis presents to her primary care physician for a medical examination required for renewal of her disability benefits. Her doctor has not seen her for more than a year. Her daughter, who accompanies the patient to the visit, appears distracted and impatient.

She is finding it more difficult to ambulate and spends more time in her wheelchair now than she had previously. It is getting more difficult to manage her daily routine. She notes that that her memory is declining and thinks she may be missing doses of her medication. She needs assistance with most ADLs and reports that she signs her disability check over to her daughter, who then pays the patient's bills. She tells her mother that there is not any money left over. The patient's daughter lives with the patient and does not work. She helps the patient on occasion but admits that it has been difficult to take care of her mother because she has her own personal problems.

When asked if her daughter helps her at home, she discloses that her daughter is an alcoholic who blames her mother for many of her own problems. The patient is at home by herself most of the time. She admits that her daughter is financially dependent on her yet threatens to put her in a nursing home if she complains. On examination you note that the patient has signs of being in active heart failure. You also note that she has a stage 2 sacral pressure ulcer and that her Mini-Mental State Examination score is 26/30.

Discussion

The patient has been nonadherent with her cardiac medications. Accessing her pharmacy has been difficult secondary to her mobility impairment, memory loss, and heart failure symptoms. She needs assistance in IADLs and some ADLs but cannot rely on her daughter, who is her primary care giver. The daughter's alcohol addiction and mental health issues make her an unfit caregiver. Her neglectful caregiving has resulted in the patient being mostly wheelchair bound and more vulnerable to developing a sacral pressure ulcer. Her daughter's behavior is also consistent with emotional and financial abuse. She is threatening her with nursing home placement as a means to control her mother financially. A referral to APS should be made because there is suspicion of dependent adult abuse.

This patient should be admitted for acute exacerbation of heart failure. After optimizing her medical conditions, the team should then begin assessing whether she can safely return to her existing home situation. This requires a capacity assessment to ensure she fully understands her options on discharge and can choose a health care proxy. Clearly her daughter is currently unable to provide the needed care for her mother. This patient warrants an in-depth social work evaluation. She requires home care to help with ADLs. Ideally she would be given a personal emergency response device to wear. She could be referred to a community social service agency for monitoring of the home situation and, in some cases, financial management services as well. A referral to a visiting nurse service would be helpful to manage the sacral wound and to monitor her heart failure symptoms and oversee her medication adherence.

The daughter's alcohol abuse and mental health problems need to be addressed as well. Referral to the appropriate resources for ongoing psychiatric care is crucial, especially if the patient intends to return home. An evaluation for suspected financial abuse should be completed.

If the daughter is unable or unwilling to address her alcohol addiction, then the patient may decide to seek an alternative housing arrangement. If the patient is deemed to lack capacity, then guardianship might be considered if the daughter is not able or willing to meet her caregiving responsibilities.

Case 2

A 79-year-old woman with a past medical history of hypertension, depression, and osteoarthritis presents for a geriatric medicine consultation with complaints of memory loss. The patient's son, who is developmentally delayed, brought her for evaluation because he does not believe the neurologist's assessment. The patient has stopped taking all of her medications. She reports that her memory has been declining over the past 5 years. Her primary physician sent her to a neurologist, who prescribed donepezil for her memory loss.

She lives alone and manages all her ADLs and most IADLs. She has an accountant who manages her finances and a cleaning lady who visits her once a week. She is currently working with a lawyer on a living will and assuring that her cognitively impaired son, who is unable to work and currently living in adult group home for people with disabilities, will be financially secure.

Nine months later, she presents a day early for her appointment accompanied by her son. She reports that over the past few months, her memory loss has continued to worsen and her son has had to take over managing her medications. When asked about her medications, the patient and her son can only reliably say that she has been taking her donepezil on a daily basis. They both were uncertain about how or why she took her other medications that included aspirin, atorvastatin, and lisinopril. Her son tells you that she was treated for a cough by her primary care physician and was given codeine some time ago that she may or may not still be taking. She was also given zolpidem for sleep, which he sometimes administers when she has insomnia because he now lives with the patient to assist her.

On physical examination, she has uncontrolled blood pressure with a Montreal Cognitive Assessment score of 23/30 (with 26 or greater considered a normal score). Her laboratory data are unremarkable and MRI reveals cerebral atrophy with significant ischemic white matter changes.

Discussion

The patient was initially assessed to have mild cognitive impairment but presents with worsening memory loss and functional impairment. The patient's son, who is developmentally delayed, has been managing her medications but does not have the full ability to provide for the patient's needs. This is an example of neglect that is unintentional. Her son's intentions were good but his learning impairment rendered him unable to fulfill the duties he took on. A referral should be made to APS so that social workers can evaluate their needs and offer appropriate resources.

An important first step of her evaluation is to reconcile her medication regimen. Then a complete medical evaluation to determine any treatable or reversible causes of her functional decline, which may include infection, metabolic derangements, and vitamin deficiencies, should follow.

The patient's home situation needs to be evaluated. Ideally home care would be instituted to assist the patient with adherence to medications. The patient's capacity should be assessed. The team should reach out to other family or friends who may be able to provide support. If there are no other means of internal support, she may have to move to an assisted living facility or board and care home for assistance. If feasible, she would benefit from a geriatric care manager to oversee her care needs. Advanced directives, power of attorney, and arrangements for her son should be clarified as soon as possible given her cognitive decline. An elder law attorney referral would be a helpful intervention. A capacity evaluation will determine what types of decisions she has the capacity to make. This may range from her preference in living arrangements to managing finances.

Case 3

An 84-year-old man with a history of atrial fibrillation, stroke with dysarthria and left hemiparesis, diabetes, hypertension, and mild vascular dementia presents to an emergency room after a fall transferring from his wheelchair to bed in the nursing home. His daughter, who is visiting from out of state, accompanies him. The nursing home notes that accompany the patient state that he is independent in feeding and grooming. Per nursing home documentation, his blood sugars and blood pressure readings have been in an acceptable range. There is no documentation of his weight in the past 3 months. This is his third fall in the past 2 months.

His daughter reports that she is shocked to see how much weight he has lost since she last saw him 3 months ago. She also feels that his mental status has declined. He appears sad and withdrawn. She noted that without her encouragement and assistance he would not eat his meals. He would eat ice cream if she brought it to him. He was not wearing his dentures and was not sure where they were. On occasion she noted him coughing after taking his pills.

The patient is in a wheelchair, frail and cachectic. He is wearing soiled clothes and smells of urine. The patient has overgrown nails with onychomycosis. He shows signs of dehydration with sunken eyes and dry mucous membranes and his heart rate is tachycardic. He has an infected stage 3 sacral ulcer with unstageable heel eschars.

Laboratory results are consistent with hypernatremia, with a sodium level of 150 and acute kidney injury.

Discussion

This patient has multiple signs of potential neglect. He has had a significant decline from his baseline and now has signs of poor hygiene, inadequate nutrition, multiple pressure ulcers, and has suffered recurrent falls.

This patient needs inpatient evaluation of an infected sacral decubitus ulcer and possible aspiration risk. The fact that he has multiple pressure ulcers could indicate lack of proper wound care and positioning required for patients with impaired mobility and skin breakdown. The presence of ulcers on the heels and knee, areas that should be easily protected by good nursing care, makes neglect even more suspect in this case. Malnutrition could also be exacerbating his skin breakdown and raises the question of adequate nutrition. Additionally his pulmonary status calls into question whether he was given a proper aspiration diet and whether proper feeding techniques were used in the nursing home.

During his hospitalization, the patient's case was reported to the hospital social work as well as APS, and the family was counseled about the role of the long-term care ombudsman.

SUMMARY

Because neglect is the most common form of elder abuse, identifying patients who are vulnerable to neglect allows clinicians to intervene early and potentially prevent situations that can escalate and lead to harm or even death. Health care workers have a unique opportunity to uncover these unfortunate situations and in many cases may be the only other contact isolated vulnerable patients have with the outside world. Responding appropriately and quickly when neglect is suspected and using a team approach can improve the health and well-being of older victims of neglect.

REFERENCES

1. Fulmer T, Paveza G, Abraham I, et al. Elder neglect assessment in the emergency department. J Emerg Nurs 2000;26(5):436–43.
2. The Administration on Aging. The National Elder Abuse Incidence Study: final report. National Center on Elder Abuse, Administration on Aging; 1998. Available at: www.ncea.aoa.gov/ www.aoa.gov.
3. Lachs MS, Pillemer K. Elder abuse. Lancet 2004;364(9441):1263–72.

4. Ahmad M, Lachs MS. Elder abuse and neglect: what physicians can and should do. Cleve Clin J Med 2002;69(10):801–8.
5. Lachs MS, Williams CS, O'Brien S, et al. The mortality of elder mistreatment. JAMA 1998;280(5):428–32.
6. Collins KA. Elder maltreatment: a review. Arch Pathol Lab Med 2006;130(9): 1290–6.
7. Acierno R, Hernandez MA, Amstadter AB, et al. Prevalence and correlates of emotional, physical, sexual, and financial abuse and potential neglect in the United States: the national elder mistreatment study. Am J Public Health 2010; 100(2):292–7.
8. Page C, Conner T, Prokhorov A, et al. The effect of care setting on elder abuse: results from a michigan survey. J Elder Abuse Negl 2009;21(3):239–52.
9. Castle N, Ferguson-Rome J, Teresi JA. Elder abuse in residential long-term care: an update to the 2003 National Research Council Report. J Appl Gerontol 2013. [Epub ahead of print].
10. Phillipis L, Ziminski C. Populations at risk across the lifespan: population studies the public health nursing role in elder neglect in assisted living facilities. Public Health Nurs 2012;29(6):499–509. http://dx.doi.org/10.1111/j.1525-1446. 2012.010129.x.
11. Minority Staff Special Investigations Division. Abuse of residents is a major problem in US nursing homes. Committee on Government Reform. Washington, DC: US House of Representatives; 2001. Available at: http://cahr.org/reports/ 2001/abusemajorproblem.pdf.
12. Broyles K. The silenced voice speaks out: a study of abuse and neglect of nursing home residents? A report from the Atlanta Long Term Care Ombudsman Program and Atlanta Legal Aid Society to the National Citizens Coalition for Nursing Home Reform; 2000. Available at: www.atlantalegalaid.org/abuse.htm.
13. Natan B, Lowenstein A. Study of factors that affect abuse of older people in nursing homes. Nurs Manag 2010;12(8):20–4.
14. Chang AL, Wong JW, Endo JO, et al. Geriatric dermatology part II. Risk factors and cutaneous signs of elder mistreatment for the dermatologist. J Am Acad Dermatol 2013;68(4):533.e1–10.
15. Agency for Healthcare Policy and research. Treatment of Pressure Ulcers. Clinical Practice Guidelines number 15. AHCPR Publication No. 95-0652, Rockville, MD: US Department of Health and Human services, Public Health Service; 1994.
16. American Medical Association (AMA). Diagnostic and treatment guidelines on elder abuse and neglect. Arch Fam Med 1993;2:371–88.
17. Lachs M, Pillemer K. Abuse and neglect of elderly persons. N Engl J Med 1995; 332:437–43.
18. Breckman R, Adelman R. Strategies for helping victims of elder mistreatment. Newbury Park (CA): Sage; 1988.
19. Collins KA, Presnell SE. Elder neglect and the pathophysiology of aging. Am J Forensic Med Pathol 2007;28(2):157–62.
20. Dong X. Elder abuse as a risk factor for hospitalization in older persons. JAMA Intern Med 2013;173:911–7. http://dx.doi.org/10.1001/jamainternmed.2013.238.
21. Fulmer T, Paveza G, VandeWeerd C, et al. Dyadic vulnerability and risk profiling for elder neglect. Gerontologist 2005;45(4):525–34.
22. Fulmer T, Paveza G, Vandeweerd C, et al. Neglect assessment in urban emergency departments and confirmation by an expert clinical team. J Gerontol A Biol Sci Med Sci 2005;60(8):1002–6.

23. Fulmer TT. Mistreatment of elders. Assessment, diagnosis, and intervention. Nurs Clin North Am 1989;24(3):707–16.
24. Joshi S, Flaherty JH. Elder abuse and neglect in long-term care. Clin Geriatr Med 2005;21(2):333–54.
25. Lindbloom EJ, Brandt J, Hough LD, et al. Elder mistreatment in the nursing home: a systematic review. J Am Med Dir Assoc 2007;8(9):610–6.
26. Mosqueda L, Burnight K, Liao S. The life cycle of bruises in older adults. J Am Geriatr Soc 2005;53(8):1339–43.
27. Strasser SM, Fulmer T. The clinical presentation of elder neglect: what we know and what we can do. J Am Psychiatr Nurses Assoc 2007;12:340. http://dx.doi. org/10.1177/107839030606298879.
28. Wiglesworth A, Austin R, Corona M, et al. Bruising as a marker of physical elder abuse. J Am Geriatr Soc 2009;57(7):1191–6.
29. Wiglesworth A, Mosqueda L, Mulnard R, et al. Screening for abuse and neglect of people with dementia. J Am Geriatr Soc 2010;58(3):493–500.
30. del Carmen T, Lachs M. Detecting, Assessing and Responding to Elder mistreatment. Current Diagnosis and Treatment 2nd Edition 2014;517–23.

Case Series of Sexual Assault in Older Persons

Patricia M. Speck, DNSc, APN, FNP-BC, FAAFS, FAAN[a],*,
Margaret T. Hartig, PhD, APN, FNP-BC, FAANP[b], Wendy Likes, PhD, DNSc, APN, FNP-BC[b],
Trimika Bowdre, PhD, MPH[b], Amy Y. Carney, PhD, APRN, FNP-BC, FAAFS[c],
Rachell A. Ekroos, MSN, ARNP-BC, AFN-BC, DF-IAFN[d], Ron Haugen, DNP, FNP-BC, PMH-BC[e],
Jill Crum, BSN, RN, SANE-A[f], Diana K. Faugno, MSN, RN, CPN, SANE-A, SANE-P, FAAFS[f]

KEYWORDS

- Sexual assault • Rape • Elder rape • Elder sexual assault • Institutional rape
- Community-dwelling elders • Institutional dwelling elders

KEY POINTS

- Older persons are sexually responsive and enjoy a variety of sexual activities.
- Older raped persons face the same shame and self-blame seen in younger populations of victims.
- Trauma focused and patient centered care following rape empowers victims of all ages.
- Cognitive decline in older persons influences reporting and interviewing strategies.
- Physiologic changes in genital structures of older persons influences injury patterns.
- Abusers of older and vulnerable adults are likely in a trusted relationship with the victim.

INTRODUCTION AND LITERATURE REVIEW

The face of America is aging. For the first time in history, people aged 65 years and older will outnumber children younger than 5 years.[1] There are many changes associated with aging, such as chronic disease, frailty, and dependency, which are beyond

Disclosure statement: no author has a conflict of interest disclosure.
[a] The University of Alabama at Birmingham School of Nursing Department of Community Health Outcomes & Systems, 1720 Second Avenue South, Rm 300, Birmingham, AL 35294-1210, USA; [b] University of Tennessee Health Science Center College of Nursing, 920 Madison Avenue, 10th floor, Memphis, TN 38163, USA; [c] School of Nursing, California State University, 441 La Moree Road, San Marcos, CA 92078, USA; [d] Center for Forensic Nursing Excellence International, 10624 S Eastern Avenue, A-793, Henderson, NV 89052, USA; [e] Synergy, LLC, 207 W, McKay Street Ste A, Carlsbad, NM 88220, USA; [f] Eisenhower Medical Center, 39000 Bob Hope Drive, Rancho Mirage, CA 92270-3221, USA
* Corresponding author.
E-mail addresses: pmspeck@uab.edu; pmspeck@gmail.com

the scope of this case series. Older persons have expectations of self-determination, especially with sexual behavior.[2] Alas, society views older adults as asexual,[3] but research[4,5] has shown that older adults are sexually responsive and enjoy a variety of sexual activities. The benefit of healthy sexuality provides a sense of normalcy to the lives of older adults,[6] which cannot be replaced with friendships or other social interaction.[7–9]

However, generally trusting of their environment and people, the older population lacks sexual knowledge, minimizes sexual violence via beliefs in myths, and generally, is unprepared for the sexual risks of today[10] (Trimika L Bowdre, PhD, 2013, unpublished data). Older patients do not report traumatic sexual histories, current practices, or needs[11,12] (Trimika L Bowdre, PhD, 2013, unpublished data); hence, older adults face vulnerability from sexual relationships, intimate or domestic partner violence,[13] and diseases.[14] Social stigma, internalized shame and self-blame, increased beliefs in myths coupled with a lifetime of resilience and adaptation, all contribute to the lack of reporting sexual abuse or assault in older women.[13] Social determinants of health and traumatic (eg, sexual violence) or excessive stress in life course experiences for some older persons result in "maladaptation to chronic stressors,"[15,16] creating a chronic allostatic load.[17] Morbidity and mortality increase in older victims of various forms of violence (including sexual assault)[18–20]; however, not all who are subjected to intentional and unintentional traumas succumb to disability, frailty, or death, even with serious chronic stressors.[15] Therefore, because little is known about the impact of sexual violence on older women,[13] "targeting the antecedents of [ie, traumatic events preceding] allostatic loads at critical periods (e.g., sexual abuse and rape) and implementing programs that cultivate resiliency is essential to improving public health"[15] in the older victimized population.

Programs that educate the community about offenders and reduce high-risk situations with criminal background checks, supervision, and advocacy[21] or identify risk factors (alcohol abuse, dependency, and history of abuse, income divergence) have the potential to identify offenders in institutional settings.[22,23] Training providers about different dementias and associated sexual behavior patterns assists in the recognition of signs of sexual assault[19,24] when older persons cannot or will not speak about the event.

Building educational curriculum along with infrastructure development within systems and institutions enhance reporting,[17,23,25] and are all necessary for quick discovery and recovery from sexual trauma in the older person, hence, avoiding increased institutional admissions[26] in semiskilled and skilled facilities (eg, nursing homes) after elder maltreatment. When cognitive capacity is diminished, complex teams of professionals representing unique systems, such as legal and health care professionals, as well as social and institutional teams, must collaborate openly to benefit the older person and their families throughout the investigative process.[11,27]

Aging is a process determined by genetics, environment, and lifestyle. Myths abound about older persons and their value to the community. Literature remains limited in helping practitioners understand the long-term societal consequences of abuse in elders,[28] although evidence is emerging. Older victims with dementias experiencing medical forensic evaluations immediately after sexual assault experience emotional shock as an acute traumatic reaction and express confusion that may mimic worsening cognition, even triggering memories from childhood assaults. In some elders, sexual assault is a precursor for increased mortality and early death.[29] Research continues to focus on recognition of the forensic markers of injury,[3,29] and understanding consent and capacity limitations after sexual assault,[30] instead of the overall global or societal impact.[28]

INTERVIEWS

Trauma-focused care assists the victim to regain feelings of safety and is empowering when communities of skilled trauma-focused providers keep the patient and family members informed, provide medical treatment, and encourage routine daily activities.[31] Shock and trauma can make trauma-focused interviewing difficult, because patients do not process information consistently or in a predictable manner.[31] Mental health and alterations in mental status are a result of an individual's chaotic life or multiple traumas experienced throughout a person's life trajectory. Normally challenging to health care providers, the mental health and alterations in mental status expose complexities, which are routinely confounded during investigations of sexual violence of older persons.[17,32]

> *Trauma-Informed Care is a strengths-based framework that is grounded in an understanding of and responsiveness to the impact of trauma, that emphasizes physical, psychological, and emotional safety for both providers and survivors, and that creates opportunities for survivors to rebuild a sense of control and empowerment.[33]*

Cognitive decline can influence reporting and valid testimony by older persons after physical or sexual violence.[29,32,34] Closed-ended direct questions, such as those used in a structured interview for a 12-year-old (or younger) that are not threatening or leading, help those with diminished verbal skills disclose the criminal act.[31,33] For others with limited verbal capacity, trauma care specialists skilled in therapeutic interviewing use drawings or dolls and even physical response by the victim to inform the investigation. Trauma-informed methods, used with the permission of the older person, continually evaluate the older person's capacity, which gives the older person an opportunity to return to a safe place, abandon resistance to the process, and cooperate.

Use of the Hudson taxonomy[35] to interview older persons after evaluation for capacity supports the older person's constitutional rights to confidentiality and autonomous decision making, including whether they want to decline participation in the medical legal evaluative process.[30] Some cases include disclosure to children and grandchildren who are horrified that their loved one was raped. Although sexuality in a parent or grandparent is a passing thought before sexual assault, children often are more fearful than the parent or grandparent about safety, after a sexual assault.[36] Therefore, children and grandchildren may actively encourage the older person to move from a familiar setting, such as their home, which may not be in the best interest or the desire of the individual victim. Patient-centered care focuses on desires of patients, even when there is diminished capacity. Legal support for the older victim may be necessary when the older person's desires conflict with family members' desires or providers' recommendations.

Older persons with a diagnosed cognitive impairment may experience accelerated dementia after a sexual assault. Sentinel recognition of the decline may occur first by a caretaker or family member, who is a mandated reporter. Increased cognitive impairment could represent increased stress from the disruption of a safe environment and a subsequent chronic allostatic load, which can lead to death.[16,37–39]

Physical symptoms, such as physical lethargy, may be the only symptom in patients with significant cognitive decline.[19,37] Like child sexual abuse, those who are unfamiliar to the elder rarely have access to a dependent older person unless they are in a formal care institution.[37] Even then, other residents with cognitive decline and mental health issues, along with caretakers, perpetrate most sexual assaults.[37] With the presence of dementia, the sexual assault forensic evaluator (SAFE) evaluates for suspicion of abuse. The evaluation is a lengthy assessment of cognition and consent, using available tools, previous medical records and reports from relatives. Surveys useful in evaluating cognitive decline include the Mini-Mental State Examination.

When a sexual event is discovered between older persons requiring institutional care, family members may be conflicted between embarrassment and protecting the rights of the elder desiring to fulfill sexual needs.[40] If there is suspicion of nonconsent or a delay in recognition, or if there is existing posttraumatic stress disorder history, the stress of the event may result in a muted response by the older person. This response may manifest as withdrawal, agitation, fear, sleeplessness, confusion, and anger.[16,37,40] Establishing a safe and secure environment using trust-building methods assists the older person in recovery. The trauma-informed interview that formulates compassionate, yet direct and simple, instructions and questions, with adequate response time, also helps the older person in the accounting of the event.[33,37] In the older cognitively and physically disabled person, a documented change in mental status can be used by prosecution to support the sexual assault charge.[37,41,42]

Being sensitive to, and documenting, sudden cognitive changes assists in the evaluation of the incident to determine if an allegation of sexual abuse is indicated. After determining intellectual and emotional capacity of the older person, specifically whether the older person can consent to sexual activity, the sexual assault assessment follows. When providers miss the subtle signs of abuse or assault, older persons do not receive treatment interventions. Sequelae or other symptoms, such as fear, flashbacks, anxiety, and hypervigilance,[37] persist, and perceptions of danger with activities of daily living, such as bathing with help, become unbearable. Without treatment and improved feelings of safety, the constant unrelenting allostatic load from the anxiety alone during waking hours may contribute to the older person's death[15,16,19,37,38] or decline. Specialized mental health services are necessary for the sexually abused elder with and without dementia.

Genital Structures

Older persons have physiologic changes that promote injury with coitus, including sexual organ atrophy, diminished hormone levels, diminished erections of poor quality, and reduced desire for coitus. Changes in women specifically include thinning vaginal mucosa, a delay or reduction in lubrication, and vasocongestion, leading to dyspareunia and bleeding during coitus. Orgasmic contractions are painful in some,[40] which may also facilitate injury during a sexual assault. In addition, the vagina narrows and shortens with age, making it more susceptible to injury.[3] Comorbid conditions and medications may also contribute to the loss of vaginal lubrication. If the older woman is on topical estrogens and practices coitus on a regular basis, injury may be less severe or nonexistent. Topical estrogens facilitate restoration of the vaginal epithelium and increase vaginal blood flow but may not improve overall sexual function.

Physical limitations influence the amount of cooperation from the older person, and health professionals may fail to recognize or distinguish obvious intentional injury from normal physical limitations with aging.[43] Furthermore, medical forensic examinations have not determined the significance of injury found on the older person's genitalia after sexual assault.[44] The aging of female genitalia is characterized by thinning tissue, friability, and loss of adipose and connective tissue support, as well as loss of pubic hair.[40,45,46] Female genitalia after menopause continue to lose form in structure and tissue, resulting in vulvar atrophy.[3,40,46,47] Circulating estrogenic hormone levels with hormone replacement therapy or topical estrogen supplementation and regular sexual activity influence the vulvar and vaginal genital appearance and injury in older healthy women.[48]

There is some evidence that estrogen is protective not only in consensual intercourse but also in forced intercourse; estrogen changes the tissue appearance if used throughout the healing process.[49,50] The Hymen Estrogen Response Scale (HERS, Speck) has proven validity (Patricia M. Speck, DNSc, APN, FNP-BC, DF-IAFN, unpublished data) and is undergoing reliability studies. Early analysis of the HERS research data show a high probability that the tool is reliable among sexual assault nurse examiners and non–sexual assault nurse examiners.[51] Specifically, the design of the tool estimates the visible signs of the effect of estrogen on the hymen, vagina, and vulva[51] by assigning a number to the color (red to white), lubrication (amount and quality), distensibility (capacity to stretch), thickness (rugae), and sensitivity (pain response to palpation). Future studies should consider incorporation of the HERS tool in evaluation of injury in women of all ages.[48] In addition to atrophy-related injuries, the older woman is more susceptible to dermatitis of the vulva, perineum, and buttocks caused by increased incidence of urinary incontinence.[52] Exposure to urinary moisture makes the skin more susceptible to friction injury. Tissue regeneration capacity is compromised in the older woman and leads to delayed healing from sustained injuries.

Previous studies addressed anogenital trauma and found older women, compared with reproductive-aged younger women, to have a statistically significant increase in numbers of injury in both nongenital and anogenital locations.[37] The injuries included lacerations, abrasions, bruises, and edema.[19] Erythema was fewer,[19] possibly because of slower physiologic responses in the old-old female victim. The injury sites varied, but generally were the labia minor, fossa navicularis, and posterior fourchette,[50,53] which are not unlike injuries found in younger women. Conversely, 1 study found more vaginal injury in the older woman.[54] Others have posed that without estrogen, atrophic changes in many women are vulnerable to injury with penetration, with or without coital consent.[40,45,46] A review of the literature indicates that not only do injuries occur more frequently in older menopausal women but these injuries are also more severe.

Offenders

There are centuries of research about sexual offenders; however, only recently has motivation emerged as a possible typology, including opportunistic, pervasive anger, sexual, and vindictive motivations.[37,55,56] Sexual perpetrators may include "stranger or acquaintance, unrelated care provider, incest, marital or partner, and commonly, resident-to-resident in elder care settings."[57] Three subtypes under marital and incestuous sexual abuse and assault include long-term domestic abuse, recent onset within a long-term marriage, and sexual victimization within a new marriage.[57] "Incestuous elder abuse involves cases perpetrated by adult children, other relatives and quasi-relatives."[57] The purpose of this article is to present cases that reflect common relationships with older persons; however, with each case, mixed offender typologies exist, as does the motivation to offend. The predation toward sexual offenses is an individual focus (eg, the personal decision toward sexual predation and an unsolicited sexual relationship) and is single minded, unpredictable, and compelled by the assailant's thinking errors.[37,55,58,59]

Case Studies

We have created a series of cases to show perpetrator schemes, traumatic reactions from victims of criminal sexual acts, and interventions to care for the victims. The case series is representative of, but not unique to, actual cases and is divided into 2 groups,[35] which include dwellers in institutional settings (eg, hospitals, skilled nursing homes, supervised group homes, and assisted-living facilities) and domestic settings with community dwellers (eg, living with family members, living alone, unsupervised group homes).

INSTITUTIONAL DWELLERS (HOSPITALS, SKILLED NURSING HOMES, SUPERVISED GROUP HOMES, AND ASSISTED-LIVING FACILITIES)
Case 1: A Hospitalized 84-Year-Old Woman Complaining of Rape

Mary, an 84-year-old white woman, had a 20-year history of coronary artery disease. Her surgical history included 4 coronary bypass surgeries and implantation of pacemaker 2 years previously. She presented to the emergency room (ER) with her son and daughter-in-law with complaints of dyspnea. She was admitted to the intensive care unit (ICU) for management of congestive heart failure. After 5 days in the ICU, she was medically stable; however the nurses reported that Mary was experiencing paranoid hallucinations in the last 24 hours. Before transfer to the step-down unit, Mary complained of rape to a female nurse at 04:00 AM. Hospital security was notified, resulting in notification of the jurisdictional law enforcement entity and dispatch of the Advanced Practice Forensic Nurse (APFN) SAFE. Mary's son and power of attorney (POA) provided consent for an examination. Mary was visibly distressed and screaming that no one believed her. The APFN SAFE positioned herself in a chair below the head of Mary's bed and began a conversation to evaluate Mary's cognitive abilities. Mary was not oriented to day or time, but did know she was in a hospital. She knew that her son was present and that he supported the evaluation. When asked what happened, Mary excitedly stated, "They tied me down and I pulled the ropes off!" A male RN assigned to Mary later confirmed that Mary was screaming incoherently and pulled out her intravenous (IV) and urinary catheter. He also reported observing blood on Mary's bedding and gown but she would not let him assess for the source of the bleeding. He immediately requested help from a female nurse to assess Mary. With both nurses in the room, Mary yelled, "That's the man that raped me!" and pointed her finger at the male nurse. The female nurse then called for security and asked the male nurse to leave the room. When asked if she would agree to have the APFN SAFE examine her, Mary agreed. The examination revealed atrophic vulva with urethral injury (**Fig. 1**).

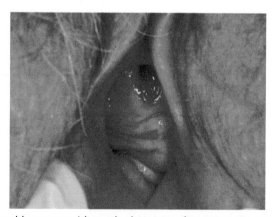

Fig. 1. An 84-year-old woman with urethral trauma after traumatic removal during reactions to paranoid hallucinations. (*Courtesy of* Eisenhower Medical Center; with permission.)

There was no visible injury to the prepuce, clitoris, labia major, labia minor, hymen remnants, vagina, or anus. Samples collected were transferred to law enforcement for forensic laboratory analysis. The analysis was negative for male DNA.

Analysis of evidence

This is a complex case, requiring the skills of an interprofessional team. Information from several sources was used to understand the events. In hospitals with resources, the Forensic Program and Risk Management (FP/RM) teams use root cause analysis to review the incidence reports. In this case, a disoriented ICU patient created genital and arm trauma when she pulled out the IV and urinary catheter. Employees followed all policies and procedures related to safety and reporting, and the FP/RM team awaited the legal outcome of the investigation. Circumstantial findings, including urethral injury and IV insertion site injury, received heavier weight in decision making by the legal community. Forensic analysis of samples did not reveal DNA from the vulva or the vagina. Therefore, charges against the male nurse did not materialize.

Discussion

It is common to find older persons who report sexual victimization in their younger years. There is an association of child sexual abuse with abuse in later years, placing the older person at higher risk.[60] When institutional systems have dedicated forensic and risk management professionals, with strict protocols for evaluation of incidences that may involve criminal acts, the process protects both patients and personnel. In this case, the conclusion of both legal representatives and the APFN SAFE is that the disoriented patient pulled the catheter out, resulting in urethral tear and bruising witnessed by the APFN SAFE. This injury may have precipitated an earlier memory of sexual assault. The forensic nurse in sexual assault care documented the injury, collected samples from the site, and determined that the location of the injury was nonspecific and that the history was consistent with forced removal of a urinary catheter.

In this case, the patient's son explained that his mother had a history of child sexual abuse and subsequent domestic violence, including sexual assault. The patient was cooperative and allowed for evaluation and sample collection. The analysis for prostate specific enzyme as well as DNA was negative. Law enforcement investigation was noncontributory, and charges were not filed in this case.

Treatment

A urogynecologist was consulted and recommended topical estrogen cream for 5 days.

Case outcome

Mary's transfer from the ICU to a step-down unit for cardiac care resulted in full recovery within 48 hours from the psychotic episode, without additional medical intervention.

Case 2: An Unconscious 65-Year-Old Woman in a Skilled Nursing Home

Francis, a 65-year-old woman, had been a resident of a skilled nursing home for the past 10 years. In a vegetative state since arrival at the nursing home, Frances received scheduled tube feedings and medications. At 6:00 AM, the staff nurse walked into her room to find a male maintenance worker in bed with Frances spooning her from behind. The staff nurse described how the male coworker calmly got out of the bed, zipped up his pants while turning his back to her, and left the room without speaking. The staff nurse immediately called the charge nurse, security, and an ambulance to transport Frances to the hospital. On her way to the nursing home, the charge nurse called Frances' sister, who was guardian and POA. Frances' sister called the local police before she drove to the nursing home. The sister, who believed that Frances was unaware of the events, declined to have Frances transported to a hospital; however, she wanted Frances protected medically from potential infections. Therefore, the APFN SAFE was called in to provide a medical forensic evaluation. The APFN SAFE arrived with an advocate, who spoke to Frances' sister to explain services. Once consent for the sister was received, the APFN SAFE began the medical forensic evaluation and sample collections. Frances' sister remained in the room and requested that the advocate also stay. The APFN SAFE systematically inspected Frances' body from head to toe and positioned Frances in a left-lateral recumbent position to view the anogenital areas (her contractures prevented supine frog-leg positioning). Vulvar adhesions of the labia major obstructed the view of the vulvovestibular structures and areas, including the labia minor, urethra, introitus, fossa navicularis, hymen, and distal vagina. Weeping serosanguineous fluid was observed from an approximately 1 to 2 cm area of the posterior fourchette margins of the labial adhesion, extending approximately 1 cm further onto the perineum, as shown in **Fig. 2.**

Examination of the anus showed a traumatic hemorrhoid, slight weeping of serosanguineous fluid, active bleeding from several fissures, and feces stains. Samples were collected from posterior mons, the anterior and posterior adhesions, perineum, and perianal folds; all actively weeping or bleeding areas were avoided. An anoscope examination showed a laceration at 3 o'clock, which extended through the dentate line into the rectum (this is at 12 o'clock in the supine position). A visible hair and rectal fluids distal to the anoscope were collected. Collecting distal to the anoscope orifice reduced the chance of contamination of samples. All samples collected for the forensic laboratory were transferred to a law enforcement officer, who then transferred them to the forensic laboratory for analysis. The APFN SAFE documented in the patient's chart a recommendation to provide medical prophylaxis for sexually transmitted infections (STIs), including human immunodeficiency virus (HIV), along with her contact information in case the medical director had any questions or concerns.

Analysis of evidence

Frances was unable to consent to any sexual activity, and she had an established legal guardian and POA (her sister), who gave permission for the medical forensic evaluation. There was an eyewitness to elements of the event. The forensic laboratory evaluation discovered male DNA from the anal fold samples collected by the APFN SAFE.

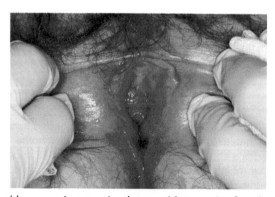

Fig. 2. A 65-year-old woman in a nursing home with posterior fourchette and perineum laceration from rape by resident. (*Courtesy of* Eisenhower Medical Center; with permission.)

This finding, in addition to hair from the rectum, and the documented injuries provided evidence that anal penetration had occurred.

Discussion

Sexual predators often choose environments to work or visit where they have access to victims who are vulnerable or unsupervised. As release of sexual offenders from prisons increases (because of increasing medical needs of older incarcerated men), some are moving into nursing homes.[61] Frances was dependent on the care of others, as shown by the collaboration between her sister (guardian and POA) and the nursing home. However, unbeknown to her sister, Frances could react to a trauma, such as anal pain. Even when noncommunicative and with the appearance of a persistent vegetative state, recovered patients speak about consciousness and awareness of surroundings and activities. In this case, nursing homes that choose to provide 24/7/365 care have a responsibility to protect those unable to speak for themselves. However, during austere times in governmental, not-for-profit, or commercial enterprises, personnel are often the first expense released, and nursing homes are notorious for staffing turnover. In this case, the state investigatory agencies were satisfied with the personnel/patient ratios as well as the policies and procedures for handling sexual assault cases. However, because the sister called police, there were strong recommendations for retraining personnel about mandatory reporting when there is suspicion of sexual assault or abuse.

In this case, DNA evidence is incriminatory for a non–health care provider, because there is no legal reason for the worker to access genitalia of a resident's body. Because there was no reason for the maintenance worker to be in Frances' room, much less a reason to be in her bed, the only hope for the charged worker was that samples collected were void of DNA evidence. However, there was male DNA detected from the anal fold sample in this case. Samples were then compared with the worker's DNA sample, subsequently identifying a match. There was also an eyewitness to circumstantial elements of the assault, placing the worker with Frances at the time reported. Although the eyewitness could not see the assault, placing the worker in Frances' bed and describing actions taken on discovery creates strong correlation between the injury and DNA deposits. In this case, there was a witness to the event. If there had been no eyewitness, cause and mechanism of injury would be difficult to determine without a clear history. Without a witness, the untrained health care provider might label the detected injury as vigorous wiping during perineal care, and no evaluation of the rectum would occur. Vigorous wiping may also be a sign of assault, and many offenders have described sexual pleasure through vigorous rubbing, injuring tissue and creating pain in vulnerable older persons.[37] Recognition of clinical presentations by health care providers[24] after a penetrating injury (as in sexual assault) should lead to an appropriate diagnostic evaluation. State laws require the reporting of elder abuse suspicions, including sexual crimes. Reports to law enforcement agencies should lead to investigation, including sample collection and analysis by the forensic laboratory in the hopes of recovering DNA and identifying the offender.

Treatment

Frances' sister discussed benefits and risks of prophylactic medications, including HIV, for Frances with the APFN SAFE and Medical Director. The sister accepted the prophylactic antibiotics and declined HIV postexposure prophylaxis (PEP).

Case outcome

Frances died in her sleep 2 weeks after the sexual assault. In fragile patients, such as Frances, the allostatic load from trauma may have contributed to her rapid decline and death.[15,16,37,38] The crime of sexual assault without a witness (Frances was deceased and unable to confront the accused [a Constitutional guarantee under the 6th Amendment, also called the Confrontation Clause]) resulted in no prosecution. Even the staff nurse witness did not see the actual injury of penetration, and the opinion of the medical evaluator was conjecture. Furthermore, there are no laboratory findings linking her death to lethal allostatic loads, and the sheriff and prosecutor declined to consider Frances' cause of death as anything but natural. The suspect did not return to work.

Case 3: A 68-Year-Old Man Living in a Supervised Group Home

Edward was a 68-year-old man living in a state-registered, supervised group home for intellectually challenged older adult men. He worked daily in a local not-for-profit organization stuffing envelopes. His parents had died several years previously, as had his brother, who was his primary caretaker. He had made several new friends after moving into the group home. Recently, the supervisor for his home had received a new location assignment and moved out. Edward did not like the new supervisor, Jerry. At work, Edward told his boss that Jerry smoked "funny stuff" and said, "Jerry makes me do things that are bad." Edward's boss called Adult Protective Services (APS) to investigate. An APS worker came to Edward's work to talk to him. Edward told the APS worker, "I can't tell because Jerry will hurt me." Recognizing that Edward was afraid of Jerry, the APS worker used Trauma-Informed Care (TIC) principles to assess the event and help Edward receive the support necessary.[33] TIC acknowledges the universality of trauma, particularly to those vulnerable through dependency or diagnosis. By spending time with Edward, the APS worker was able to help Edward feel safe enough to tell what happened. Edward stated, "Jerry makes me smoke and drink and then he takes off my clothes and puts his mouth on my dingy <beginning to cry>... then last night he put his dingy in my number 2 hole <sobbing>." The APS worker used TIC principles to inform Edward that he was brave to tell[33] and that Jerry would not return to his home.

In the meanwhile, APS called law enforcement, and law enforcement dispatched the advocate and the APFN SAFE to the clinic, where they all met. After consenting to the medical forensic evaluation, Edward requested his friend from the home stay with him during the examination. Interviews of all men in the group home are APS policy after a sex crime report, and APS agreed to bring the men to the clinic for interviews and an examination if needed based on the interview. The men, including Edward's friends, were transported to the clinic, each with a different law enforcement officer and advocate. APS workers conducted their interviews and requested medical forensic evaluations of 2 other group home residents. During this time, Edward became comfortable with his advocate and APFN SAFE and agreed to complete medical forensic evaluation without his friend in the room. Unbeknown to Edward, the examination could not include other potential victims, because of the possibility for contamination of histories through suggestibility. Therefore, it was imperative that all group home residents be interviewed as quickly as possible to avoid suggestibility and contamination of the men's personal experiences when they returned home. Edward's examination did not show any visible physical injury. Edward declined evaluation using an anoscope. Absence of injury does not mean that an assault did not occur. Considering Edward's disclosure coupled with Jerry's presence at the group home, samples were collected for forensic evaluation. This evaluation included samples that could later be evaluated for lubricant, saliva, and seminal or touch DNA from the penis corona, frenulum, and the anal folds. Law enforcement facilitated the transportation of the samples to the forensic laboratory, where saliva was detected on samples from all 3 of the residents examined at the clinic. After all of the patients left the clinic, a law enforcement officer informed the APFN SAFE that that Jerry was on the sex offender registry in another state, where he had sexually assaulted several men living in group homes. On release from jail earlier that month, he had settled in Edward's community but had not reported to his parole officer.

Analysis of evidence

Evidence of a crime in supervised homes against vulnerable persons may or may not include DNA. In this case, Edward's history and laboratory detection of saliva from the samples provided by the APFN SAFE provided the evidence necessary for a parole violation judgment with immediate incarceration. Jerry would also face a new trial for sexual assault against Jerry and 2 other group home residents.

Discussion

Offenders often seek preferred sexual partners through their work or location. The need for supervision in adult group homes was pressing and in this case, the owners did not wait for the criminal background clearance, becoming complicit in the crime against Edward. Had they waited, the identification of Jerry as a sex offender would have denied Jerry employment, and Edward and his friends would not have become victims. Patient-centered care is critical for healthy integration and recovery from the sexual assault experience, regardless of dependency or vulnerability. Using trauma-focused care frameworks[31] for working with vulnerable populations with few resources creates a supportive atmosphere.

Treatment

Edward was offered, and his guardian ad litem accepted, prophylactic antibiotics, including PEP. Psychological trauma-focused care continued in the group home for 12 weeks for all residents of the group home and individually for 2 of the men, who had histories of assault in the past.

Case outcome

Edward did not develop any disease, nor did he have destructive or disruptive behavioral changes with the other residents. The residents saw Edward as a hero, who protected them from "bad" things that Jerry did while he lived with them.

Case 4: A 70-Year-Old Woman Residing in an Assisted-Living Facility

Carol had recently moved to an assisted-living facility, for assistance in preparing meals as well as light housekeeping, where several of her widowed girlfriends resided. Carol performed all personal care activities of daily living, washed and ironed her own clothes, and enjoyed the activities in the facility. The building had been experiencing electrical problems, and a crew worked over a 2-week period to restore electricity to all parts of the building. Carol was carrying her laundry up to her apartment when one of the electrical workers asked if he could use her restroom. She said yes, opened her door and walked in front of the worker into her apartment. Once in her apartment, he grabbed her arm and hair from behind and quickly shoved her into the bedroom, demanding her jewelry and money. When she tried turning around to tell him she had neither, he hit her in the face and told her to shut up. She covered her face with her hands as he grabbed her hair and 1 shoulder, threw her on the bed, and ripped off some of her clothes. He turned her over so that she was face down and penetrated her anally. He then proceeded to penetrate her orally, anally again, and then, vaginally. During the vaginal penetration, Carol lost consciousness, and therefore, she could not provide any additional history. Her girlfriend found her barely responsive on her bedroom floor alone. The police were called, and an ambulance transported Carol to the hospital. At the hospital, an APFN SAFE responded with the patient advocate.

Once she was stabilized, emergency department (ED) nurses educated in the forensic nursing basics of preserving evidence delivered all 4 × 4 pads and perineal pads used during the stabilization procedures, specifically during catheterization preparation. In addition, the ED nurses folded Carol's sheets from the ambulance and placed them in a paper bag, sealed it, and placed the bag in a secure closet. After the medical tests were completed, the APFN SAFE used a trauma-focused approach to speak with Carol about her options. Carol wanted the man who raped her to be arrested, but she could not remember what he looked like and could not remember going to the hospital. She was reassured that some of her memory might return in bits and pieces, and when it did, she could keep a diary of the memories. In the meanwhile, law enforcement would be investigating the crime from evidence from her apartment. Carol said, "I am confident that all that can be done is being done," and thanked the APFN SAFE.

To make Carol as comfortable as possible during the examination process, the APFN SAFE first removed paper bags that had been placed on Carol's hands by the ED nurse to avoid losing evidence transferred from the assailant. Samples from her hands and under her fingernails were collected and photographs were taken. The bags from the hands were secured with the samples for analysis by the forensic laboratory. The APFN SAFE then began a head-to-toe medical forensic examination, which included photographic documentation of all findings. This documentation included sample collection and photographic documentation of:

- One laceration repair spanning 15 stitches over the left sagittal and temporal areas, with visible traumatic alopecia
- A large hematoma contusion over the left brow and periorbital area, without displacement of the ocular globe or cranial nerve deficit
- Large hematoma on left maxillary and mandibular area (**Fig. 3**), without dislocation of teeth
- In the oral cavity, a torn upper frenulum, petechia on the soft palate, and dried brown yellow matter on her lips and around her mouth with blue bruising and a hematoma on the mucous membrane of her left upper lip and cheeks bilaterally (see **Fig. 3**)

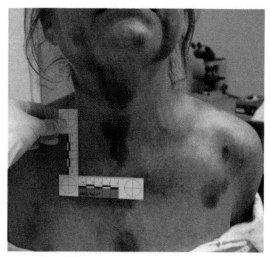

Fig. 3. A 70-year-old community-dwelling independent woman in hospital after physical and sexual assault. (*Courtesy of* Eisenhower Medical Center; with permission.)

After thorough evaluation of the oral cavity, sample collection, and photographic documentation, gentle oral hygiene was provided. Physical and emotional trauma can disorient the older person in unfamiliar locations, like the hospital. To continue to reorient the older patient, the APFN SAFE sought continuous confirmation that Carol wanted to participate in the process of the medical forensic evaluation. Carol was resolute to continue. Carol's neck had evidence of strangulation injuries, and the APFN SAFE continued with the evaluation documenting and collecting samples from:

- Linear reddish-brown bruises on the right side of the neck to trachea, extending to central supraclavicular notch (see **Fig. 3**)
- Blue and red bruising on the right shoulder, arms, and centrally between clavicles, and red contusions over the left and right chest and around the central breast (**Fig. 4**)
- Red and blue abrasions and contusions across the upper and lower back extending to the central coccyx area and both sides of the buttocks (**Fig. 5**)
- The inner left and inner right thigh had 5 purplish-red round contusions (~2 cm each)
- The anogenital examination showed (1) a large hematoma of the right labia major (**Fig. 6**), a catheter in the urethra, and red bruising and dried brownish matter on distal vaginal area; a posterior fourchette laceration at 6 o'clock, actively bleeding; hymeneal swelling and perihymeneal bruising 3, 6, and 9 o'clock
- Before labial traction, serosanguineous fluid was noted with necrotic white tissue at 11 o'clock with fresh blood (**Fig. 7**). With full labial traction, active bleeding from the anus was observed at 11 o'clock, adjacent to a traumatic hemorrhoid or hematoma at 12 to 3 o'clock in the supine position.

Samples were collected from all anogenital structures and adjacent to any wounds (not from the wound), packaged, and secured accordingly. The APFN SAFE also collected, packaged, and secured the sheet that was under Carol during the medical forensic evaluation.

Analysis of evidence
Carol's injuries were significant and might be life threatening. Of note is a lack of obvious pattern injuries under the contusions and hematomas; this is because ecchymotic spread masks pattern injuries. With time, the blunt trauma clears and

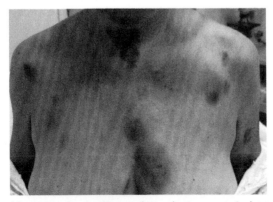

Fig. 4. A 70-year-old community-dwelling independent woman in hospital after physical and sexual assault. (*Courtesy of* Eisenhower Medical Center; with permission.)

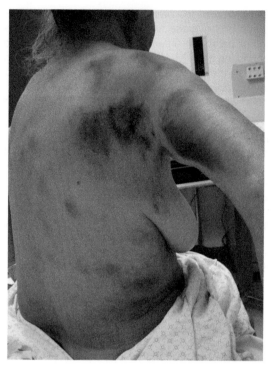

Fig. 5. A 70-year-old community-dwelling independent woman in hospital after physical and sexual assault. (*Courtesy of* Eisenhower Medical Center; with permission.)

the pattern emerges, necessitating serial photographs throughout the healing of the injuries by the APFN SAFE. The amount of evidence from a physical and sexual assault case such as this is significant and requires skillful triage by the forensic laboratory. Life-saving medical interventions have been known to mask or destroy trace evidence left during an assault. The samples taken from various locations did not show DNA. Although Carol could not remember what the man looked like, the project supervisor reported to police that there was only 1 technician assigned to work in the location of Carol's apartment. This man had subsequently been brought in for questioning. The law enforcement officer had samples collected from the man's hands

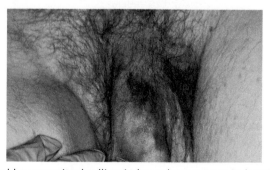

Fig. 6. A 70-year-old community-dwelling independent woman in hospital after physical and sexual assault. (*Courtesy of* Eisenhower Medical Center; with permission.)

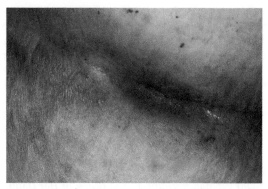

Fig. 7. A 70-year-old community-dwelling independent woman in hospital after physical and sexual assault. (*Courtesy of* Eisenhower Medical Center; with permission.)

and genitalia as well as collection of the clothes he was wearing, especially undergarments. Just as an assailant's DNA may be found on a victim, the victim's DNA may also be found on the assailant. Sample collection from the suspect resulted in Carol's DNA being found on his genitalia (under his foreskin and on the scrotum) and in his underwear.

Discussion
Violent and disorganized assailants tell us that victims like Carol are nothing and they have difficulty seeing Carol as another human being.[37] There are different offender typologies and, based on the disorganized scene, this assailant had evidence of evasive anger and vindictive motivations.[37,55,56] Carol did not have complete memory of the experienced event, because of a lacerated head trauma and possible concussion.[62] The strangulation injuries could also account for her lack of memory, especially if there was a significant hypoxic event.[62,63] Even without serious physical injury, reconstruction of experienced memory after trauma occurs over time. In older persons who have physiologic changes that challenge memory, the event may never fully return.[62] Depending on the TIC received over the following few weeks, Carol had the capacity to recall all of the experience. Coordinated community responses to sexual abuse and sexual assault can improve the well-being and safety within communities in which rapists target the older person because they are vulnerable.[37,55,56]

Treatment
Carol was admitted to the hospital overnight for observation because of clinical findings consistent with concussion, and hypoxic from a strangulation act. Neurologic checks with neck measurements occurred every 2 hours and assessment of Carol's breathing patterns were monitored. The hospitalist ordered ice packs for all injury areas. Prophylactic recommendations included antibiotics, immunizations for hepatitis B and tetanus (TDAP [tetanus, diphtheria, and pertussis]) and PEP for HIV.

Case outcome
The assailant's defense was "Of course her DNA is on me, I worked in her apartment so everywhere I touch, her DNA will be there!" Carol testified in a grand jury hearing, important because in the event of death, her testimony could be used to satisfy the Sixth Amendment Confrontation Clause, in lieu of her presence during a trial of the accused. Although she was injured and recovering, Carol's pretrial recorded testimony was valuable and recorded on film. The prosecutor understood the increased

risk for death for older persons[37] after sexual violence, because, like injured children, they are subject to persistent and increased allostatic loads after criminal assault and sexual assault.[15,16,37,38] In this case, Carol died before trial. During trial, Carol's pretrial testimony was entered as evidence, and the APFN SAFE was instrumental in helping explain the extent of the injuries inflicted and why Carol was unable to remember all elements of her experiences after the traumatic event. The APFN SAFE's comprehensive medical forensic evaluation and documentation of the patient's injuries and words, as well as treatment recommendations, were exempt from hearsay under the medical diagnosis and treatment exemption. The accused received a sentence of 25 years to life by jury trial.

DOMESTIC COMMUNITY DWELLERS
Case 5: An 88-Year-Old Woman Residing in the Home of Her Daughter

Hattie, an 88-year-old woman, was no longer able to financially support herself and moved in with her daughter approximately 18 months previously. Her daughter Alice and son-in-law Joe agreed to have Hattie stay with them and they built a mother-in-law suite. Alice's siblings were concerned that Alice and Joe's motivation was financial and not for Hattie's well-being.

Nine months later, Alice and Joe reported that Hattie had fallen and had a broken hip. After hospital treatment, Hattie returned to Alice's house, unable to walk unassisted. She was regularly visited by friends and home health care providers, and talked on the telephone with members of her church. She also found joy watching basketball on TV, and never missed a game of her favorite team. Alice developed breast cancer and while undergoing chemotherapy was not able care for her mother. Therefore, Joe began taking care of Hattie. Alice died 4 months later. Within 2 months of Alice's death, Joe began to sexually abuse Hattie. One night, Hattie called the police and reported that Joe had just "raped me again." A police officer responded, and she was transported to the ER. A law enforcement officer, APS worker, and APFN SAFE met the hospital social worker in the waiting room. Hattie met the Sexual Assault Response Team members and apologized for getting everyone out late at night, but that she was "sick and tired of him messing with me!" Hattie told her story of Joe "having sex with me whenever he wanted," and stated, "I'm trapped in his house, unable to get up, and, quite frankly, I'm ashamed."

Criteria for Incest in Elder Sexual Abuse
Incestuous elder abuse involves cases perpetrated by adult children, other relatives, and quasi-relatives

Analysis of evidence

The medical forensic evaluation by the APRN SAFE focused on the areas identified by Hattie. Hattie's memory was intact, and she consented for the medical forensic evaluation. An alternative light source was used in the external evaluation of Hattie's body for dried fluids and injury detection without out any positive findings. Samples were collected from the lips, perioral area, neck, and breasts for forensic analysis. When positioning Hattie for the genital examination, she said, "I look ugly down there because of what he did." The APFN SAFE acknowledged her concern and, using TIC, delayed the examination to explore the statement.[33] Hattie had said that since he started "doing this to me," she now has to wear a diaper. Hattie then said she was ready to continue and verbalized comfort in the supine position with her feet in the stirrups. Padding was placed underneath her previously injured hip to provide support and promote comfort. A glistening discharge was present, as was a strong urine odor; there was visible urethrocele and linear and diffuse less than 1 mm punctate petechia on vestibular and vaginal tissues (**Fig. 8**). No lacerations to the vulvar or introitus was observed. Speculum evaluation showed fluid in the posterior fornix. Samples were collected from the cervical os and posterior fornix with a wet mount prepared for visualization under a microscope. The wet mount showed motile sperm, which was photographed for the medical record.

Discussion

Although considered old-old, Hattie had normal mental capacities and chose to stay with her son-in-law after her daughter's death. Her physical capacities diminished with regard to ambulation, and she spent most of her time in bed, dependent on her son-in-law for care and on the phone for socialization. His criminal actions met the criteria established by early researchers for incest.[57] Planning safe care for dependent elders who live with relatives requires comprehensive assessment and collaborative decision making by those legislated to protect the older person; safe care could entail removing the abuser or transferring the patient to a facility. As for the emotional abuse that likely was part of the preincest behavior to diminish her as a person, it is likely he planted thoughts about her looks as a very old woman and said her genitals were "ugly." He may have even injured her initially, creating pain and possibly other injury. Incestuous sexual abuse in the older adult is a common cause of sexual abuse,[37,64] and little is understood about the emotional reaction of older adults with normal cognition.[15]

Hattie's body dysmorphic thinking was concerning, particularly if she became obsessed with adopting his view about her "ugly" genitals. Body dysmorphic disorder (BDD) is a thinking compulsion with an unknown cause; however, biological and environmental factors influence the development of symptoms, and suicide ideation and attempts are a significant outcome.[65–67] Persistent thoughts about the perceived flaw reflects neurobiological and life course experience. Although common with victims of child maltreatment,[66] including sexual assault, dysmorphic disorders are absent in current literature addressing elders or their life course experience.

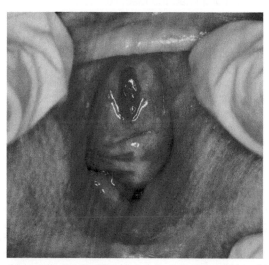

Fig. 8. An 88-year-old community-dwelling dependent woman, victim of incest. (*Courtesy of* Eisenhower Medical Center; with permission.)

Because the son-in-law was the care provider, his DNA might be present regardless of sexual assault. The presence of sperm would be more difficult to explain from the posterior fornix or cervix. When found, a DNA match would compound evidence of his crimes.

Treatment
Hattie declined prophylactic treatments.

Case outcome
The APS caseworker encouraged Hattie to leave her son-in-law's home. She was temporarily admitted to a nursing home owned by her church, where she died 6 months after she reported the sexual abuse.

Case 6: A 65-Year-Old Woman with Spastic Cerebral Palsy Living with Her Sister in the Community on Weekends

Mary lives in a skilled nursing facility during the week and spends the weekends with her sister Joy at Joy's apartment. Mary required intermittent but continuous attention for her physical and intellectual ability deficits. She took medications for a seizure disorder and suffered from malnutrition from long-term tube feedings. Mary was small for her age and had contractures that prohibited wheelchair transport, so she was transported in a cushioned tray. She had vulvar and vaginal atrophy and a chronic perineal diaper rash from postmenopausal urinary incontinence. Mary communicated with facial gestures, vocal sounds. and pointing with her right hand. She attended a day care program for adults with disabilities. Mary's sister had a new boyfriend, who also visited during the weekend. Joy was preparing Mary's feeding, and she heard Mary making unusual noises. When she entered the room, the boyfriend was sitting down in a chair near Mary and when he was questioned, said that Mary just started making noises. Joy asked her sister what happened, and Mary pointed to her mouth and grunted. Mary was also crying. The sister smelled Mary's mouth and turned to the boyfriend and screamed at him to "Get out!" He left and Joy called the police. The APFN SAFE joined the police at Joy's apartment and completed the medical forensic examination on site. When Mary was asked what happened, she again pointed to her mouth, grunted, and began to cry.

Analysis of evidence
Mary had movements consistent with spastic cerebral palsy, contractures of all limbs, and was in a t-shirt and diapers, with a blanket covering her body. Her communication was limited, yet effective. Samples were collected from the cheeks, perioral cavity, lips, and pharyngeal crypts. Additional samples were collected from the neck and both breasts. The medical forensic evaluation also included inspection of the genitalia and anogenital samples. The diaper was collected along with the t-shirt and sheet. The forensic laboratory found DNA on the oral swabs and amylase on her nipple and both breast samples. There was no detection of injury.

Discussion
Mary's demeanor immediately after the event, as described by Joy and recorded by the APFN SAFE, and Mary's level of cooperation with the medical forensic evaluation would be considered and could corroborate an active lack of consent to sexual activity. In addition, her care providers would be witnesses to her interactive capacities during daily living activities to support her choices as well as behavioral outcomes since the intentional sexual trauma.

Consent for sexual activity is an important issue for adults with disabilities. Mary's is a complex case, in that the state has guardianship for Mary as a dependent adult. Had Mary wanted a relationship, it is likely that the state, as guardian, would evaluate her capacity to engage in a relationship willingly through assent. She certainly gave permission through her gestures and cooperation for the medical forensic evaluation.

Treatment

Mary accepted HIV PEP. She was up to date with all immunizations. Without physical injury, the cognitive-behavioral therapists focused on behavioral manifestations of the acute and long-term effects of the sexual assault.[68]

Case outcome

Joy, although initially supportive of her sister, Mary, turned her support to her boyfriend, who stood trial for the sexual assault of Mary. Mary was unable to testify on her own behalf, and Joy was actively undermining the prosecution of her boyfriend. An APS case opened after a complaint from the prosecutor, who found that Joy was living with the boyfriend. Joy was found to be a passive perpetrator, and the label of passive perpetrator ensured that Mary could no longer visit Joy on the weekend. The presence of semen and DNA in Mary's mouth resulted in a conviction of the boyfriend, and he received a 20 years to life sentence. A conviction for obstruction of justice by Joy resulted in a suspended sentence and probation for 10 years.

Case 7: A 78-Year-Old Woman Residing Alone

Betty, a 78-year-old widow, with mild vascular dementia to multiple strokes, lived in a community-subsidized apartment. Her 4 children and their families lived in town near Betty. Betty developed a relationship with a 45-year-old male neighbor, who had an intellectual disability, and she paid him every week to have sex with her. The children began compensating their mother's living expenses when she did not have enough money to purchase groceries and cigarettes throughout the month. On questioning, they learned about the "sex for money scheme" (1 child's words) with the neighbor. Betty denied any exploitation, and called the neighbor her "boyfriend" and said they like to play cards and smoke. Betty agreed to the comprehensive evaluation by the APFN SAFE. Betty declined a support person or a child's support during the interview, against the wishes of her son and POA, because as she said, "I have some things to say that my children might not like." Betty agreed to seek the input of her son after the interview. Betty started the interview by saying, "I can have sex with who I want, and I can pay them if I want... My children don't like my boyfriend because he is not my race, and he's a little slow...but he is nice to me – very nice!" With that, the APFN SAFE proceeded to complete an evaluation of Betty's cognition using the AD8 Dementia Screening Interview (http://www.alz.org/documents_custom/ad8.pdf) to determine if Betty was competent to consent to sexual activity. Results were consistent with her diagnosis of early dementia using the Mini-Cog (http://www.alz.org/documents_custom/minicog.pdf) and Memory Impairment Screen (http://www.alz.org/documents_custom/mis.pdf), which are measures of cognition and recall. Betty agreed to complete a medical forensic evaluation, and the APFN SAFE found atrophic vulvar and vaginal tissue, a pouting urethra, moisture from incontinence, with minor injury in the posterior fourchette, fossa navicularis, and petechia in the visible vaginal tissue (**Fig. 9**). Removal of the speculum showed a prolapsed cervix (**Fig. 10**) and Betty responded, "Don't worry, I have to push it up in there all the time." Betty declined sample collection because "My boyfriend is not going to jail just because I want to have sex."

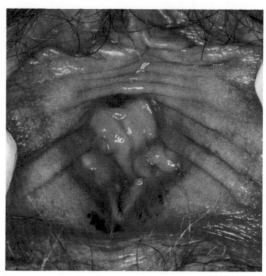

Fig. 9. A 78-year-old community-dwelling woman after consensual coitus with minor vulvar injury. (*Courtesy of* Eisenhower Medical Center; with permission.)

Analysis of evidence

This case is complex, because exploitation, both financially and sexually, is rooted in comprehension and autonomy of the patient. Therefore, an analysis of capacity and competence showed that Betty could and did exercise autonomy in the area of sexuality. The findings in the vestibular and vaginal areas relate to genital atrophy in older menopausal women, and there is a propensity toward injury from sexual activity, albeit consensual. The financial payment, although foolhardy and irritating to the children, was not exploitation.

Eisenstadt v Baird, 405 US 438 (1972) is a US Supreme Court case establishing the right of unmarried people to possess contraception on the same basis as married couples and by implication and confirming subsequent Supreme Court decisions, the right of unmarried couples to engage in potentially nonprocreative sexual coitus.

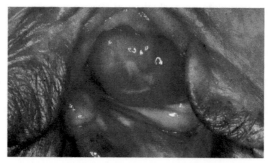

Fig. 10. A 78-year-old community-dwelling woman with prolapsed cervix after consensual coitus. (*Courtesy of* Eisenhower Medical Center; with permission.)

Discussion

The evidence for exploitation is rooted in capacity of consent and assent, and in adjudicated competency.[30] Capacity is the "ability to understand the nature and effects of one's acts,"[69,70] in which consent and assent to coital relationships is rooted in understanding the benefits and risks. On the other hand, competency is defined as "characteristics which render a witness legally fit and qualified to give testimony in court."[69] In this case, Betty was deemed competent. Betty volunteered information about her relationship with the boyfriend, which showed an appreciation of the situation. Of concern was the intellectual disability of Betty's boyfriend, which required an assessment of his competency and capacity for autonomy. It was determined that both parties were capable of making decisions for themselves. The privacy guarantee in nonprocreative intercourse for those with early dementia and diminished cognitive abilities is viewed legally through a series of Supreme Court decisions beginning with Eisenstadt v Baird (1972). In this case, both Betty and her boyfriend were happy with their relationship. Betty and the boyfriend agreed that Betty would stop paying him after they have sex, but she expressed sadness and fear that he would stop coming to her apartment.

Treatment

A consultation with the family health care provider resulted in a recommendation of topical estrogen cream periodically to avoid the minor injuries to the atrophic tissues during coital activity.

Case outcome

At the time of the investigation, Betty was in the early stages of multi-infarct dementia, and within the year, had deteriorated after a series of larger strokes, resulting in admission to a nursing home. The boyfriend continued to remain with her during the day until she died of a stroke.

Case 8: Mary Is a 72-Year-Old Woman Who Lives Alone in a Federally Subsidized Apartment

Mary, a 72-year-old woman who lived alone in a federally subsidized apartment, took the public transportation to the hospital to report a sexual assault that occurred the previous night. Mary told the nurse that her "private area is burning and hurting so bad this morning" that she took her facial cold cream and put it on her private parts. The APFN SAFE was called for an evaluation. The nurse examiner talked with Mary, who stated, "I know they are trying to get me. Over the past several weeks, they have been tazing me through the walls in my apartment. They come in at night and steal my food out of the refrigerator… and they are the ones who raped me last night! I told the manager about all of this, but he does nothing. I came here because I could not take the pain of these rapes anymore!" Mary also reported that she had diabetes, high blood pressure, and a history of schizophrenia. She went to the free clinic when she needed help. She took medications for diabetes only, but said "I haven't had any pills for a while"; she took Tylenol for pain and used ice to help with the burning "down there." She took 4 Tylenol pills that morning.

Analysis of evidence

Mary agreed to an examination and signed the written consent for the medical forensic evaluation. Persons are considered competent until deemed incompetent by a formal evaluation. Mary initially declined sample collection for both medical and forensic analysis, stating, "it hurts too much," but she agreed to allow the examination, collection of samples, and photography of the injured areas, if any. Inspection of the anogenital area occurred with Mary in a lithotomy position. The APFN SAFE observed a copious discharge, consistent with a persistent yeast infection (**Fig. 11**). Labial traction showed minor superficial tears in the posterior fourchette (**Fig. 12**). Mary said, "my private parts (meaning the vulva and vestibule) are red and on fire!" The APFN SAFE deferred the speculum insertion. Her underwear was also collected, secured in a paper bag, and transferred to law enforcement.

Description of findings
Mary had a thick white coating of exudate from the mons pubis to the buttocks. The labia major and perineum were erythematous, with caked white areas covering the vestibule. She had diffuse satellite lesions, classic for fungal infections. She reported pain with inspection and palpation and stated, "It burns." All hospital laboratory tests were negative before Mary was released. There was no objective evidence to support a recent sexual assault history.

Treatment
Mary's treatment included an antifungal cream and referral to a primary care provider to address her chronic medical issues. Mary received the standard protocol for sexually transmitted infection prophylaxis after sexual assault. Mary received instructions to follow up for cultures at the clinic, and an appointment was made for her. Mary's case is complex and required several interventions in the community, so after the hospital personnel met Mary's medical needs, the hospital released Mary to law enforcement. The hospital social worker arranged for transportation to the clinic and then contacted community services to provide meal deliveries immediately. After the APFN SAFE notified APS, an investigation into Mary's capacity to remain in the community opened. Law enforcement and APS took Mary to her apartment to assess the condition of the apartment. Mary had no utilities, so APS called the Salvation Army to implement utility assistance emergency funding. Mary was also a hoarder. APS spoke with the manager about Mary, her capacity to care for herself, and her living conditions. A referral was made to a psychiatrist for a capacity evaluation.

Discussion of case
Mary's is a common presentation for persons with mental illness involving delusional thinking. Her probable history of sexual assault in the past and her history of homelessness would shape the care providers' plan as they helped Mary through TIC. When older women seek help for care of genital complaints, it is imperative that

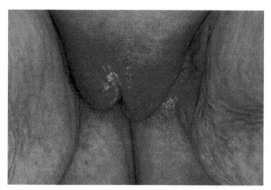

Fig. 11. A 72-year-old community-dwelling woman with vulvar yeast and history of uncontrolled diabetes mellitus. (*Courtesy of* Eisenhower Medical Center; with permission.)

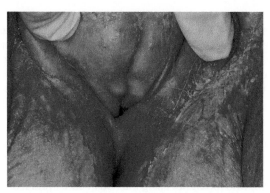

Fig. 12. A 72-year-old community-dwelling woman with vulvar yeast and history of uncontrolled diabetes mellitus. (*Courtesy of* Eisenhower Medical Center; with permission.)

providers do not discount that a sexual assault occurred recently, particularly if there is a complaint. Failure to collect evidence is tantamount to failing to draw blood to detect cardiac enzymes after a myocardial infarction. Although DNA is not proof of evidence in all cases, collecting DNA in a timely matter is an important component of all investigations.

Outcome of the case
Mary entered therapy with a trauma-focused cognitive-behavioral therapy counselor. The DNA test was negative on the vaginal swabs. The case was closed.

Case 9: A 70-Year-Old Vietnam Veteran Residing in an Unsupervised Group Home
John was a recovering alcoholic, with long-standing posttraumatic stress disorder (PTSD). He had been homeless for more than 20 years when a local veterans group provided him with trauma-focused group therapy. He admitted frequently that he felt safer on the streets than with other men in homeless shelters. He said, "They don't understand me anyway." He continued to attend trauma-focused cognitive-behavioral therapy and live on the streets, continuing to use alcohol and drugs. When a bed came available, the counselor invited him to stay in the unsupervised group home. Living on the streets had taken their toll on John, and the previous winter was the worst on record. He had begun to lose weight and, with his small frame, he became vulnerable as a target for robbery and sexual assault. His decision to move into the home was because he wanted safety and warmth. On the first night in the home, a physically larger resident came to his bedroom, held him down, and sexually assaulted him. The next day while in a group, John's angry behavior resulted in a separate conference with the counselor. Still angry and wanting to leave the group for the streets, he told the counselor about the assault. When asked, John agreed to tell police. The counselor asked a community health worker to escort John and provide support. The 2 men went to the hospital for a medical forensic evaluation by an advanced practice nurse specializing in forensic nursing care.

Analysis of evidence
John was fearful but consented to the medical forensic evaluation after speaking with the community health worker who accompanied him to the hospital. The medical forensic examination showed that John was a thin, small-framed man, with a 45-year history of alcohol and drug use. He complained of bleeding from his rectum

when asked if he hurt anywhere. The APFN SAFE decided to look at the anogenital area first to address John's report that he was still bleeding. On examination, the anal area had a swollen bleeding anus with a fissure at 11 to 12 o'clock that terminated at the dentate line in the supine position (**Fig. 13**). Sitting in the ED had served to apply pressure to the area, and John's bleeding had stopped. Samples were collected from the dried blood in the perianal area, anal folds, and anal verge. The forensic laboratory confirmed that a second male's DNA was present in samples from the perianal area.

Discussion

Addiction and comorbid mental health vulnerabilities are complex confounders in preparing a case for prosecution. They are equally complex for the never-served in the health care system, who tend to be homeless, incarcerated, adolescent males, the addicted and others, who report not using the health care system until there is a catastrophic event.[71] With proper support from his friends, and his commitment to continue in trauma-focused behavioral health interventions,[72] John had a good chance for healthy integration of the event and the ability to pursue positive health-seeking behaviors.

Treatment

John accepted medical treatment options offered and including CDC guideline recommendations for PEP for STIs, including HIV.[14] Orders were placed for immunizations including TDAP, pneumococcus, and hepatitis B virus. In the meantime, discharge teaching included an increase of fiber in his diet, continuation of ointment on the anal wound daily, and instructions to return to the clinic to document healing after 2 weeks. At that time, a referral appointment would be made to a primary care provider skilled in addiction treatment and PTSD to help John reach a higher level of wellness.

Case outcome

After evaluation for competency, the accused was confined to a mental health hospital for paranoid schizophrenia until stabilized on medication. He was charged with sexual assault, and pled guilty. As a convicted felon, he was moved to a secure jail facility for protection. John continued to attend group sessions, where he led groups for other

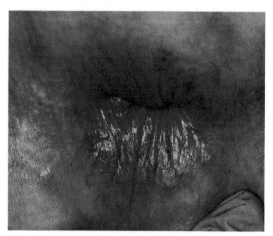

Fig. 13. A 66-year-old community-dwelling male veteran sexually assaulted with anal injury. (*Courtesy of* Eisenhower Medical Center; with permission.)

veterans struggling with PTSD. He continued employment in the agency that supported him after the sexual assault and throughout his struggles on the streets as a homeless veteran.

REFERENCES

1. National Institutes on Aging. Why population aging matters: A global perspective. 2011. Available at: http://www.nia.nih.gov/sites/default/files/WPAM.pdf. Accessed August 24, 2014.
2. Tarzia L, Fetherstonhaugh D, Bauer M. Dementia, sexuality and consent in residential aged care facilities. J Med Ethics 2012;38(10):609–13.
3. Poulos CA, Sheridan DJ. Genital injuries in postmenopausal women after sexual assault. J Elder Abuse Negl 2008;20(4):323–35.
4. Eldred S, West L. HIV prevalence in older adults. Cancer Nurs 2005;101(9): 20–3.
5. Hillman J. Sexuality and aging. New York: Springer; 2012.
6. Lindau ST, Schumm LP, Laumann EO, et al. A study of sexuality and health among older adults in the United States. N Engl J Med 2007;357(8):762–74.
7. DeLamater JD, Sill M. Sexual desire in later life. J Sex Res 2005;42(2):138–49.
8. Inelman EM, Gasparini G, Enzi G. HIV/AIDS in older adults: a case report and literature review. Geriatrics 2005;60(9):26–30.
9. Lichtenberg PA. Sexuality and physical intimacy in long-term care. Occup Ther Health Care 2014;28(1):42–50.
10. Lea SJ, Hunt L, Shaw S. Sexual assault of older women by strangers. J Interpers Violence 2011;26(11):2303–20.
11. Connolly MT, Breckman R, Callahan J, et al. The sexual revolution's last frontier: how silence about sex undermines health, well-being, and safety in old age. Generations 2012;36(3):43–52.
12. Duffin C. Taking the risky out of frisky. Nurs Older People 2008;20(5):6–7.
13. Cook JM, Dinnen S, O'Donnell C. Older women survivors of physical and sexual violence: a systematic review of the quantitative literature. J Womens Health (Larchmt) 2011;20(7):1075–81.
14. Centers for Disease Control. Hepatitis C: expansion of testing recommendations, 2012. 2012. Available at: http://www.cdc.gov/nchhstp/newsroom/docs/HCV-Testing-Recs.pdf. Accessed August 24, 2014.
15. Juster RP, McEwen BS, Lupien SJ. Allostatic load biomarkers of chronic stress and impact on health and cognition. Neurosci Biobehav Rev 2010;35(1):2–16.
16. Repetti RL, Taylor SE, Seeman TE. Risky families: family social environments and the mental and physical health of offspring. Psychol Bull 2002;128(2): 330–66.
17. Acierno R, Lawyer SR, Rheingold A, et al. Current psychopathology in previously assaulted older adults. J Interpers Violence 2007;22(2):250–8.
18. Bright CL, Bowland SE. Assessing interpersonal trauma in older adult women. J Loss Trauma 2008;13(4):373–93.
19. Brown K, Streubert GE, Burgess AW. Effectively detect and manage elder abuse. Nurse Pract 2004;29(8):22–7, 31; [quiz 32–3].
20. Fisher BS, Regan SL. The extent and frequency of abuse in the lives of older women and their relationship with health outcomes. Gerontologist 2006;46(2): 200–9.
21. Oktay JS, Tompkins CJ. Personal assistance providers' mistreatment of disabled adults. Health Soc Work 2004;29(3):177–88.

22. A perfect cause. Predators in America's nursing homes: registered sex offenders residing in nursing homes 2005 report. 2005. Available at: http://www.aperfectcause.org/APerfectCause-PredatorsinAmericasNursingHomes-2005Report.pdf. Accessed August 24, 2014.

23. Ramsey-Klawsnik H, Teaster PB. Sexual abuse happens in healthcare facilities–what can be done to prevent it? Generations 2012;36(3):53–9.

24. Chihowski K, Hughes S. Clinical issues in responding to alleged elder sexual abuse. J Elder Abuse Negl 2008;20(4):377–400.

25. Rosen T, Lachs MS, Pillemer K. Sexual aggression between residents in nursing homes: literature synthesis of an underrecognized problem. J Am Geriatr Soc 2010;58(10):1970–9.

26. Rovi S, Chen PH, Vega M, et al. Mapping the elder mistreatment iceberg: US hospitalizations with elder abuse and neglect diagnoses. J Elder Abuse Negl 2009;21(4):346–59.

27. Ramsey-Klawsnik, Holly. Elder sexual abuse: research findings and clinical issues. Introduction. Journal of Elder Abuse & Neglect (0894-6566) 2008; 20(4):301.

28. Dong X, Simon M, Mendes de Leon C, et al. Elder self-neglect and abuse and mortality risk in a community-dwelling population. JAMA 2009;302(5):517–26.

29. Burgess AW, Clements PT. Information processing of sexual abuse in elders. J Forensic Nurs 2006;2(3):113–20.

30. Speck PM, Chasson S. Informed consent and sexual assault. In: Giardino AP, Starling SP, Rotolo SL, et al, editors. Sexual assault across the life span: a comprehensive clinical reference. 2nd edition. St Louis (MO): STM Learning; 2014, in press.

31. van Ommeren M, Saxena S, Saraceno B. Mental and social health during and after acute emergencies: Emerging consensus? 2005. Available at: http://www.who.int/mental_health/media/mental_and_social_health_in_emergency.pdf. Accessed August 24, 2014.

32. Speck PM, Kennedy BL, Henry ND, et al. Analysis of possible sexual assault or abuse in a 67-year-old female with early dementia post-brain attack. Adv Emerg Nurs J 2013;35(3):217–39.

33. Hopper EK, Bassuk EL, Olivet J. Shelter from the storm: trauma-informed care in homelessness services. 2010. Available at: http://homeless.samhsa.gov/ResourceFiles/cenfdthy.pdf. Accessed August 24, 2014.

34. Burgess AW, Hanrahan NP, Baker T. Forensic markers in elder female sexual abuse cases. Clin Geriatr Med 2005;21(2):399–412.

35. Anetzberger GJ. An update on the nature and scope of elder abuse. Generations 2012;36(3):12–20.

36. Hillman JL. Clinical perspectives on elderly sexuality. New York: Plenum; 2000.

37. Burgess AW. Elderly victims of sexual abuse and their offenders. 2006. Available at: https://www.ncjrs.gov/pdffiles1/nij/grants/216550.pdf. Accessed August 24, 2014.

38. McEwen BS. Sex, stress and the hippocampus: allostasis, allostatic load and the aging process. Neurobiol Aging 2002;23(5):921–39.

39. Wicklund M, Petersen RC. Emerging biomarkers in cognition. Clin Geriatr Med 2013;29(4):809–28.

40. Phanjoo AL. Sexual dysfunction in old age. Adv Psychiatr Treat 2000;6(4):270–7.

41. Haddad PM, Benbow SM. Sexual problems associated with dementia: part 1. Problems and their consequences. Int J Geriatr Psychiatry 1993;8(7):547–51.

42. Taler G, Ansello EF. Elder abuse. Am Fam Physician 1985;32(2):107–14.

43. Lamonica P, Pagiaro EM. Sexual assault intervention and the forensic examination. In: Hammer RM, Moynihan B, Pagliaro EM, editors. Forensic nursing: a handbook for practice. Sudbury (MA): Jones and Bartlett; 2006. p. 547–78.
44. Anderson S, McClain N, Riviello RJ. Genital findings of women after consensual and nonconsensual intercourse. J Forensic Nurs 2006;2(2):59–65.
45. Clark M, Newman BS, Speck PM. Sexual assault among older adults. In: Giardino AP, Starling SP, Rotolo SL, et al, editors. Sexual assault across the life span: a comprehensive clinical reference. 2nd edition. St Louis (MO): STM Learning, in press.
46. Faugno DK, Speck PM. Basic anogenital and oral anatomy. In: Ledray L, Burgess AW, Giardino AP, editors. Medical Response to Adult Sexual Assault. St Louis (MO): STM Learning; 2011. p. 15–52.
47. Muram D, Miller K, Cutler A. Sexual assault of the elderly victim. J Interpers Violence 1992;7(1):70–6.
48. Speck PM, Patton SB. Hymen morphology updated: classifying estrogen effect across the life span. Presented at: International Association of Forensic Nurses, 15th Annual Scientific Assembly 2007. Salt Lake City (UT), October, 2007.
49. McCann J, Miyamoto S, Boyle C, et al. Healing of nonhymenal genital injuries in prepubertal and adolescent girls: a descriptive study. Pediatrics 2007;120(5): 1000–11.
50. Speck PM. Hymen injury in elderly consensual partners. Presented at: American Academy of Forensic Science, 60th Annual Scientific Assembly 2007. Washington, DC, February, 2008.
51. Speck PM, Lee ED. Hymen Estrogen Response Scale (HERS) reliability study [Abstract]. End Violence Against Women International and Office for Victims of Crime Notebook. 2011:28–29.
52. Farage MA, Maibach HI. Morphology and physiological changes of genital skin and mucosa. Curr Probl Dermatol 2011;40:9–19.
53. Jones JS, Rossman L, Diegel R, et al. Sexual assault in postmenopausal women: epidemiology and patterns of genital injury. Am J Emerg Med 2009; 27(8):922–9.
54. Del Bove G, Stermac L, Bainbridge D. Comparisons of sexual assault among older and younger women. J Elder Abuse Negl 2005;17(3):1–18.
55. Carabellese F, Candelli C, Vinci F, et al. Elderly sexual offenders: two unusual cases. J Forensic Sci 2012;57(5):1381–3.
56. Shipley SL, Arrigo BA. Sexual offenses against adults. In: Sturmey P, McMurran M, editors. Forensic case formulation. Chichester (United Kingdom): John Wiley; 2011. p. 195–213.
57. Ramsey-Klawsnik H, Teaster PB, Mendiondo MS, et al. Sexual predators who target elders: findings from the first national study of sexual abuse in care facilities. J Elder Abuse Negl 2008;20(4):353–76.
58. Roberto KA, Teaster PB. Sexual abuse of vulnerable young and old women: a comparative analysis of circumstances and outcomes. Violence Against Women 2005;11(4):473–504.
59. Safarik ME, Jarvis JP, Nussbaum KE. Sexual homicide of elderly females: linking offender characteristics to victim and crime scene attributes. J Interpers Violence 2002;17(5):500–25.
60. Bonomi AE, Anderson ML, Rivara FP, et al. Health care utilization and costs associated with childhood abuse. J Gen Intern Med 2008;23(3):294–9.
61. Government Accounting Office. Long term care facilities: information on residents who are registered sex offenders or are paroled for other crimes. 2006.

Available at: http://www.gpo.gov/fdsys/pkg/GAOREPORTS-GAO-06-326/pdf/ GAOREPORTS-GAO-06-326.pdf. Accessed August 24, 2014.

62. Cabeza R. Hemispheric asymmetry reduction in older adults: the HAROLD model. Psychol Aging 2002;17(1):85–100.

63. Faugno D, Waszak D, Strack GB, et al. Strangulation forensic examination: best practice for health care providers. Adv Emerg Nurs J 2013;35(4):314–27.

64. Ramsey-Klawsnik H, Teaster PB, Mendiondo MS, et al. Sexual predators who target elders: findings from the first national study of sexual abuse in care facilities. J Elder Abuse Negl 2008;20(4):353–76.

65. Anxiety and Depression Association of America. Body dysmorphic disorder. n.d. Available at: http://www.adaa.org/understanding-anxiety/related-illnesses/ other-related-conditions/body-dysmorphic-disorder-bdd. Accessed August 24, 2014.

66. Didie ER, Tortolani CC, Pope CG, et al. Childhood abuse and neglect in body dysmorphic disorder. Child Abuse Negl 2006;30(10):1105–15.

67. Phillips KA. The presentation of body dysmorphic disorder in medical settings. Prim Psychiatry 2006;13(7):51–9.

68. Butler AC, Chapman JE, Forman EM, et al. The empirical status of cognitive-behavioral therapy: a review of meta-analyses. Clin Psychol Rev 2006;26(1): 17–31.

69. Black HC. Black's law dictionary. St Paul (MN): West; 1991.

70. Lynch V. Forensic nursing. St Louis (MO): Elsevier Mosby; 2006.

71. Speck PM, Connor PD, Hartig MT, et al. Vulnerable populations: drug court program clients. Nurs Clin North Am 2008;43(3):477–89, x–xi.

72. Mason AE, Boden MT, Cucciare MA. Prospective associations among approach coping, alcohol misuse and psychiatric symptoms among veterans receiving a brief alcohol intervention. J Subst Abuse Treat 2014;46(5):553–60.

Medical Implications of Elder Abuse: Self-Neglect

 CrossMark

Carlos A. Reyes-Ortiz, MD, PhD[a], Jason Burnett, PhD[a,b,c],
David V. Flores, PhD, LMSW, MPH, CPH[a,b,c], John M. Halphen, MD[a,b,c],
Carmel Bitondo Dyer, MD, AGSF[a,b,c],*

KEYWORDS

- Self-neglect • Squalor • Geriatric assessment • Capacity

KEY POINTS

- Self-neglect is the most common report received by Adult Protective Service Agencies.
- Self-neglect is associated with multiple medical comorbidities and increased mortality.
- Comprehensive geriatric assessment coupled with capacity assessment is the best practice for case identification and evaluation.
- Medical and social interventions are indicated in cases of self-neglect.
- Self-neglect is a significant public health issue, and policies are needed to address the clinical needs of this vulnerable population.

CASE STUDY: "THE POSSUM HOUSE"

Mrs L.J. is a 79-year-old white widowed woman, who lives in a one-story house with her 40-year-old daughter. Mrs L.J. worked as a secretary but has been unemployed for about 20 years. She has a family history of abuse by her father and her deceased husband. Her medical diagnoses include hypothyroidism, gastrointestinal reflux disease, hypertension, urinary incontinence, arthritis, fatigue, and a history of breast cancer. She complains of falling, vision problems caused by cataracts, and tooth pain when eating. She denies any alcohol, tobacco, or illicit substance use. She has refused to see her physician for more than a year. Adult Protective Services (APS) was concerned about an unhealthy and dangerous environment, and referred her to the Texas Elder Abuse and Mistreatment Institute (TEAM) for a physical and mental evaluation. TEAM is a consortium of medical and academic institutions, APS, and

[a] Division of Geriatric and Palliative Care, Department of Internal Medicine, University of Texas Medical School, 6431 Fannin Street, Houston, TX 77030, USA; [b] Texas Elder Abuse and Mistreatment Institute, 3601 North MacGregor Way, Houston, TX 77004, USA; [c] Harris Health System, 2525 Holly Hall, Houston, TX 77054, USA
* Corresponding author. Division of Geriatric and Palliative Care, Department of Internal Medicine, University of Texas Medical School, 5656 Kelley Street, COS 101, Houston, TX 77026.
E-mail address: carmel.b.dyer@uth.tmc.edu

Clin Geriatr Med 30 (2014) 807–823
http://dx.doi.org/10.1016/j.cger.2014.08.008
0749-0690/14/$ – see front matter © 2014 Elsevier Inc. All rights reserved.

law enforcement groups working collectively to investigate, assess, and assist victims of elder abuse and self-neglect.[1,2]

Home Environment

The visit to Mrs L.J.'s home revealed an overgrown lawn, trash around the property, and lack of upkeep (eg, holes in the roof) in an otherwise clean, pleasant neighborhood. She has been living in her house for more than 30 years and has been reported to the homeowners association, the Houston Police Department, and the local Society for the Protection of Cruelty to Animals (SPCA) on multiple occasions. She recently went to jail for multiple unpaid city warrants for her refusal to clean up piles of trash in her back yard.

Most of the interior of the house was inaccessible because of clutter and old boxes that stood 4 feet high. The home was roach-infested and smelled of trash and urine. Piles of articles, cans, and old food were noted throughout the residence. There was a mattress in the middle of the living room floor, and both the daughter and mother slept in the same bed. An open-faced electrical heater sat approximately 1 foot from the mattress, creating a significant fire hazard. Roaches crawled around the piles of trash in the home and on Mrs L.J. herself, including through her hair. Multiple animals lived in the house including 2 cats, a parrot, and a wild pregnant possum who had taken up residency in an old shopping cart full of cans in the kitchen. When asked if she would like for animal control to be called to remove the wild animal, she replied, "I think it's better if she stays in the kitchen...she's like my pet!" The sink was filled with dirty dishes, roaches, and cat food. There was moldy food in the refrigerator, and its temperature was inappropriate for food storage. The bathroom was unusable because of roof collapse. Mrs L.J. and her daughter used a nearby bucket when they needed to use the bathroom. A significant plumbing leak was present from an inaccessible rear bathroom, and stagnant water was pooling in the back of the house.

Social Support

Mrs L.J. was isolated and had rare contact with individuals other than her daughter. The daughter reported having technical training; however, she worked as a cashier and was the sole income provider. She exhibited some evidence of developmental delay.

Clinical Impressions and Capacity Assessment

During the TEAM visit Mrs L.J. wore a dirty nightshirt, had marginal personal hygiene, and was lying on a mattress about 6 inches off the ground. Vital signs were normal. Multiple dental caries were visible on her teeth. There were no obvious signs of physical trauma. She had a history of bilateral breast removal and weakness in the legs, but otherwise her physical examination was normal. She could rise from the mattress to a standing position, but with considerable effort. She used a cane to brace herself while getting up, but almost stumbled head-first into the wall.

Mrs L.J. was awake and oriented to person, place, and time. She was often tangential and lost her train of thought. Her Confusion Assessment Measurement score was negative for delirium.[3] She did not complete the Geriatric Depression Scale or the Clox 1 test for executive function, owing to a combination of suspicion of the interviewers and inability to answer the more challenging questions.[4,5] Her St Louis University Mental Status score was 23 out of 30 (normal range 27–30) and her Clox 2 score 6 out of 15 (normal range 12–15), which showed cognitive impairment with severe executive control dysfunction.[5,6] She failed the Kohlman Evaluation of Living Skills test (KELS) with a score of 8 out of 16 (score of $5\frac{1}{2}$ or less indicates client is capable of living independently), indicating a need for assistance or supportive services to live safely in the community.[7,8]

Her connection to low-value items was consistent with hoarding behavior.[9,10] Mrs L.J. also exhibited a suspicious personality trait and paranoid thoughts. These cognitive deficits suggested a diagnosis of dementia, Alzheimer disease.[9]

Mrs L.J. lacked the capacity to remain living independently in the community, based on the following[11,12]:

- Failure to take appropriate steps to rectify her situation by accepting assistance provided by APS (animal control, extermination or cleaning services)
- Unable to recognize dangerous situations related to the electric heater and its proximity to combustibles
- Failure to recognize the dangers of having a wild animal living in her home (physical harm, parasites, or transmission of *Salmonella*)[13]
- Unable to recognize the degree of insect infestation and its risks for health
- Failure to recognize squalor and the degree of work required to improve conditions, in addition to her inability to clean the home

Recommendations and Outcome

Mrs L.J. was referred for guardianship and transfer to an assisted living facility for supervision of activities of daily living and self-care. She received medical follow-up and physical and occupational rehabilitation. She was able to take her parrot to the facility and enjoyed socialization with other residents, which helped to alleviate some of her anxiety related to hoarding and loss of other pets. Mrs L.J.'s daughter willingly moved to a group home nearby to her mother, and visits her daily.

BACKGROUND
Definitions

Self-neglect is defined by the National Committee for the Prevention of Elder Abuse and the National Adult Protective Services Association as

> ...an adult's inability, due to physical or mental impairment or diminished capacity, to perform essential self-care tasks including (a) obtaining essential food, clothing, shelter, and medical care; (b) obtaining goods and services necessary to maintain physical health, mental health, or general safety; and/or (c) managing one's own financial affairs.[14]

A self-neglecting elder has been also defined as a person who exhibits at least 1 of the following: (1) persistent inattention to personal hygiene and/or environment; (2) repeated refusal of some/all indicated services that can reasonably be expected to improve quality of life; (3) self-endangerment through the manifestation of unsafe behaviors (eg, persistent refusal to care for a disease).[15]

Personal and/or domestic squalor, used extensively in the literature to describe elder self-neglect, has also been phrased to include "the aged recluse,"[16] "senile breakdown,"[17] "lack of cleanliness,"[18,19] "Diogenes syndrome,"[20] "social breakdown in the elderly,"[21,22] "squalor syndrome,"[23,24] or "gross self-neglect."[25]

To characterize the severity of this condition, 3 domains of self-neglect indicators have been identified: (1) personal hygiene (eg, dirty hair and clothing, poor condition of nails and skin); (2) impaired function (eg, decline in cognitive function and activities of daily living); and (3) environmental neglect (eg, evidence of subject's inability to clean the house and yard, and manage material goods acquired over the years).[26] Mrs L.J. was affected by all domains.

Clinical Findings

The etiology of self-neglect is unknown, but may be associated with premorbid personality traits (aloof, detached, suspicious, quarrelsome), behaviors (reclusive, hoarding), or disorders (obsessive-compulsive, paranoid, schizoid).[20,21,27–30] Indeed, hoarding (accumulation of rubbish or syllogomania), is considered an important clinical characteristic of the self-neglect syndrome,[28–30] and has been linked to obsessive-compulsive disorder.[10,31] For example, in an English study including referral cases living in squalor conditions in the community, hoarding was present in 51% of households.[28] In an Australian survey conducted in 12 community health centers, hoarding occurred among 72% of subjects living in unclean conditions.[10,19,30] As in the case with Mrs L.J., hoarding behavior results in stacks of trash and other objects that significantly reduce the total living space and present risks for falls, fire, and safety, and interfere with daily tasks such as cleaning, cooking, sleeping, and socialization.[10,31]

The development of executive dysfunction, a condition whereby an individual is unable to translate simple tasks into complex, goal-directed behaviors such as cooking, dressing oneself, and performing basic housework, has been proposed as an important etiologic factor in elder self-neglect.[32,33] Related to this, some cases of severe domestic squalor or self-neglect have been found to have frontal lobe dysfunction or frontal lobe dementia.[11,30,34]

Risk factors for the development of self-neglect include old age, male gender, cognitive impairment, depression, delirium, medical illness (stroke, hip fracture), functional and social dependence, stressful events (eg, bereavement), history of social isolation, and alcohol and substance abuse.[11,29,33,35] For example, in a cohort study, the New Haven Established Population for Epidemiologic Studies in the Elderly (EPESE), cognitive impairment (odds ratio [OR] 4.63, 95% confidence interval [CI] 2.32–9.23) and clinically significant depressive symptoms (OR 2.38, 95% CI 1.26–4.48) were independent predictors of self-neglect after 9 years of follow-up.[36]

Mental disorders are commonly described in elders with severe self-neglect. These disorders include schizophrenia, dementia, alcohol abuse, and psychosis, with dementia being the most common.[17,20,30,37–39] In a community study of people living in squalor, 70% of the individuals were classified as having an ICD-10 mental disorder. Identifiable psychiatric illnesses are more common among younger individuals who manifest self-neglect.[19,28,38]

Self-neglect, like other geriatric syndromes, is associated with significant comorbidity, including hypertension, dementia, diabetes mellitus, arthritis, stroke, depression, urinary incontinence, and delirium.[33] Self-neglecting elders may exhibit greater functional limitations when compared with other elders in cross-sectional or longitudinal studies.[17,27,40,41] Individuals with severe self-neglect were often described as having sensory impairment.[17,20,27] As a consequence of living in squalor conditions, self-neglecting elders may have altered nutritional status, which includes multiple nutritional deficiencies such as iron, folate, vitamin B_{12}, vitamin C, β-carotene, α-tocopherol, serum proteins/albumin, calcium, and vitamin D.[20,42]

Outcomes

Self-neglect is an independent risk factor for death. Indeed, in the New Haven EPESE study, self-neglecting elders had an increased risk of 13-year all-cause mortality (OR 1.7, 95% CI 1.2–2.5) when compared with other members of the cohort.[35] Also, in the Chicago Health and Aging Project (CHAP), self-neglecting elders had an increased risk of 1-year mortality (hazard ratio [HR] 5.82, 95% CI 5.20–6.51), which remained significant over the entire 9-year follow-up period, but was greatly reduced starting in year 2 (HR 1.88; 95% CI 1.67–2.14).[43]

Self-neglecters may make increased use of health services because of the severity of self-neglect and the accompanying comorbidity or health complications. Thus there is an increased risk for nursing home placement,[44] and hospice,[45] hospital,[46] and emergency department utilization.[47] However, once self-neglecters are brought into the health care system, they are no more expensive than other similar patients.[48]

Acute hospitalization of patients who self-neglect has often resulted in worse outcomes in comparison with patients treated in the outpatient setting for the same conditions.[17,20,27] In addition, self-neglect is also associated with other geriatric syndromes such as dementia, depression, or urinary incontinence.[33,39] Nonadherence to treatments has been found to be a problem in the elder self-neglect population. Turner and colleagues[49] reported that 90% of 100 elder self-neglecters were nonadherent with at least 1 medication, and even more were nonadherent with approximately 4 medications. Nonadherence was associated with the number of prescribed medications and lower objective physical function.

MODEL
Etiology of Elder Self-Neglect

After more than 10 years of practice by TEAM, Dyer and colleagues[33] developed a biopsychosocial path model proposing causal links between health conditions and the development of elder self-neglect. In addition to clinical practice, case studies and findings from a large descriptive study of more than 450 APS clients with self-neglect informed this model.[33] The TEAM model depicted in **Fig. 1** illustrates the path from certain illnesses to self-neglect within specific social contexts. The syndromes or diagnoses included in the top box may be due to a variety of reasons

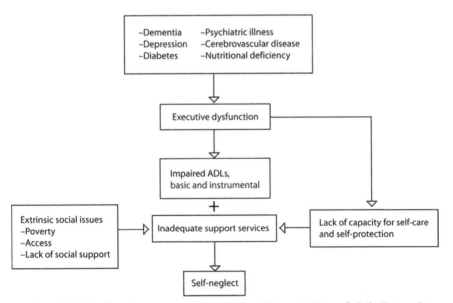

Fig. 1. Model of self-neglect among the elderly. ADLs, activities of daily living. (*From* Dyer CB, Goodwin JS, Vogel M, et al. Characterizing self-neglect: a report of over 500 cases of self-neglect seen by a geriatric medicine team. Am J Public Health 2007;97:1675; with permission.)

including poor self-management skills, limited or fragmented health care, reduce resources, psychiatric illnesses, delusional disorders, and substance abuse.[10,11,15] Resulting memory impairment and or lack of executive function may then reduce the older adult's ability for self-care and self-protection, requiring social, medical and functional interventions[6] to impede the onset of elder self-neglect.

In many instances family members step in to address these deficits, and provide the assistance needed. For instance, family members may move their loved one to an assisted living facility, provide in-home help, or reduce their work load to help the individual at home. Individuals who develop functional deficits without the memory deficits or executive dysfunction may themselves voluntarily stop driving, move to a senior center, or hire assistance. Self-neglect occurs when seniors fail to recognize their deficits or lack the social support or financial resources to accomplish activities of daily living.[33]

Work by Dong and colleagues, Dyer and colleagues, Mosqueda, Lachs, and others have demonstrated that this model holds true in different jurisdictions.[40,41,50–55] There are various disparities in social services across the United States that may contribute to the prevalence of elder self-neglect. Services in rural areas differ significantly from those in urban settings. In rural areas there may be more cohesive communities, whereas in urban settings more medical resources and social resources may be available to individuals who develop executive memory problems or executive dysfunctions. APS agencies also differ across the country. For example, in the state of Texas there is a relatively large protective service organization, organized at the state level and integrated into the fabric of the social community and health care community. In many jurisdictions, the expertise of the medical practitioners in addressing self-neglect cases differs. There are also variances in state statutes regarding the definitions and remedies.

Many aspects of the TEAM model[33] have been tested, but more work is needed to determine the ideal timing and type of interventions.

ASSESSMENT
Approach

When a clinician evaluates a suspected self-neglecter, he or she will attempt to determine the ways in which one is not taking care of oneself, the cause, and what support would help meet the identified needs.

It is necessary to seek information about the circumstances of the elder and his or her functional abilities from all available sources. More accurate information may be available from neighbors, bank tellers, apartment building managers, and others, than is available from the elder. Visiting the self-neglecter in his or her usual living environment is often more informative than seeing the patient in the clinical environment. At the home, more accurate information about the living conditions can be gathered, providing more evidence of how patients are functioning in their everyday environment.[56] Self-report in these cases is often grossly incorrect and misleading.[57]

A comprehensive geriatric assessment with medical, functional, and social history is considered best practice. This information, when added to that from alternative credible sources, may help determine the self-neglecter's appreciation of the circumstances. A clinician such as a physician or nurse practitioner should conduct a physical examination and screen for depression, delirium, dementia, and functional abilities.[58] The goal is to identify physical or mental conditions that interfere with their understanding and function.

There are key questions to be answered when evaluating self-neglect, which have been developed based on the literature and TEAM's clinical experience.

To live independently without supervision, the self-neglecter must be able to arrange to have the following needs met if he or she cannot perform them independently: activities of daily living (dressing, bathing, toileting, feeding oneself, moving about their home); instrumental activities of daily living (managing finances, preparing meals, performing housework, using the telephone, shopping, use of transportation, taking medications, or managing medical issues); protection from harm (from strangers or nonstrangers); and a reasonably safe and hygienic living environment.[59,60]

Important considerations include whether the elder is able to make decisions about his or her needs, and is able to take reasonable steps to meet these needs. Some with capacity may simply decide not to address their needs. For instance, an impoverished individual may want a better home environment, but elect to stay in a dilapidated home with pets.

Capacity Assessment

All adults are presumed to have full capacity to live independently. Finding one incapacitated in some or all areas is a joint medical and judicial decision, based on expert clinical opinion. The state definitions of incapacity are usually based on the functional abilities of the person to meet, or arrange to meet, the essential requirements for physical health, safety, or self-care (American Bar Association/American Psychological Association, 2006).[61] Other questions posed during a TEAM evaluation are noted in **Tables 1** and **2**.

The cognitive domains thought to be important to independent living are: attention; working memory; short-term memory; long-term memory; receptive language; expressive language; understanding of basic quantities and making simple calculations; verbal reasoning; visual-spatial reasoning; and executive function.[60] Stated more concisely, the person must have the ability to make decisions, and carry out decisions, with respect to his or her needs.[11] A person's decision-making capacity requires the ability to receive and understand relevant information, reason through the options, communicate a choice, and appreciate the situation.[62] Appreciation of the patient's own circumstances is critical to patient's decision making. An adequate memory is needed for this appreciation.

Executive function has been found to be a necessary cognitive ability for independent functioning in the community. This ability allows the individual to plan, direct, sequence, organize, monitor, and supervise his or her own behavior.[32,63–65] It is possible to have an intact memory, but fail to live independently with success because of poor executive function, a necessary capability when taking reasonable steps to carry out individual decisions and intentions.[33] Screening instruments may test for this ability, but observation of how well the individual is able to carry out intentions without supervision may be a better test for this.

The assessment approach described here, including answering the questions in **Tables 1** and **2**, should provide the needed information for the clinician to arrive at an opinion about the patient's capacity to live independently without supervision. It should also help the clinician to identify unmet needs and possible interventions to support the patient besides guardianship.

INTERVENTIONS
Adult Protective Services

Research conducted over the last decade has increased the understanding of how varying health conditions, both chronic and acute, can lead older adults to neglect themselves.[33,40,66,67] Less known is how to effectively intervene in this population,

Table 1
TEAM checklist for determining capacity

Key Question	ADL	IADL	Housing	Self-Protection
Does the person understand their circumstances?	(T/F) Despite adequate resources, the person is failing to perform an ADL and does *not understand this fact*	(T/F) Despite adequate resources, the person is failing to perform an IADL and does *not understand this fact*	(T/F) Despite adequate resources, the person is exposed to an unsafe/unsanitary/inadequate housing condition and does *not understand this fact*	(T/F) Despite adequate resources, the person is the victim of abuse, neglect, exploitation, or self-neglect, and does *not understand this fact*
Is the person failing to self-care and self-protect?	(T/F) Despite adequate resources, the person is failing to perform an ADL and does *not take appropriate steps to correct the problem*	(T/F) Despite adequate resources, the person is failing to perform an IADL and does *not take appropriate steps to correct the problem*	(T/F) Despite adequate resources, the person is exposed to an unsafe/unsanitary/inadequate housing condition and *does not take appropriate steps to correct the problem*	(T/F) Despite adequate resources, the person is the victim of abuse, neglect, exploitation, or self-neglect, and does *not take appropriate steps to correct the problem*

The documentation should be made of each finding to justify a "T" response. The documentation should include the source of the alleged fact (personal observation, information from a third party, and so forth). Effort should be taken to find multiple sources of information for each significant finding. Care should be taken to try to determine if the person is arranging for assistance or if assistance is being provided without the person arranging for it. What we would like to know is how well persons would take care of themselves if arranging for their own care and protection. Developed by John M. Halphen.

Abbreviations: ADL, activities of daily living (toileting, feeding, dressing, grooming, physical ambulation, bathing); IADL, instrumental activities of daily living (ability to use telephone, shopping, food preparation, housekeeping, laundry, arrange for transportation, ability to handle finances, responsible for taking own medications); T/F, true or false.

whose members are known to eschew conventional medical and social intervention. The complexities in the often unique biopsychosocial profiles of elder self-neglecters limit the effectiveness of standard medical interventions, and there is a need for more comprehensive approaches.

When the suspicion of elder self-neglect is raised, clinicians can substantiate these suspicions through a comprehensive geriatric assessment as already noted, and/or by making a referral to APS. Including APS services provides a more comprehensive understanding of the causes for the unmet needs of the older adult. In fact, interprofessional teams of health care and social services professionals are recommended for effective treatment and intervention in elder self-neglect. These teams provide a comprehensive assessment and treatment approach designed to meet the intermixed medical, social, mental health, and behavioral problems that facilitate self-neglect and impede effective treatment.[2] Intervention using the interprofessional team approach has reported success in reducing self-neglect behaviors and risk factors such as depression, impairments in activities of daily living, and lack of self-perceived social support.[68,69]

Clinical Interventions Teams

The inclusion of other disciplines is important and reduces the treatment burden of the primary care provider. The traditional "treat and release" approach may not be effective for reducing or preventing elder self-neglect. Older adults who neglect themselves often fall along a continuum of able self-care, which includes progressive categories such as autonomous, collaborative, structured, and subordinate. Autonomous individuals are those who are able to self-manage on their own with minimal need for external support. Collaborative individuals also self-manage on their own, but the clinicians and external support are jointly involved in the decision making. Structured individuals are those who have very limited ability to adequately engage in self-management and thus require even more active external support. Subordinate individuals are those who have very modest patient discretion and require very controlling and supervisory environments to manage their health conditions.[70] Older adults with limited mental capacity or executive functioning fall into the structured and subordinate groups that require more supervisory care. Evidence shows that elder self-neglecters with mental health issues simultaneously neglect multiple life domains, and thus may fall into the structured and subordinate categories that require more supervision.[71] In this instance it is important for the clinician to first determine which factors may be limiting adequate self-care and whether these deficiencies can be reversed.[33] Depending on the findings, temporary or long-term provider or guardianship services will be warranted to protect the older adult from further self-neglect and harm.

Recent evidence suggests that self-neglect is not always associated with mental health problems, whereas mental health problems are not always associated with elder self-neglect; therefore, other avenues of intervention are needed.[71] Some elder self-neglecters are cognitively capable of performing self-care behaviors, but lack the physical ability necessary for managing their health.[33,71] Just as medication nonadherence in this population was associated with low physical functioning and the number of medications prescribed, interventions aimed at improving physical functioning and reducing the number of medications in this population could lead to better health outcomes and a reduction in self-neglect behaviors.[49]

Moreover, many self-neglecters may not have the necessary problem-solving skills to effectively manage their health and mental health conditions. Studies show that low-socioeconomic older adults have reduced problem-solving skills, which may limit the

Table 2
TEAM report

Domain	Information
Biographic data	Date client seen: Client name: Client address: Client DOB:
Adult Protective Services (APS)	Reason for the visit: APS concerned that... History of the problem (years): Allegations (concerns of APS and others): Prior History with APS:
History	Medical/surgical history of the patient (unaided awareness of medical circumstances): Medical/surgical history, from other sources: The medications the patient is aware of, and why they are taken (patient's unaided awareness of medical circumstances): The medications the patient actually takes, from other sources: Social history according to the patient: Social history from other sources:
Examination	Physical examination (conducted by MD or NP): Sensory issues: Delirium: CAM: Depression: GDS score and does it report depression?: SLUMS or MMSE: Score: Level of education: Where were the problems on the MMSE: CAGE: GET-UP-AND-GO:

ADL capacity	Is the person failing to perform an ADL and *not understanding this fact?* Describe:	Is the person failing to take reasonable steps under the circumstances (considering resources) to correct the problem? Describe:
IADL capacity	Is the person failing to perform an IADL and *not understanding this fact?* Describe:	Is the person failing to take reasonable steps under the circumstances (considering resources) to correct the problem? Describe:
Housing capacity	Is the person failing to secure safe/sanitary/adequate housing conditions and *not understanding this fact?* Describe:	Is the person failing to take reasonable steps under the circumstances (considering resources) to correct the problem? Describe:
Self-protection capacity	Is the person the victim of abuse, neglect, exploitation, or self-neglect and *not understanding this fact?* Describe:	Is the person failing to take reasonable steps under the circumstances (considering resources) to correct the problem? Describe:
Outcomes	ASSESSMENT: RECOMMENDATIONS: PLAN: Describe plan discussed in Interdisciplinary Team conference:	

Abbreviations: ADL, activities of daily living (toileting, feeding, dressing, grooming, physical ambulation, bathing); CAGE, Cut-Annoyed-Guilty-Eye (alcoholism screening test); CAM, Confusion Assessment Method; GDS, Geriatric Depression Scale; GET-UP-AND-GO, mobility assessment test; IADL, instrumental activities of daily living (ability to use telephone, shopping, food preparation, housekeeping, laundry, arrange for transportation, ability to handle finances, responsible for taking own medications); MD, physician; MMSE, Mini Mental State Examination; NP, nurse practitioner; SLUMS, St Louis University Mental Status.

effectiveness of traditional medical care that tends to focus more on the disease rather than the individual.[72] This fact does not diminish the importance of treating disease, but indicates the need for alternative interventions that both treat disease and improve the ability of the elder self-neglecter to self-manage, as many live isolated and alone in the community. Chronic disease self-management programs in older adults have been widely successful for improving the overall health and self-care behaviors of older adult populations with very similar biopsychosocial profiles to that of elder self-neglect.[73] Specifically, teaching physical and mental health–related problem-solving techniques has resulted in reductions in depression and improvements in overall chronic disease self-management in low-income, home-bound older adults.[74]

Medical Interventions

There is no standard prescription for intervening in elder self-neglect. These cases are often medically complicated. Historically these patients may be recalcitrant and nonadherent to proposed interventions. In the past, many have considered intervention in cases of self-neglect to be impossible or futile; however, evidence supports the ability to intervene and improve outcomes in this population.[69,71] The feasibility of intervening in elder self-neglect has been demonstrated by Burnett and colleagues,[75] who conducted a randomized clinical trial (RCT) in 50 community-living elder self-neglecters and reported clinically significant increases in vitamin D levels over a 10-month period. Likewise, in a separate RCT, Burnett and colleagues[68] compared APS usual care versus APS usual care with multidisciplinary team (MDT) medical recommendations, based on review of comprehensive geriatric assessment data. Implementing the recommendations provided by the MDT demonstrated statistically reliable reductions in elder self-neglect behaviors at 6-month follow-up in comparison with APS usual care.

In sum, the traditional approaches to successful aging outlined in Robert Butler's "longevity prescription" will likely not work in elders who neglect themselves.[76] Instead, nontraditional and more comprehensive approaches are likely necessary for effectively intervening in this population. Nevertheless, it is a challenge and obligation of health care professionals to determine the best interventions for improving the overall health and well-being of vulnerable self-neglecting older adults.

FUTURE IMPLICATIONS FOR POLICY

Although elder self-neglect is a comparatively new focus in aging research, there is sufficient evidence regarding its pervasiveness and deleterious outcomes[14,33,35,43] to warrant the development of national, state-wide, and community-level policy and legislation around this issue (**Fig. 2**).

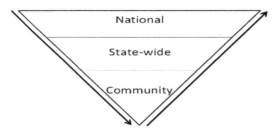

Fig. 2. Top-down approach to elder self-neglect policy development and impact, showing a feedback loop for how policy at the federal level can affect lower-level policy decisions leading to actions that then provide evidence for changing policy at the upper levels. (Designed by Jason Burnett.)

On a national level, much of the legislation and policies in aging focus on violence.[77] Thus, elder self-neglect does not meet the requirement for inclusion even though self-neglect is the most common report to APS agencies nationwide. Recent evidence suggests that elder self-neglecters will, by default, be covered by these policies and legislation because of the increased likelihood of subsequent abuse. Unfortunately, subsequent abuse occurs approximately 3 years after the substantiation of elder self-neglect, and for many frail older adults with reduced physiologic and psychological reserves such a latency period can be detrimental.[78] Broader and more inclusive legislation and policies, in addition to elder self-neglect specific policies and legislation, are needed to advance the field. This approach will require expanding the funding of federal programs such as the US Centers for Disease Control and Prevention, the National Institute on Aging, the Agency for Healthcare Research and Quality, the Administration on Community-Living, and APS, in addition to other federal organizations with interests in aging. Doing so will allow for the expansion of research capacity, which should focus on developing universal definitions and improving the detection, prevention, treatment, and management of elder self-neglect.

Consistent policies regarding reporting of elder self-neglect to state Adult Protective Service Agencies would be highly beneficial for establishing less biased national prevalence and incidence measures. Likewise, establishing policies for the use of standardized assessments to substantiate elder self-neglect would also help reduce inconsistent findings in this population. Accurate data would strengthen research findings regarding risk factors and effective treatment modalities across the country. In addition, policies for establishing medical and social service collaborations similar to the TEAM is of particular importance for the treatment and management of the comprehensive needs in vulnerable elder self-neglecters.

In 2012, Dong[77] provided a comprehensive discussion regarding the future directions of elder abuse and included self-neglect, which included the role of the community in helping to advance the understanding of self-neglect. There was little discussion, however, about the need for policies related to clinical settings. The US Joint Commissions have already established mandatory screening for elder abuse and neglect for emergency department patients who present with injury or advanced medical circumstances. It is unclear as to whether this mandate includes self-neglect, despite the evidence that elder self-neglecters frequently visit the emergency department.[47] Health care settings are primed for policies that promote screening and prevention. These settings have the potential to be the first line of prevention, and could make available a copious amount of biopsychosocial data to establish the etiology of elder self-neglect and identify the most robust risk factors.

Policies at all levels are needed to facilitate research development. There is a direct need for advancing the study of elder self-neglect beyond the epidemiology and to focus on the development of intervention and prevention. Future well-designed longitudinal trials should be used to understand effective ways to prevent and treat elder self-neglect. The ultimate goal is to improve the health of vulnerable older adults and to inform policy-makers and legislators at the community, state-wide, and national levels regarding the best way to limit associated societal costs and other public health burdens.[53]

REFERENCES

1. Dyer CB, Gleason MS, Murphy KP, et al. Treating elder neglect: collaboration between a geriatrics assessment team and adult protective services. South Med J 1999;92:242–4.

2. Dyer CB, Heisler CJ, Hill CA, et al. Community approaches to elder abuse. Clin Geriatr Med 2005;21:429–47.

3. Inouye SK, VanDyck CH, Alessi CA, et al. Clarifying confusion: the confusion assessment method. A new method for detecting delirium. Ann Intern Med 1990;113:941–8.

4. Yeasavage JA, Brink TL, Rose TL, et al. Development and validation of a geriatric depression screening scale: a preliminary report. J Psychiatr Res 1983; 17:37–49.

5. Royall DR, Cordes J, Polk MJ. CLOX: an executive clock-drawing task. J Neurol Neurosurg Psychiatr 1998;64:588–94.

6. Tariq SH, Tumosa N, Chibnall JT, et al. Comparison of the Saint Louis University mental status examination and the mini-mental state examination for detecting dementia and mild neurocognitive disorder–a pilot study. Am J Geriatr Psychiatry 2006;14:900–10.

7. Kohlman-Thomson L. Kohlman evaluation of living skills. 3rd edition. Bethesda (MD): American Occupational Therapy Association; 1992.

8. Burnett J, Dyer CB, Naik AD. Convergent validation of the Kohlman evaluation of living skills (KELS) as a screening tool of older adults' capacity to live safely and independently in the community. Arch Phys Med Rehabil 2009;90:1948–52.

9. American Psychiatric Association. Diagnostic and statistical manual of mental disorders. 5th edition. Arlington (VA): American Psychiatric Publishing; 2013.

10. Poythress EL, Burnett J, Naik AD, et al. Severe self-neglect: an epidemiological and historical perspective. J Elder Abuse Negl 2006;18:5–12.

11. Naik AD, Lai JM, Kunik ME, et al. Assessing capacity in suspected cases of self-neglect. Geriatrics 2008;63:24–31.

12. Naik AD, Teal CR, Pavlik VN, et al. Conceptual challenges and practical approaches to screening capacity for self-care and protection in vulnerable older adults. J Am Geriatr Soc 2008;56(Suppl 2):S266–70.

13. Oates SC, Miller MA, Byrne BA, et al. Epidemiology and potential land-sea transfer of enteric bacteria from terrestrial to marine species in the Monterey Bay region of California. J Wildl Dis 2012;48:654–68.

14. Teaster PB, Dugar TA, Mendiondo MS, et al. The 2004 survey of state adult protective services: abuse of adults 60 years of age and older. The National Center on elder abuse; 2007. Available at: http://www.ncea.aoa.gov/Resources/Publication/docs/APS_2004NCEASurvey.pdf. Accessed January 24, 2014.

15. Pavlou MP, Lachs MS. Self-neglect in older adults: a primer for clinicians. J Gen Intern Med 2008;23:1841–6.

16. Granick R, Zeman FD. The aged recluse- an exploratory study with particular reference to community responsibility. J Chronic Dis 1960;12:639–53.

17. Macmillan D, Shaw P. Senile breakdown in standards of personal and environmental cleanliness. Br Med J 1966;2:1032–7.

18. Leake CD. Senile lack of cleanliness. Geriatrics 1967;22(7):76.

19. Snowdon J. Uncleanliness among persons seen by community health workers. Hosp Community Psychiatry 1987;38:491–4.

20. Clark AN, Mankikar GD, Gray I. Diogenes syndrome: a clinical study of gross neglect in old age. Lancet 1975;1:366–8.

21. Ungvari GS, Hantz PM. Social breakdown in the elderly. I. Case studies and management. Compr Psychiatry 1991;32:440–4.

22. Radebaugh TS, Hooper FJ, Gruenberg EM. The social breakdown syndrome in the elderly population living in the community: the helping study. Br J Psychiatry 1987;151:341–6.

23. Shah AK. Senile squalor syndrome. What to expect and how to treat it. Geriatr Med 1990;20(10):26.
24. Snowdon J. Squalor syndrome. J Am Geriatr Soc 1997;45:1539–40.
25. Cybulska E, Rucinski J. Gross self-neglect. Br J Hosp Med 1986;36:21–5.
26. Kelly PA, Dyer CB, Pavlik V, et al. Exploring self-neglect in older adults: preliminary findings of the self-neglect severity scale and next steps. J Am Geriatr Soc 2008;56(Suppl 2):S253–60.
27. Wrigley M, Cooney C. Diogenes syndrome: an Irish series. Ir J Psychol Med 1992;9:37–41.
28. Halliday G, Banerjee S, Philpot M, et al. Community study of people who live in squalor. Lancet 2000;355:882–6.
29. Reyes-Ortiz C. Self-neglect as a geriatric syndrome. J Am Geriatr Soc 2006;54:1945–6.
30. Snowdon J, Shah A, Halliday G. Severe domestic squalor: a review. Int Psychogeriatr 2007;19:37–51.
31. Rasmussen JL, Steketee G, Frost RO, et al. Assessing squalor in hoarding: the home environment index. Community Ment Health J 2014;50(5):591–6.
32. Royall DR, Palmer R, Chiodo LK, et al. Declining executive control in normal aging predicts change in functional status: the freedom house study. J Am Geriatr Soc 2004;52:346–52.
33. Dyer CB, Goodwin JS, Vogel M, et al. Characterizing self-neglect: a report of over 500 cases of self-neglect seen by a geriatric medicine team. Am J Public Health 2007;97:1671–6.
34. Beauchet O, Imler D, Cadet L, et al. Diogenes syndrome in the elderly: clinical form of frontal dysfunction? Report of 4 cases. Rev Med Interne 2002;23:122–31 [in French].
35. Lachs MS, Williams CS, O'Brien S, et al. The mortality of elder mistreatment. JAMA 1998;280:428–32.
36. Abrams RC, Lachs M, McAvay G, et al. Predictors of self-neglect in community-dwelling elders. Am J Psychiatry 2002;159:1724–30.
37. Dyer CB, Pavlik VN, Murphy KP, et al. The high prevalence of depression and dementia in elder neglect. J Am Geriatr Soc 2000;48:205–8.
38. Hurley M, Scallen E, Johnson H, et al. Adult service refusers in the greater Dublin. Ir Med J 2000;93:208–11.
39. Pavlou MP, Lachs MS. Could self-neglect in older adults be a geriatric syndrome? J Am Geriatr Soc 2006;54:831–42.
40. Dong X, Simon M, Fulmer T, et al. Physical function decline and the risk of elder self-neglect in a community-dwelling population. Gerontologist 2010;50:316–26.
41. Naik AD, Burnett J, Pickens-Pace S, et al. Impairment in activities of daily living and the geriatric syndrome of self-neglect. Gerontologist 2008;48:388–93.
42. Smith SM, Mathews Oliver SA, Zwart SR, et al. Nutritional status is altered in the self-neglecting elderly. J Nutr 2006;136:2534–41.
43. Dong X, Simon M, Mendes de Leon C, et al. Elder self-neglect and abuse and mortality risk in a community-dwelling population. JAMA 2009;302:517–26.
44. Lachs MS, Williams CS, O'Brien S, et al. Adult protective service use and nursing home placement. Gerontologist 2002;42:734–9.
45. Dong X, Simon MA. Association between elder self-neglect and hospice utilization in a community population. Arch Gerontol Geriatr 2013;56:192–8.
46. Dong X, Simon MA, Evans D. Elder self-neglect and hospitalization: findings from the Chicago Health and Aging Project. J Am Geriatr Soc 2012;60:202–9.

47. Dong X, Simon MA, Evans D. Prospective study of the elder self-neglect and ED use in a community population. Am J Emerg Med 2012;30:553–61.

48. Franzini L, Dyer CB. Healthcare costs and utilization of vulnerable elderly people reported to Adult Protective Services for self-neglect. J Am Geriatr Soc 2008;56: 667–76.

49. Turner A, Hochschild A, Burnett J, et al. High prevalence of medication non-adherence in a sample of community-dwelling older adults with adult protective services-validated self-neglect. Drugs Aging 2012;29:741–9.

50. Dong X, Mendes de Leon CF, Evans DA. Is greater self-neglect severity associated with lower levels of physical function? J Aging Health 2009;21:596–610.

51. Dong X, Simon MA, Mosqueda L, et al. The prevalence of elder self-neglect in a community-dwelling population: hoarding, hygiene, and environmental hazards. J Aging Health 2012;24:507–24.

52. Pickens S, Naik AD, Burnett J, et al. The utility of the Kohlman evaluation of living skills test is associated with substantiated cases of elder self-neglect. J Am Acad Nurse Pract 2007;19:137–42.

53. Dyer CB, Franzini L, Watson M, et al. Future research: a prospective longitudinal study of elder self-neglect. J Am Geriatr Soc 2008;56(Suppl 2):S261–5.

54. McDermott S. The devil is in the details: self-neglect in Australia. J Elder Abuse Negl 2008;20:231–50.

55. Paveza G, Vandeweerd C, Laumann E. Elder self-neglect: a discussion of a social typology. J Am Geriatr Soc 2008;56(Suppl 2):S271–5.

56. Dyer CB, Pickens S, Burnett J. Vulnerable elders-when it is no longer safe to live alone. JAMA 2007;298:1448–50.

57. Burnett J, Cully J, Achenbaum WA, et al. Assessing self-efficacy for safe and independent living: a cross-sectional study in vulnerable older adults. J Appl Gerontol 2011;30(3):390–402.

58. Dyer CB, Goins AM. The role of the interdisciplinary geriatric assessment in addressing self-neglect of the elderly. Generations 2000;24:23.

59. Lawton MP, Brody EM. Assessment of older people: self-maintaining and instrumental activities of daily living. Gerontologist 1969;9:179–86.

60. Moye J, Butz SW, Marson DC, et al. A conceptual model and assessment template for capacity evaluation in adult guardianship. Gerontologist 2007;47:591–603.

61. Judicial determination of capacity of older adults in guardianship proceedings: a handbook for judges. American Bar Association and the American Psychological Association 2006. Available at: www.abanet.org/aging/docs/judges_book. Accessed January 5, 2009.

62. Appelbaum PS. Assessment of patients' competence to consent to treatment. N Engl J Med 2007;357:1834–40.

63. Cooney LM, Kennedy GJ, Hawkins KA, et al. Who can stay at home? assessing the capacity to choose to live in the community. Arch Intern Med 2004;164: 357–60.

64. Samton JB, Ferrando SJ, Sanelli P, et al. The clock drawing test: diagnostic, functional, and neuroimaging correlates in older medically ill adults. J Neuropsychiatry Clin Neurosci 2005;17:533–40.

65. Royall DR, Chiodo LK, Polk MJ. An empiric approach to level of care determinations: the importance of executive measures. J Gerontol A Biol Sci Med Sci 2005;60A:1059–64.

66. Dong X, Simon MA, Wilson RS, et al. Decline in cognitive function and risk of elder self-neglect: finding from the Chicago health aging project. J Am Geriatr Soc 2010;58:2292–9.

67. Pickens S, Ostwald SK, Pace KM, et al. Assessing dimensions of executive function in community-dwelling older adults with self-neglect. Clinical Nursing Studies 2014;2(1):17–29.
68. Burnett J, Hossain MD, Hochschild A, et al. Results from the first randomized clinical trial in elder self-neglect. Poster Presentation at the Gerontological Society of America Annual Scientific Conference. Boston (MA), November 18–22, 2011.
69. Burnett J, Pickens S, Aung K, et al. Caring for vulnerable elders reported to Adult Protective Services for self-neglect: a multidimensional approach. Poster accepted by the American Geriatrics Society 63rd Scientific Meeting, Orlando, May 12–15, 2010.
70. Barret MJ. Patient self-management tools: an overview. Oakland (CA): California Healthcare Foundation; 2005.
71. Burnett J, Dyer CB, Halphen JM, et al. Four subtypes of self-neglect in older adults: results of a latent class analysis. J Am Geriatr Soc 2014;62(6):1127–32.
72. Alexopolous GS, Raue PJ, Kiosses DN, et al. Problem solving therapy and supportive therapy in older adults with major depression and executive dysfunction. Arch Gen Psychiatry 2011;68:33–41.
73. Kiosses DN, Teri L, Velligan DI, et al. A home-delivered intervention for depressed, cognitively impaired, disabled elders. Int J Geriatr Psychiatry 2011;26:256–62.
74. Choi NG, Mayer J. Elder abuse, neglect and exploitation: risk factors and prevention strategies. J Gerontol Soc Work 2000;33:5–25.
75. Burnett J, Hochschild A, Diamond PM, et al. Results of a clinical trial to increase vitamin D deficiency in older adults who neglect themselves. Accepted for a poster presentation at the American Geriatrics Society 65th Annual Scientific Conference. Seattle (WA), May 2–5, 2012.
76. Butler RN. The longevity prescription: the 8 proven keys to a long & healthy life. New York: The Penguin Group; 2010.
77. Dong X. Advancing the field of elder abuse: future directions and policy implications. J Am Geriatr Soc 2012;60:2151–6.
78. Dong X, Simon M, Evans D. Elder self-neglect is associated with increased risk of elder abuse in a community-dwelling population: findings from the Chicago Health and Aging Project. J Aging Health 2013;25(1):80–96.

Evaluating Abuse in the Patient with Dementia

Pamela Tronetti, DO

KEYWORDS

- Elder abuse • Dementia • Interviewing • Victimization

KEY POINTS

- For patients with dementia, abuse ranges from subtle scams to outright physical violence. As dementia progresses, all forms of abuse escalate.
- The stages of dementia—mild cognitive impairment, mild dementia, moderate dementia and severe dementia—lend themselves to varied presentations of abuse.
- Knowing which types of abuse are more prominent at each stage aids the clinician in anticipating risk of abuse as well as patient and caregiver needs.
- Interviewing the victim is crucial in uncovering, documenting, and intervening in an abuse situation.
- A clinician who is skilled in drawing out the facts while remaining supportive of the patient is a key factor in ending the victimization.

HISTORICAL PERSPECTIVE

That the aged are neglected is obvious. There are books, journals, and societies devoted to the welfare of children; their number is increasing steadily. Aside from small organizations interested in particular homes for the aged, there is no general body interested in the welfare of the aged. There is no publication dedicated to this group…

—Malford Thewlis MD, The Care of the Aged (Geriatrics).[1]

Dr Thewlis, cofounder of the American Geriatrics Society, first penned this text in 1919, when the average life expectancy was 47.3 years.[2] He recognized elder abuse, but there was no formal reporting system, or even a name for it, until Burtson coined the term "granny battering" in a letter to the *British Medical Journal* in 1975.[3] That same year, the federal government released block grants to provide services for "vulnerable elders," the forerunner of adult protective services.[4] In the 1980s, researchers in the medical and social sciences sought to resolve basic questions such as "How do you define abuse?" "What is the extent of the problem?" "Who are the victims?" "Who are the abusers?" and

The author has nothing to disclose.
Parrish Senior Consultation Center, 805 A Century Medical Drive, Titusville, FL 32796, USA
E-mail address: Pamela.Tronetti@Parrishmed.com

Clin Geriatr Med 30 (2014) 825–838
http://dx.doi.org/10.1016/j.cger.2014.08.010
0749-0690/14/$ – see front matter © 2014 Elsevier Inc. All rights reserved.

geriatric.theclinics.com

"Where is abuse most likely to occur?" These answers were incorporated into the American Medical Association (AMA) guidelines for addressing elder abuse.[5]

DEMENTIA AND RISK OF ABUSE

One of the most disturbing findings during early research and guideline development was that, compared with the general population, patients with dementia were more frequent targets of abuse.[6–8] In retrospect, that conclusion seemed almost inevitable. By definition, dementia is a deterioration of intellectual function that ultimately leads to a decline in the ability to perform activities of daily living.[9] Patients with dementia have multiple cognitive impairments that include lack of insight and judgment, leaving them vulnerable to becoming victims of designing persons. As the disease progresses, the patients become more dependent on caregivers, who may or may not be equipped to handle the stress of care giving.[7,10,11]

Prevalence rates for abuse and neglect in people with dementia vary from study to study, ranging from 27.5%[12] to 55%.[13] Some studies relied on information gleaned from interviews of caregivers, others from victims of the abuse. Research based on caregivers' self-reported abusive behavior found that about half of all caregivers admitted to some form of abuse.[8,10] Another study of caregivers and care receivers detected mistreatment in 47.3% of participating dyads.[14]

A 2008 review article concluded that in general population studies, 6% of older people reported significant abuse in the past month, but 25% of vulnerable elders were at risk for abuse.[15] Vulnerable elders included those who were dependent on a caregiver due to cognitive or physical impairments. One difficulty with studies on abuse of patients with dementia is that many look at abuse as a single entity, rather than differentiating between physical, psychological/emotional abuse and neglect, although most rightly conclude that there is typically an overlap.[15–17]

Studies specifically evaluating psychological abuse indicate that psychological abuse is more common than physical abuse, ranging from 27.9% to 62.3%.[12,18] Physical abuse/violence was reported in the 1990s as ranging from approximately 6% to 12%,[19,20] although later review studies have found reports ranging from 1.4% to 23.1%.[10,11,20,21] Studies focusing on neglect show a prevalence rate of 4% to 15.8%.[14,16,20,22] Separate studies looked at financial abuse.[23,24] The prevalence of financial abuse is 30% of all substantiated elder abuse reports to adult protective services,[25] with evidence of worsening abuses as the patient becomes more helpless.[26] The prevalence of sexual abuse has been reported to be 0.6% of all substantiated reports of elder abuse.[27] However, in 2005, the National Center on Elder Abuse noted that 8.8% of abuse cases reported in nursing homes were sexual in nature.[28] According to the report, the likelihood of abuse was greater in facilities with a high percentage of residents with dementia and those with low staff ratios.[29]

Just as the term elder abuse is used broadly, many studies label participants with dementia globally, failing to specify their level of impairment.[27] Now the question arises "Are patients at different stages of dementia at higher risk for certain types of abuse?" Several studies have confirmed that as dementia progresses, so does the risk of all types of abuse.[26,30] There are also special considerations as dementia patients move from the community into assisted living facilities (ALFs) and nursing homes where institutional abuse can occur.[31–33]

Special Issues

There are some subsets of persons with dementia who are at increased risk for all types of abuse, including, but not limited to, those with a history of intimate partner violence and minorities, and those who experience prejudice, including racial and cultural prejudice.

Dementia in the Setting of Domestic Violence

Clinicians who deal with elder abuse must keep in mind that domestic violence does not end at retirement age. Domestic violence is a pattern of coercive (forceful) and controlling behavior that seeks to establish power and control over another person through fear and intimidation. It is behavior that physically harms, arouses fear, prevents an individual from doing what they wish or forces them to behave in ways they do not want. It can be physical, sexual, emotional, economic, or psychological actions or threats of actions that influence another person.[34] Being an abuser or a victim of domestic violence earlier in life is a strong predictor for becoming an abusive caregiver.[20]

Dementia in the Setting of Prejudice

As persons develop dementia, they are at increased vulnerability for abuse. This also includes persons in minority groups subject to prejudice. One specific group of people that the literature has not adequately addressed includes gay elders. For instance, lesbian, gay, bisexual, and transgendered (LGBT) individuals who are dependent because of physical or cognitive impairments are especially vulnerable to psychological abuse. Name-calling, blaming, and shaming are common. Some LGBT seniors may have closeted their sexual preferences for decades, and suffer when a caregiver threatens to "out" them to family and friends. Also, because most lesbian or gay couples are not married, there is no legal process to make sure that assets would be evenly divided if the healthy partner left the partner with dementia.[35] Meanwhile, gay caregivers also report a lack of support from medical, legal, and caregiver services.[36] Although research in the field of abuse of LGBT older adults is emerging as seen in the report "LGBT Older Adults in Long-Term Care Facilities: Stories from the Field,[37]" more attention to LGBT dementia patients and their caregivers, with particular emphasis on abuse in the home and institutional setting, would be welcome.

Defending the Caregiver

Among special considerations when caring for patients with dementia are false accusations. At some point, a clinician may find himself or herself on the other side, defending a caregiver who is being falsely accused of elder abuse. There may be a phone call at 3 AM from the police who need someone to confirm that the intruder they were called about is indeed a live-in caregiver. A jealous or vindictive relative may report a caregiver to adult protective services. The patient may accuse the family of financial abuse when actually it was the patient who spent all of his or her money while in the early stages of dementia. A mother may forget that her son visits for several hours a day and tell her neighbor that she has been alone for a week. Or a patient with dementia-related paranoia will accuse caregivers of various types of abuse. Of course, the patient's concerns must be fully evaluated at all times before allegations are deemed false. The professional's intimate knowledge of the patient, relationship with the family, and documentation will assist the dedicated caregiver during challenging situations.

STAGES OF DEMENTIA AND TYPES OF ABUSE

Researchers, clinicians, and other geriatric service professionals rely on various assessment tools to gauge the patient's level of dementia. These include the

Functional Assessment Staging Tool (FAST) and the Mini Mental Status Exam (MMSE). Sometimes the broader categories of mild cognitive impairment (MCI), and mild, moderate, and severe dementia provide a more descriptive explanation of the patient's multiple deficits.

Mild Cognitive Impairment (MCI)

MCI has been defined as "subjective and objective impairment in memory or other cognitive domains that represents a decline and is greater than expected for age, but is of insufficient severity to significantly affect activities of daily living."[38] A FAST score of 3[39] and an MMSE score of 23 to 27 are typical,[40] but should not be used diagnostically, as individuals with these MMSE scores may already have Alzheimer disease (AD) or another dementia. A thorough evaluation is required to differentiate MCI from the mild AD or other dementia. A 2013 study indicated that even MCI increases risk of abuse.[41] Most references to MCI patients and elder abuse have been in the category of financial exploitation.[42,43] One study focused on the affect of mild cognitive impairment on financial capacities such as bill paying and checkbook management. Those MCI patients who progressed to AD over a 1-year period demonstrated a dramatic deterioration in financial abilities.[44]

Financial exploitation

This is being monitored nationally. In 2010, Americans over age 60 lost about $2.9 billion to financial abuse.[45] This number includes numerous scams perpetrated by strangers,[46] such as health-related frauds in which the perpetrator poses as a legitimate medical supplier to sell bogus medical equipment services, or drugs. Sweetheart scammers create a profile on dating websites to entice the victim into an online relationship, and invariably request financial assistance. Money scams include investment scams, prize scams that require a fee for delivery, bogus charity requests, and distress calls by someone claiming to be a family member or friend who is suffering a legal or health catastrophe. Official scams via phone calls or e-mails warn of a problem with the bank account, credit card, Social Security check, or Medicare information, and ask for the victim's personal information to fix the problem.

Even though MCI patients are functional in a home setting, they may have memory difficulties, compromised executive skills, and other cognitive impairments that interfere with their ability to understand complex financial decisions and place them at risk for financial exploitation.[47,48]

Physical abuse

Very little has been written on physical abuse in patients with MCI. However, the Domestic Violence Network makes it clear that memory loss may frustrate and anger an abusive spouse.[49] Traumatic brain injury is common in abuse victims, which may lead to cognitive impairment, so there is a vicious cycle of memory loss followed by trauma and more impairment.[50]

Psychological/emotional abuse

These will continue in a domestic violence relationship.[51] Cognitive impairment may play a role of trapping the victim in a relationship, because now the victim has lost the ability to live independently even if he or she chooses to leave. An Italian study suggests that MCI patients may lose the ability to interpret facial expression, reflecting degeneration of brain structures modulating emotional processes. This may dull the patient's insight into the abusive nature of the relationship.[52] In general, victims of long-term abusive relationships have shown decreases in the perception of noxious stimuli,[53] so they learn to tolerate what others could not abide. Even new onset of cognitive impairment can increase risk of abuse,[54] so early identification of an at-risk partner is key.

Neglect/abandonment
Neglect in the strictest sense has a limited effect on a functional elder with MCI. However, because there is evidence that new cognitive impairment is associated with abuse and neglect, clinicians still need to remain alert.[30]

Sexual abuse/abusive sexual contact
Patients with mild cognitive impairment may be the victims of a coercive sexual relationship. They may also be victims of criminal sexual assault, but most often they know the perpetrator.[55]

Mild Dementia

Mild dementia is characterized by short-term memory loss and subtle but noticeable impairment in judgment.[56] Mildly impaired patients have a FAST score of 4[39] and MMSE of 20 to 24.[56] They have difficulty with complex tasks such as managing finances or medication regimens (bill and pills), are unable to work, and may have driving difficulty.

The types of elder abuse that a person with mild dementia may face include

Financial abuse. Half of all financial fraud is perpetrated by strangers, such as scam artists, gold diggers, and unscrupulous tradesmen. But family, friends, and neighbors accounted for 34% of financial abuse. This includes gifts and loans that were never repaid, coercion of impaired seniors to sign financial documents, and identity theft to obtain the senior's Medicare or Medicaid benefits or have access to bank accounts.[45] Financial abuse increases as the dementia progresses, with some families feeling justified as to their right to their elders' belongings and funds.[57,58]

Physical abuse. Physical and verbal abuse increase as dementia becomes more apparent.[26] Ninety percent of abusers are family members.[59] The traditional portrait of an abuser is that of a younger man with a history of substance abuse, violence, and dependence on the victim.[4]

However, a recent study highlighted that seemingly low-risk caregivers can become abusive. Long-time caregivers of patients with physical disabilities and mild-to-moderate dementia, who themselves have developed poor health, cognitive impairments, or depressive symptoms may start to display harmful behavior.[60] Calasanti and King's study on gender roles and caregiving noted that when women caregivers were faced with conflict (ie, "he won't bathe") they internalized the stress, because they were torn between enforcing compliance versus respecting autonomy. Men, however, prioritized the job of care giving over their wife's feelings. They believed that using force, coercion, or active restraint was an acceptable option to complete a necessary chore or assure patient safety.[61]

Psychological abuse. Spouses and caregivers of patients showing mild dementia often report frustration and anger with the patient because of repetition, atypical behaviors, and attitudes that may occur with the developing dementia. Verbal and psychological abuse increase as the dementia progresses.[62] Early intervention by clinicians is advocated, and includes counseling, providing educational caregiving books like *The 36 hour Day*,[63] enrolling caregivers in support groups, and directing them to Web sites such as cargiver.org and alz.org, which offer tips for dealing with troubling behavior.

Neglect/abandonment. In mild dementia, the patient may be unable to pay bills, plan healthy meals, manage medications, or shop efficiently. Yet it is possible that family members may be unaware of the deficits, because patients tend to minimize their symptoms and the extent of their disease. Often caregivers who are just learning of the diagnosis may unknowingly neglect the patient by not intervening soon enough to prevent a medical, financial, or legal catastrophe such as a foreclosure, utility shut off, or avoidable hospitalization. However, if the family is educated as to the patient's needs and they refuse to provide proper oversight and safeguards, then the professional must respond to this potential abuse situation.

Sexual abuse/abusive sexual contact. Patients with mild dementia may be taken advantage of sexually by spouses, significant others, or acquaintances.[55] They may also be the victims of criminal sexual assault. Because of judgment impairment, they may take risks such as allowing strangers into the home, not taking adequate precautions when out in public, or even getting lost in a strange neighborhood. They also may begin to have more disinhibited behavior.[64] This is especially true in frontotemporal dementia, which may be characterized by severe lapses in judgment, impaired social mores, and reckless choices. The very nature of the disease exposes patients to behavior that could result in financial and sexual exploitation.[65]

Moderate Dementia

At this stage, the patient requires assistance with activities of daily living. The average FAST score is 5,[39] and MMSE is 13 to 20.[56] The patient is now dependent on a caregiver. Because by definition people with moderate dementia require 24 hour care, many reside in ALFs. There are approximately 700,000 elders living in ALFs in the United States,[66] and 50% of those people have dementia.[6,31]

To elicit information about elder abuse in ALFs, one study reported on a survey of administrators and direct care workers in ALFs.[32] The results were tallied in number of estimated events per 1000 residents per year. The most common type of abuse according to the direct care workers was verbal abuse:

- Especially humiliating remarks (203)
- Swearing (173), critical remarks (163)
- Arguments with the residents (160)
- Physical abuse included throwing things at the resident (46)
- Pushing, grabbing, or pinching (41)
- "Hurting" the resident (35)
- Stealing things (44)
- Stealing money (22)
- Destroying belongings of the resident (36)

There were also reports of

- Not giving needed medication (43)
- Giving excesses medication (32)
- Withholding food (31) and fluid (25)
- Sexual abuse, including unwelcome touching (16)
- Unwelcome discussion of sexual activity (12)
- Exposure of private body parts to embarrass the patient (21)

Digital penetration was estimated to occur at a rate of less than 1 time per 1000 residents per year. The news media have provided more graphic examples, as evidenced in the 2001 Miami Herald 3-part series entitled "Neglected to Death," which cataloged horrific abuses in Florida's ALFs.[67]

The types of elder abuse that a person with moderate dementia may face include

Financial abuse. Because the patient is now dependent on someone else to intercept mail, phone calls, and e-mails, and to screen in-home workers, there is less chance of being victim to a stranger scam. They do remain at risk for financial abuse by the caregiver. This may include removing valuable items from the home, overcharging for services, demanding that the patient buy the caregiver big-ticket items such as cars or appliances, and use of the patient's credit and debit cards, telephone, Internet, and TV services.

Physical abuse. This escalates as patients' physical and mental health deteriorates. A recent study on use of physical violence against Alzheimer patients found that 17% of caregivers reported using it, but 26% of the patients reported being on the receiving end.[68] The patients studied had a diagnosis of Alzheimer dementia and an MMSE score of 16 or greater. Physical punishments are sometimes meted out for behaviors over which the patients have no control. Caregivers who do not understand, or do not want to acknowledge that the care recipient has dementia and therefore is not always responsible for their actions are at high risk of becoming abusive.[8,10,69,70] In a 2000 study, Ramsey-Klawsnik proposed categorizing abusers into 5 personality types, including the overwhelmed, the impaired, the narcissistic, the domineering or bullying, and the sadistic.[4,71] The research came from forensic investigation and interviews with victims and perpetrators. Overwhelmed caregivers were known to strike out physically under severe stress. Impaired offenders tended toward neglect. Narcissists were known to use physical abuse or threats as a means to an end, but generally tended toward financial exploitation, psychological abuse, and neglect. Domineering, bullying, and sadistic abusers perpetrated extreme physical abuse and deprivations.[71]

Psychological abuse. This type of abuse includes intimidation, humiliation, threats, and blaming the patient for what professionals would define as expected dementia behavior. Although not as dramatic as physical abuse and neglect (and often more difficult to document, report, and be accepted as a basis for an adult protective services investigation), it still significantly affects the victim, as evidenced by the increased mortality risk in community-dwelling elders who were victims of abuse or self-neglect.[29,62]

Neglect/abandonment. At this stage of dementia, neglect by a caregiver can have severe and possibly fatal consequences. At this point, the patient lacks the ability to survive independently, or even access help.[44] As noted, studies indicate a 4% to 15% rate of neglect in patients with dementia.[14,16,20,22]

Sexual abuse/abusive sexual contact. In 2006, research on elderly victims of sexual abuse indicated that patients with moderate-to-severe dementia were the most likely seniors to suffer sexual assault or abuse.[55] Other studies report that there is a high risk of sexual abuse in patients with dementia.[21,72,73] There is a growing concern for spousal sexual abuse, in which the dementia victim may be forced to have nonconsensual sex, especially by an established partner/spouse.[74,75] Research into the area of evaluating a patient's capacity to consent to sex has led to guidelines for the health care professional faced with this issue.[76]

Severe Dementia

The patient with severe dementia is at FAST stage 6 to 7,[39] with MMSE scores less than 12.[56] He or she requires total care, including decision making regarding safety, health, nutrition, and medication. A 2011 study of community-dwelling elders confirmed that the patients with severe dementia are at highest risk for physical abuse, emotional abuse, caregiver neglect, and financial exploitation.[26] But many of the severely impaired patients with dementia reside in nursing homes. Approximately 3.2 million Americans resided in nursing homes in 2008,[77] and this number is expected to grow. Of all nursing home residents, 42% to 66% have cognitive impairment, and 67% of all dementia-related deaths occur in nursing homes.[56] Patients with severe dementia and behavior problems are at highest risk for abuse.[56,78]

Several studies have looked at abuse of nursing home patients by staff. A study of 2000 nursing home patients found that 44% said they had been abused, and 95% said they had been neglected or witnessed another resident being neglected.[79] The residents who volunteered to be interviewed for this study had to demonstrate that they had "sufficient memory and comprehension to answer coherently." These more functional patients described abuse of frail and cognitively impaired roommates and friends in the facility.

A national report on abuse of residents in nursing homes noted that more than 9% of facilities were cited for abuse that resulted in danger or harm to the resident, and 1 out of every 3 nursing homes was cited for physical, sexual, or verbal abuse during the 2-year study period.[31,32]

Types of Elder Abuse That a Person with Severe Dementia May Face

Financial abuse
It is usually apparent to medical professionals that the patient has been exploited financially. However, often the damage is already done; the money is gone, and the patient loses access to higher-quality personal care because of lack of funds.

Physical abuse
This involves inflicting pain, but also isolating, confining, or restraining the patient.[15] This includes tying the patient to the bed, chair or commode, locking the patient within the house, or using medication as a restraint.[4] One study done in 2011 showed that patients with a low MMSE score were more likely to experience physical abuse as those with a higher MMSE score. The mean MMSE score for the elder abuse group was 21.9, and the mean for no elder abuse was 26.2.[26]

Psychological abuse
Similarly, there is a high rate of psychological/emotional abuse in severely demented patients. Community-dwelling elders are often threatened with placement (ie, "I swear I'm going to put you in a home!"). There is a correlation of length of time spent care giving, lower patient function, and perceived caregiver burden with elder abuse.[20,68] Some shocking displays of abuse have been discovered by hidden cameras placed by concerned family members.[80] A YouTube search for "hidden camera elder abuse" disclosed 12,600 results, many of which were graphic undercover videos of elder abuse in private homes and institutions.[81]

Neglect/abandonment
Patients with severe dementia are often the victims of neglect and abandonment.[82] This occurs when the patient is left alone, or if the caregiver is present but actively withholding care.

Sexual abuse
Although rare, sexual abuse of nursing home patients increases as the patients become more helpless. The perpetrator may be an employee, visitor, or resident of

the home.[55] Legal literature offers extensive discussions about elder sexual abuse in nursing homes,[28] and the news media paint a sordid picture, such as the *Chicago Tribune* article describing 86 cases of sexual violence in Chicago nursing homes from 2007 to 2010, with only 1 arrest.[83]

INTERVIEWING TECHNIQUES

Clinicians often speak with patients about very personal matters, such as substance abuse, embarrassing physical symptoms, and sexual concerns. To do this successfully, the patient has to be secure in the knowledge that the clinician will use this information to make life better. This skill of putting patients at ease is crucial in eliciting information from dementia patients about their abuse. Like other domestic violence victims, the elder abuse victim is overcome with conflicting emotions.[49] These may be fear of the future ("What will happen to me? What will happen to my caregiver?"), guilt, ("I should never have said anything to that nurse") shame, ("What kind of a mother am I that my son needs to hurt me?") and embarrassment ("Now the neighbors know all about it").

Some dementia patients may not comprehend the extent of abuse, or even be aware that it is a crime. They may minimize events or simply not recall them. This does not mean that they cannot be reliable witnesses, just that they may need to be evaluated appropriately to determine their level of dementia and interviewed using proper techniques. In fact there is evidence that emotional memories can be retained even in patients with dementia.[84]

General principles for interviewing older adults can be gleaned from many sources.[56,85,86]

The basic requirement is a safe, comfortable, private setting with the patient fed and rested, but not oversedated. If the patient is more lucid at certain hours of the day, the optimal interviewing time should be adjusted for this. Many patients with dementia are affected by sundowning, or alterations in cognitive function, typically occurring in the later afternoon.[56]

The key words in interviewing a victim of elder abuse, especially one with dementia, are respect and patience. The interviewer should sit at eye level/lip level, and make sure that the patient has glasses, hearing amplification, dentures, and proper attire. Good lighting is essential. The interviewer should avoid being backlit by sunlight or lamps, so as not to subject the patient to glare and eye strain. In a home setting, keep in mind that baby monitors and computers can be used to listen in on conversations.

Interviewers should start by explaining who they are, why they are there, and what they will be doing. They should ask the patient how they prefer to be addressed. They need to speak slowly and clearly, making sure that the patient can hear and understand. Only 1 question should be asked at a time, giving the patient the opportunity to absorb, process, and respond to the query. For some patients, especially with vascular dementia, processing speed is slow, and the time necessary for retrieval of information and expression is increased. In addition, if a patient is not able to answer a question, reframing it may yield more understanding and elicit a better response. For patients with receptive aphasia, the interviewer may need to use graphics or a writing tablet.

Conversely, the interviewer must make sure he or she understands the patient's answers if they have aphasia or word finding difficulty. Sometimes short-answer questions that require only a yes, no, or nod of the head are superior to those requiring complicated phrasing. The interviewer needs to avoid leading questions, which may result in the patient giving the answer they think the interviewer wants. They can, however, repeat the patient's answer to clarify their response (ie, "So, you were alone while your son was at work?").

Unless the interviewer can maintain eye contact while typing on a laptop, it may be best to take hand-written notes. Personal engagement and face-to-face conversation maintain an atmosphere of respect.

It is often helpful to start with general, disarming statements, such as "Many of my patients are having this problem. It's very common." or "Families are under such stress these days." This opens the door to allow the patient to tell their story without feeling singled out or judged.

But the medical interviewer should bear in mind that he or she is part of a team. His or her primary goal is to document the patient's level of dementia, the medical aspects of the alleged abuse, and assess the need for safe placement in a hospital or long-term care facility. Other professionals such as police officers, social workers, psychologists, or financial experts may be interviewing the patient and testifying within their area of expertise.

Documentation

Documentation of exact quotes is crucial. "He hurt my cat," followed by a written description gleaned from the patient's disjointed recollections paints the picture for law enforcement, social services, and other involved parties. Careful handwritten notes can then be dictated, with emphasis on the patient's words, the physical findings, and the memory testing and observations that clearly indicate the patient's level of dementia. Also, because the Medicare meaningful use of Electronic Medical Records (EMR) includes the ability for patients or caregivers to have Web-view access to their chart,[87] it may be prudent to place notes detailing observations and examinations for suspected elder abuse under a confidential note section of the EMR, or in a separate paper chart.

SUMMARY

Elder abuse has been documented in the geriatric literature for almost a century. There is now clear evidence that patients with dementia are especially vulnerable. Correlating the stages of dementia with the most likely types of abuse may increase the rates of detection by health care providers. Recognition of the victimization of this high-risk population is crucial for intervention and ending the abuse.

REFERENCES

1. Thewlis M. Neglect of the aged. In: Thewlis M, editor. The care of the aged (Geriatrics). 3rd edition. St Louis (MO): CV Mosby Company; 1941. p. 24–6.
2. Murphy SL, Xu J, Kochanek KD. Death: final data for 2010. Stat Report 2013; 61(4):2.
3. Bruston GR. Granny battering. BMJ 1975;3(5983):592.
4. Gorbien MJ, Eisenstein AR. Elder abuse and neglect: an overview. Clin Geriatr Med 2005;21(2):279–92.
5. American Medical Association. Diagnostic and Treatment Guidelines on Elder Abuse and Neglect. Chicago (IL): American Medical Association; 1992.
6. Dyer CB, Pavlik VN, Murphy KP. The high prevalence of depression and dementia in elder abuse or neglect. J Am Geriatr Soc 2000;48(2):205–8.
7. Hansbery MR, Chen E, Grobien MJ. Dementia and elder abuse. Clin Geriatr Med 2005;21(2):315–32.

8. Cooney C, Howard R, Lawlor B. Abuse of vulnerable people with dementia by their carers: can we identify those most at risk? Int J Geriatr Psychiatry 2006; 21(6):564–71.
9. Abrams WB, Beers M, Berkow R, editors. Merck Manual of Geriatrics. 2nd edition. Whitehouse Station (NJ): Merck & Co; 1995. p. 1146.
10. Cooper C, Sellwood A, Blanchard M, et al. Abuse of people with dementia by family carers: representative cross-sectional survey. BMJ 2009;338:b155.
11. Paveza GJ, Cohen D, Eisdorfer C, et al. Severe family violence and Alzheimer's disease: prevalence and risk factors. Gerontologist 1992;32:493–7.
12. Cooper C, Manila M, Katona C, et al. Screening for elder abuse in dementia in the LASER-AD study: prevalence, correlates, and validation of instruments. Int J Geriatr Psychiatry 2008;23(3):283–8.
13. Cooney C, Mortimer A. Elder abuse and dementia—a pilot study. Int J Soc Psychiatry 1995;10(9):735–41.
14. Wigglesworth A, Mosqueda L, Mulnard R, et al. Screening for abuse and neglect of people with dementia. J Am Geriatr Soc 2010;58(3):493–500.
15. Cooper C, Selwood A, Livingston G. The prevalence of elder abuse and neglect; a systematic review. Age Ageing 2008;37(2):151–60.
16. Compton SA, Flanagan P, Gregg W. Elder abuse in people with dementia in Northern Ireland: prevalence and predictors in cases referred to a psychiatry of old age service. Int J Geriatr Psychiatry 1997;12:632–5.
17. Pot AM, Dyck R, Jonker C, et al. Verbal and physical aggression against demented elderly by informal caregivers in the Netherlands. Soc Psychiatry Psychiatr Epidemiol 1996;31:156–62.
18. Yan E, Kwok T. Abuse of older Chinese with dementia by family caregivers: an inquiry into the role of caregiver burden. Int J Geriatr Psychiatry 2011;26(5):527–35.
19. Pillemer K, Suitor JJ. Violence and violent feelings: what causes them among family caregivers? J Gerontol 1992;47(4):165–72.
20. Coyne AC, Reichman WE, Berbig LJ. The relationship between dementia and elder abuse. Am J Psychiatry 1993;150(4):643–6.
21. Downes C, Fealy G, Phelan A, et al. Abuse of Older People with Dementia: A Review. Dublin (Ireland): NCPOP, University College Dublin; 2013.
22. Cooney C, Wrigley M. Abuse of the elderly with dementia. Ir J Psychol Med 1996;13(3):94–6.
23. Rowe J, Davies KN, Baburaj V, Sinha RN. FADE AWAY—the financial affairs of dementing elders and who is the attorney? J Elder Abuse Negl 1993;5(2):73–9.
24. Setterlund D, Tilse C, Wilson J, et al. Understanding financial elder abuse within families: exploring the potential of routine activities theory. Ageing and Society 2007;27(4):599–614.
25. National Center on Elder Abuse. The national elder abuse incidence study. Final report to the Administration on Children and Families and Administration on Aging. Washington, DC: US Department of Health and Human Services; 1998. 23(4).
26. Dong X, Simon M, Rajan K, et al. Association of cognitive function and risk for elder abuse in a community-dwelling population. Dement Geriatr Cogn Disord 2011;32(3):209–15.
27. Acierno R, Hernadez M, Amstadter A, et al. Prevalence and correlates of emotional, physical, sexual, and financial abuse and potential neglect in the United States: the National Elder Mistreatment Study. Am J Public Health 2010; 100(2):292–7.
28. Hawks RA. Grandparent Molesting: Sexual Abuse of Elderly Nursing Home Residents and its Prevention. Marquette Elder's Advisor 2012;8(1):159–97.

29. NCEA. Nursing Home Abuse: risk prevention profile and checklist. 2005. Available at: elderabusecenter.org. Accessed January 5, 2014.
30. Lachs MS, Pillemer K. Elder abuse. Lancet 2004;364:1263–72.
31. Gibbs L, Mosqueda L. Confronting elder mistreatment in long-term care. Ann Longterm Care 2004;12(4):30–5.
32. Castle N. An examination of resident abuse in assisted-living facilities. Research Report 2013. p. 3–39. Available at: https://www.ncjrs.gov/pdffiles1/nij/grants/241611.pdf. Accessed August 4, 2014.
33. Abuse of residents is a major problem in US nursing homes. Committee on Governmental Reform, Special Investigations Division, Minority Staff Report prepared for Rep. Henry A. Waxman. Washington, DC: US Government Printing Office; 2001.
34. Adapted from Florida Coalition against Domestic Violence. What is domestic violence? Available at: www.fcadv.org. Accessed October 14, 2013.
35. Mistreatment of lesbian, gay, bisexual, and transgender (LGBT) elders. Research brief: LGBT elders. National Center on Elder Abuse. Available at: http://www.centeronelderabuse.org/docs/ResearchBrief_LGBT_Elders_508web.pdf. Accessed November 16, 2013.
36. Moore WR. Lesbian and Gay Elders: Connecting Care Providers Through a Telephone Support Group. Journal of Gay & Lesbian Social Services 2002;14(3):23–41.
37. Available at: www.lgbtlongtermcare.org. Accessed February 23, 2014.
38. Epstein-Lubow G. Dementia. In: Wachtel T, editor. Geriatric clinical advisor: instant diagnosis and treatment. Philadelphia: Mosby Elsevier; 2007. p. P54–7.
39. Reisberg B, Jamil IA, Kahn S, et al. Staging dementia—principles and practice of geriatric psychiatry. Hoboken (NJ): John Wiley & Sons; 2010. p. 162–9.
40. Petersen RC, Stevens JC, Ganguli M, et al. Practice parameter: early detection of dementia: mild cognitive impairment (an evidence-based review): of the American Academy of Neurology. Neurology 2001;56:1133.
41. Kishomoto Y, Terada S, Takeda N, et al. Abuse of people with cognitive impairment by family caregivers in Japan (a cross sectional study). Psychiatry Res 2013;209(3):699–704.
42. Okonkwo O, Wadley VG, Griffith HR, et al. Awareness of deficits in financial abilities in patients with mild cognitive impairment: going beyond self-informant discrepancy. Am J Geriatr Psychiatry 2008;16(8):650–8.
43. Griffith HR, Belue K, Sicola A, et al. Impaired financial abilities in mild cognitive impairment: a direct assessment approach. Neurology 2003;60(3):449–57.
44. Treibel KL, Martin R, Griffith HR, et al. Declining financial capacity and mild cognitive impairment; a one-year longitudinal study. Neurology 2009;73(12):928–34.
45. Roberto KA, Teaster PB. The Met Life Study of Elder Financial Abuse: Crimes of Occasion, Desperation, and Predation Against America's Elders. New York: Met Life Mature Market Institute; 2011.
46. Top 10 scams targeting seniors. National Council on Aging. Available at: http://www.ncoa.org/enhance-economic-security/economic-security-Initiative/savvy-saving-seniors/top-10-scams-targeting.html. Accessed November 16, 2013.
47. Widera E, Steenpass V, Marson D, et al. Finances in the older patient with cognitive impairment "He didn't want me to take over." JAMA 2011;305(7):698–706.
48. Johnson K. Financial crimes against the elderly. Problem-oriented guides for police. Guide number 20. 2004. p. 1–88. Available at: http://www.popcenter.org/problems/crimes_against_elderly/. Accessed August 4, 2014.

49. Aravanis S. Late life domestic violence: what the aging network needs to know. Issue brief. Washington, DC: National Center on Elder Abuse; 2006. p. 1–13.

50. Jackson H. Traumatic brain injury: a hidden consequence for battered women. Prof Psychol Res Pract 2002;33(1):39–45.

51. Flannery RB. Domestic violence and elderly dementia sufferers. Am J Alzheimers Dis Other Demen 2003;18(1):21–3.

52. Spoletini I, Marra C, Dilulio F, et al. Facial emotional recognition deficit in amnestic mild cognitive impairment and Alzheimer disease. Am J Geriatr Psychiatry 2008;16(5):389–98.

53. Strigo IA, Simmons AN, Matthews SC, et al. Neural correlates of altered pain response in women with posttraumatic stress disorder from intimate partner violence. Biol Psychiatry 2010;68:442–50.

54. Lachs MS, Williams C, O'Brien S, et al. Risk factors for reported elder abuse and neglect: a nine year observational cohort study. Gerontologist 1997;37(4):469–74.

55. Burgess AW. Elderly victims of sexual abuse and their offenders. 2006. p. 1–37. Available at: https://www.ncjrs.gov/pdffiles1/nij/grants/216550.pdf. Accessed August 4, 2014.

56. Available at: www.alz.org/stages and behavior. Accessed December 3, 2013.

57. Conrad KJ, Iris M, Ridings JW, et al. Self-report measure of financial exploitation of older adults. Gerontologist 2010;50(6):758–73.

58. King C, Wainer J, Lowndes G, et al. For love or money: intergenerational management of older Victorians' assets. Protecting Elders Assets Study. Melbourne (Australia): Monash University; 2011. p. 1–46.

59. National Center on Elder Abuse. The National Elder Abuse Incident Study: final report. Washington, DC: Westat, Inc; 2011. Available at: http://www.ncoa.org/public-policy-action/elder-justice/faqs-on-elder-abuse.html. Accessed August 4, 2014.

60. Beach SR, Schultz R, Williamson G, et al. Risk factors for potentially harmful informal caregiver behavior. J Am Geriatr Soc 2005;53(2):255–61.

61. Calasanti TM, King N. Taking women's work like a man: husband's experiences of care work. Gerontologist 2007;47:516–27.

62. Dong XQ, Simon M, Evans D. Elder or self-neglect and abuse and mortality risk in a community dwelling population. JAMA 2009;302(5):517–26.

63. Mace NL, Rabins PV. The 36 hour day: a family guide to caring for people who have Alzheimer disease, related dementias, and memory loss. 5th edition. Baltimore (MD): The Johns Hopkins University Press; 2011.

64. Joller P, Gupta N, Gill SS. Approach to inappropriate sexual behaviour in people with dementia. Can Fam Physician 2013;59(3):255–60.

65. Snowden JS, Neary D, Mann DM. Frontotemporal dementia. Br J Psychiatry 2002;180:140–3.

66. Caffrey C, Sengupta M, Park Lee E, et al. Residents living in residential care facilities: United States, 2010. NCHS Data Brief 2012;91:1–8.

67. Barry R, Sallah M, Marbin Miller C. Neglected to death; three part series. Miami Herald 2011. Available at: http://www.miamiherald.com/news/special-reports/neglected-to-death/. Accessed October 13, 2013.

68. VandeWeerd C, Paveza GJ, Walsh M, et al. Physical mistreatment in persons with Alzheimer's disease. J Aging Res 2013;2013:920324.

69. Brodaty H. Family caregivers of people with dementia. Dialogues Clin Neurosci 2009;11(2):217–28.

70. Miller LS, Lewis MS, Williamson CE, et al. Caregiver cognitive status and potentially harmful caregiver behavior. Aging Ment Health 2006;10(2):125–33.

71. Ramsey-Klawsnik H. Elder abuse offenders: a typology. Generations 2000;2: 17–22.
72. Teitelman JL, Copolillo A. Sexual abuse among persons with Alzheimer's disease: guidelines for recognition and intervention. Alzheimers Care Today 2002;3(3):252–7.
73. Burgess AW, Phillips SL. Sexual abuse and dementia in older people. J Am Geriatr Soc 2006;54(7):1154–5.
74. Benbow SM, Haddad P. Sexual abuse of the elderly mentally III. Postgrad Med J 1993;69:803–7.
75. Ramsey-Klawsnik H. Elder sexual abuse: preliminary findings. J Elder Abuse Negl 1991;3(3):73–90.
76. Lichtenberg PA, Strzepek DM. Assessments of institutionalized dementia patients' competencies to participate in intimate relationship. Gerontologist 1990; 30(1):117–20.
77. US Department of Health and Human Services, Centers for Medicare and Medicaid Services. Washington, DC: Nursing Home Data Compendium; 2009.
78. Johannesen M, LoGiudice D. Elder abuse: a systematic review of risk factors in community dwelling elders. Age Ageing 2013;42(3):292–8.
79. Broyles K. The silenced voice speaks out: a study of abuse and neglect of nursing home residents. A report from the Atlanta Long-Term Care Ombudsman Program and Atlanta Legal Aid Society to the National Citizens Coalition for Nursing Home. 2000. Available at: http://www.atlantalegalaid.org/abuse.html. Accessed August 4, 2014.
80. Brooke C. Caught on camera, dementia patient's abuse by care staff: family of 89-year-old hid CCTV device in her room. MailOnline 2012. Available at: http:// www.dailymail.co.uk/news/article-2112563/Care-home-workers-caught-camera-beating-frail-dementia-sufferers-SPARED-jail.html. Accessed December 12, 2013.
81. Available at: www.youtube.com. Accessed December 12, 2013.
82. National Center on Elder Abuse. The 2004 survey of state adult protective services: abuse of elders 60 years of age and over. 2006. Available at: http:// www.ncea.aoa.gov/Resources/Publication/docs/APS_2004NCEASurvey.pdf. Accessed October 13, 2013.
83. Jackson D, Marx G. Nursing home sexual violence: 86 Chicago cases since July 2007—but only one arrest. Chicago Tribune. 2010. Available at: http://articles. chicagotribune.com/2010-01-26/health/ct-met-nursing-home-rape-20100126_ 1_rainbow-beach-care-center-faith-pavilion-state-records. Accessed January 15, 2014.
84. Wiglesworth A, Mosqueda L. People with dementia as witnesses to emotional events. Report to the Department of Justice 2011. Available at: https://www. ncjrs.gov/pdffiles1/nij/grants/234132.pdf. Accessed August 4, 2014.
85. Communicating with older adults: an evidence-based review of what really works. Washington, DC: The Gerontological Society of America; 2012. Available at: http://www.agingresources.com/cms/wp-content/uploads/2012/10/GSA_ Communicating-with-Older-Adults-low-Final.pdf. Accessed August 4, 2014.
86. Mosqueda L. Geriatric Pocket Doc; a resource for the non-physician. Irvine (CA): Center of Excellence on Elder Abuse and Neglect. University of California Irvine School of Medicine; 2012.
87. Eligible professional meaningful use core measures: measures 13. Eligible professional meaningful use set objectives number 12. Available at: https://www. cms.gov/ehrincentiveprograms. Accessed November 16, 2013.

Mental Health/Psychiatric Issues in Elder Abuse and Neglect

Claudia Cooper, PhD, MSc, BM*, Gill Livingston, MD

KEYWORDS

- Dementia • Abuse • Mental health • Neglect

KEY POINTS

- Elder abuse and neglect more frequently occur in people with dementia, particularly those with significant neuropsychiatric symptoms, compared with the older general population.
- People who screen positive for elder abuse are more likely to report depression, anxiety, and harmful use of alcohol.
- Those who are most dependent on others for care, especially when challenging behaviors cause the delivery of this care to be difficult and stressful, are particularly vulnerable.
- People who provide care to others are more likely to act abusively if they are depressed, experience anxiety, or have alcohol use disorders.
- Mental health services are often involved in the management of abuse, through assessing the capacity of people to decide whether to leave or report abuse, counseling them on how to handle abusive situations, and managing the psychological effects of abuse.
- Interventions to increase detection are urgently needed; potential barriers to reporting that should be considered when designing these interventions are reviewed.

PSYCHIATRIC RISK FACTORS FOR ABUSE

Dementia

People with dementia are particularly vulnerable to abuse because of impairments in memory, communication abilities, and judgment that make it difficult for them to avoid, prevent, or report the abuse. Many are reluctant to report abuse perpetrated by those on whom they depend.

Ninety percent of patients with dementia develop neuropsychiatric symptoms, including psychosis, overactivity, aggression, depression, and anxiety.[1] People who have neuropsychiatric symptoms are likely to be at increased risk of abuse. These symptoms and resultant challenging behaviors, including agitation, can cause frustration for carers. Some carers, especially those working long hours or who have

Division of Psychiatry, University College London, Charles Bell House, Riding House Street, London W1W 7EJ, UK
* Corresponding author.
E-mail address: claudia.cooper@ucl.ac.uk

Clin Geriatr Med 30 (2014) 839–850
http://dx.doi.org/10.1016/j.cger.2014.08.011   geriatric.theclinics.com
0749-0690/14/$ – see front matter © 2014 Elsevier Inc. All rights reserved.

psychiatric symptoms themselves (as discussed later), may react abusively. Abuse seems to be particularly prevalent in 24-hour care facilities, perhaps because of the high level of cognitive and neuropsychiatric morbidity among older people living in care homes (most of whom have dementia), together with the nature of the relationships between people with dementia and professional care workers compared with family carers. Although family relationships may be difficult and challenging, a family member acting as caregiver usually has a knowledge and understanding of the patient that predates the dementia. By contrast, the professional carer may only have known the person since they developed dementia, and thus may have less understanding of the person behind the illness. This unfamiliarity can contribute to a decrease in empathy and respect for that person's humanity, thus removing social and emotional barriers to abusive behavior.

Prevalence estimates are influenced, and possibly underestimated, by the fact that many people with dementia are unable, frightened, or embarrassed to report abuse. A wide range of prevalence figures are reported in the literature, possibly because of the different populations studied and the methods used to measure abuse.[2] No research study, to the author's knowledge, has asked older people with dementia to self-report abuse. Thus, although health care professionals who suspect or have evidence of abuse will ask people with dementia whether they feel safe, have fears, or recall abuse, and many people with dementia can give at least a partial account of their experiences, the number of people with dementia who would report abuse if asked is unknown. In this section we review the evidence that there is an association between abuse and neglect and dementia in studies interviewing family carers, professional carers and finally in studies that have used objective measures of abuse.

Family carers reporting abuse

A survey was conducted of family carers of people with dementia referred to older people's mental health team services in London (United Kingdom) and the surrounding area. Based on the Modified Conflict Tactics Scale, nearly half of the carers reported any abusive acts within the past 3 months and a third reported that abusive acts were happening "at least sometimes."[3] Using the severe violence subscale of the Conflict Tactics Scale, a previous study found that 5% of carers reported physical abuse in the year since diagnosis.[4] In other studies involving carers of people with dementia, 37% to 55% reported any abuse.[5–8] The act of abuse does not imply intent, and in many cases the carers may not have viewed their own actions in this light.

Evidence from these studies showed that people with dementia and neuropsychiatric symptoms were most likely to experience abuse from carers. In the CARD (Carers and Relatives of People with Dementia) study, carer abusive behavior was associated with neuropsychiatric symptoms in the person with dementia, and in particular with aggression toward the carer, but not with severity of dementia.[9] Cooney and colleagues[6] interviewed 82 Irish family carers of people with dementia and found significant associations between carer-reported verbal abuse and behavioral problems in the person with dementia. It is noteworthy that carers will admit to actions such as hitting, yelling, and rough handling of a loved one. Clinicians should therefore not shrink from asking about abusive behaviors in a direct and empathetic manner.

Professional carers reporting abuse

Professionals working with people with dementia have also reported high rates of abusive behavior. In one study that used a valid and reliable measure to examine elder abuse by professionals, 16% of a random sample of nurses and care attendants who had been working at one of several long-term care facilities in Taiwan for at least 6 months reported committing significant psychological abuse.[10] Other studies have shown that approximately 80% of nursing home staff had observed abusive behavior in the past year,[11,12] but only 2% of these instances were reported to the nursing home management.[13] This finding suggests that, unsurprisingly, professional carers are reluctant to report abuse, perhaps because of fears regarding loss of employment.

To find out more about the types of abusive situations that arise in care homes, the authors recently held qualitative focus groups with 36 care workers from facilities caring for people with dementia in London. The participants reported that situations with potentially abusive consequences were common, but deliberate abuse was rare. Some common potentially abusive circumstances were described as residents waiting too long for personal care or being denied care necessary to ensure they had enough to eat, were moved safely, or were not emotionally neglected. Some care workers acted in potentially abusive ways because they did not know of a better strategy or understand the resident's illness, and some workers made threats to coerce residents to accept care, or restrained them. In once instance, a resident at high risk of falling was required to walk because care workers thought he would forget the skill otherwise. Most care workers said they would be willing to report abuse anonymously.[14] Anonymous reporting may be an important next step in elder abuse research with professional carers, because until abuse can be accurately measured, the capacity to evaluate interventions to reduce its occurrence will be limited.

Objective Measures of Abuse

Objective measures of abuse, which identify signs of abuse such as a person being fearful, or having cuts or bruises, are less sensitive than self-report measures. A couple of large studies have used the Minimum Data Set for Home Care (MDS-HC) abuse screen, an objective measure, to report correlates of abuse in people receiving home care services. In the largest European survey of home care recipients to date (4000 people aged $\geq$65 years receiving health or social community services), those screening positive for abuse were more likely to be cognitively impaired, be depressed, have delusions, and be actively resisting care.[15] In a study that used this screen in 701 people aged 60 years and older seeking community-based home care services in Michigan between November 1996 and October 1997, participants' alcohol abuse, psychiatric illness, and short-term memory problems were significantly associated with signs of potential elder abuse.[16]

Depression and Anxiety

Several studies encompassing general older populations, clinic-based samples, and people with and without comorbid dementia have found that older people who are abused or neglected are more likely to be depressed than those who are not.[15,17–22] This relationship is likely to be bidirectional. Being a victim of abuse or neglect may be a stressor leading to depression, whereas being depressed may also lead to a greater vulnerability to abuse and neglect as a result of, for example, low self-esteem, poor concentration, and decreased motivation, leading to a lesser likelihood of reporting abuse. Although self-neglect is not considered a type of abuse in many research definitions, it is the most commonly reported form of elder mistreatment in the United States and is associated with increased morbidity and mortality.[23] One US study of 2812 older adults in the Established Populations for Epidemiologic Studies of the Elderly (EPESE) cohort found that cognitive impairment and symptoms of depression predicted the reporting of self-neglect to Adult Protective Services.[24]

Anxiety is recognized clinically to be a sign of elder abuse but has been less frequently studied as a potential associate of abuse in research studies. In the National Elder Mistreatment Study, participants who reported depression, anxiety, or irritability that limited their activities were more likely to report emotional abuse but not physical or sexual abuse, although the study probably had limited power to detect an association with sexual abuse, which is a rarer outcome.[25]

Alcohol Use Disorders

Mosqueda and Dong[23] reported a case study of a 70-year-old woman who neglects herself and dies despite multiple contacts with the medical community. They comment that, although no population-based study has examined the relationship between alcoholism and self-neglect, common sense and the investigators' clinical experience, which is also this article's authors' experience, suggest that the harmful use of alcohol is correlated with self-neglect. In the Caring for Relatives with Dementia (CARD) study, the alcohol intake of neither the care recipient with dementia nor the family carer correlated significantly with the amount of abusive behavior reported by the carer toward the care recipient.[26] Although the association between alcohol and aggression is well-known, these findings probably reflect the very low levels of alcohol use among carers of people with dementia, many of whom are older people (**Box 1**).

PSYCHIATRIC MORBIDITY IN PERPETRATORS

Reay and Browne[27] described a sample of 9 carers who had physically abused their elderly dependents and 10 who had neglected them. Heavy alcohol consumption and depression were associated with the act of physical abuse, whereas the perpetrators of neglect had significantly higher anxiety scores. Harmful use of alcohol predisposes to aggressive behavior, disinhibition, depression, vulnerability, and decreased self-care, and therefore its identification as a risk factor for perpetrating abuse is not surprising. Greenberg and colleagues[28] found that among 204 financially dependent adult children found to be abusing their elderly, dependent parents, 44% had alcohol or drug use problems.

At a regional level, Jogerst and colleagues[29] found that state-reported domestic elder abuse was significantly associated with a higher rate of any illicit drug use in certain regions in the past month. Their analyses indicated that this was due to an association with higher use of marijuana and cocaine rather than alcohol. This finding might reflect the fact that more abuse occurs in areas with higher crime incidence and poorer standards of living because people are living in more stressful circumstances,

Box 1		
Why psychiatric symptoms and disorders increase the risk of abuse and neglect		
Dementia	Impaired memory	Vulnerability
	Impaired judgment	Dependency
	Loss of personhood	Social isolation
Challenging behaviors	Resisting care	Decreased self-care
	Difficult relationship with carers	Decreased communication
	Aggression	
Depression	Decreased motivation	
	Decreased self-esteem, self-confidence	
Harmful alcohol use	Aggressive behavior, disinhibition, depression	

or that more health and community workers are working in areas with more compared to less social deprivation, and therefore more abuse is discovered. These findings suggest that if substance abuse is occurring in the home of an older person, this contributes directly to a more risky environment.

Family Carers of People with Dementia

Most research on the mental health of carers and elder abuse has involved family carers of individuals with dementia.[19] In the CARD study, the authors used the revised Modified Conflict Tactics Scale to explore what determined whether family carers of people with dementia self-reported abusive behavior. Interviews of 220 of these carers, who were consecutively referred to 4 mental health teams for older people in London (United Kingdom) and the surrounding area, showed that those who were more anxious and depressed were more likely to act abusively. Among the carers who were psychologically distressed, those who felt more burdened by caring or who used less helpful coping strategies, acted abusively.[26] This finding may be because their difficulties remained emotionally and practically unresolved.

As shown in one previous study,[17] caring for someone who is abusive was the strongest predictor of carer abuse. Abusive behavior may be a continued feature of an earlier aggressive relationship,[30] or it may be a symptom of dementia, with some carers shouting or occasionally hitting back in response to being abused.

Carer abusive behavior increased over a year, and this increase was strongly associated with an increase in depression and anxiety symptoms.[31] Perhaps carers who felt they had lost the person they knew to dementia were more anxious and depressed, and also more likely to abuse. Alternatively, carer anxiety and depression may have been associated with a lack of confidence in their ability to care, and thus a greater use of abusive rather than more helpful strategies for managing difficulties. Anxiety and depression also may have lowered the ability of carers to manage difficulties that arose, and therefore they were more likely to feel overwhelmed and react abusively. Although none of these explanations excuse abusive behavior, they can help clinicians understand the origin, and therefore prevent or intervene in situations of abuse at earlier stages.

Family members may become carers for many different reasons. The authors asked carers in the study what led to them becoming the primary carer, and then categorized the answer according to whether the reason was predominantly positive, neutral, or negative.[32] Nineteen family carers (17.1%) said they were the main carer because of the high quality of their relationship with the care recipient and their willingness to assume or suitability for the carer role. A further 22 (19.8%) said they were the main carer because of other potential carers' negative relationship with the care recipient and unwillingness to assume or lack of suitability for the role. Carers who gave the latter explanation tended to be more anxious at baseline, and to report higher rates of abusive behavior toward the care recipient a year later.

DETECTING AND MANAGING ABUSE IN PEOPLE WITH PSYCHIATRIC AND COGNITIVE ILLNESS
Detection

Even trained professionals underestimate the prevalence of elder abuse, and report that lack of confidence and knowledge regarding defining, diagnosing, and reporting abuse are important barriers to managing abuse effectively.[33] Only a minority routinely ask about abuse. This finding is important, because asking people about abuse helps detect it and identify it at an earlier stage, because many people, even those with dementia, will be able and willing to report it. Basing detection of abuse only on objective evidence means a high bar by which time people are, for example, bruised, dirty, or have pressure sores.

As discussed later, detection of abuse may be particularly challenging in people with dementia or other psychiatric illnesses.

Detecting abuse in a person with dementia and challenging behavior

In 2 UK studies and one Romanian study, health and social care professionals,[34] home care workers,[35] and medical students[36] were asked whether different strategies a family carer might use to manage a person with dementia who exhibited challenging behaviors, including wandering and refusing care, were abusive. In the UK studies, most professionals and students ($\geq$80%) considered trapping the person in an armchair using a table over the lap as abusive, but fewer than two-thirds considered locking the person in the house alone all day and fewer than one-fifth considered accepting when the person chose to be unclean, to be abusive strategies. Among Romanian home care workers, only 43% considered trapping the person in an armchair using a table over the lap as abusive, 23% considered locking the person in the house alone all day as abusive, and none of the workers considered accepting when the person chose to be unclean to be abusive.

Although the expert panel used standard World Health Organization criteria, which reflected United Kingdom and Romanian guidelines, to judge whether the strategies surveyed were abusive, views about what constitutes abuse vary among countries. For example, the item of accepting the choice of the person with dementia to be unclean was rated as abusive, because if a person does not have the capacity to understand what implications being unclean will have on their health, well-being, and social interactions, then a carer has a duty to act in the person's best interests, and not to do so is neglectful. However, a recent Australian study using the same vignette categorized this item as nonabusive, in line with the local state guidelines that it is the older person's choice to be clean.[37]

Making judgments about what constitutes abuse may be more complex in people with dementia, who lack the capacity to make decisions for themselves. Challenging behaviors often present dilemmas for health care professionals, wherein acting against a person's wishes to prevent abuse, such as by washing without consent, feels like an act of abuse itself. Family carers often feel they have to choose between 2 undesirable choices, such as locking a person in the house alone versus risk having the person wander. The clinical's role is to help carers find alternative options, such as day care or respite.

Assessing Capacity

A fundamental issue in managing the abuse of people with dementia and other psychiatric illnesses is whether they have the capacity to make decisions about how to manage the abuse. An older person with capacity may decline assistance and refuse interventions deemed appropriate by an abuse investigation, such as moving to alternative accommodations. People with capacity have the right to make decisions that involve risk. Services have a responsibility in these circumstances to ensure that such risk is recognized and understood by all concerned, and minimized whenever possible. An open discussion should occur between the individual and the agencies about the personal risks involved. In people who lack the capacity to make decisions regarding the abuse, usually because of dementia but sometimes because of other serious mental illness, decisions must be made in their best interests, taking into account their current views and previous known wishes.

Treating Psychiatric Symptoms

Providing interventions for mistreated older adults may reduce the emotional consequences of abuse, such as depression and anxiety. No specific evidence base exists to inform this work, but psychological therapy to allow discussion of the impact of abuse is likely helpful. Decreasing isolation may help treat psychological symptoms, rebuild confidence, and reduce the risk of revictimization. Psychological or other interventions may also be indicated for abusers, especially when it is a family member. Family therapy may be appropriate occasionally.

Supporting Carers

Social services seek the least disruptive, safest option for the older person in managing abuse. When the abuse is less severe, support services may be increased or the carer may be referred for support to attempt to alleviate the situation.

It is logical that if abuse of people with dementia often arises from carer stress, then interventions to reduce this stress may reduce abusive behavior (**Fig. 1**). Results from studies exploring the relationships between carer distress and elder abuse suggest that carers' psychological morbidity and dysfunctional coping strategies are potential targets for elder abuse prevention.[3] Coping style can change,[38] and psychological interventions promoting emotion-focused coping have reduced carer anxiety.[39] In addition, treatment to reduce neuropsychiatric symptoms such as aggression may also help, although limited evidence exists of effective and safe treatments of these symptoms.[40,41] A handful of studies have sought to reduce abuse in this way, but as yet no randomized controlled trials provide good evidence that this approach works.

A recent randomized controlled trial evaluated the START (STrAtegies for RelatTives) intervention, which sought to reduce depression and anxiety symptoms in family carers of people with dementia. Abusive behavior by carers was a secondary outcome. The program evaluated an 8-session manual-based coping intervention delivered by supervised psychology graduates. It consists of psychoeducation

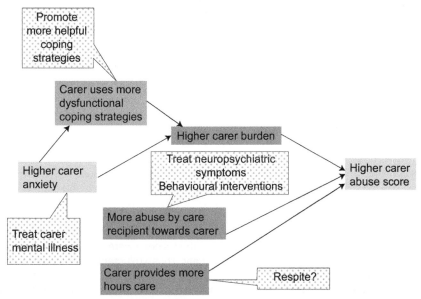

Fig. 1. How could family carer abuse be reduced? Dotted boxes denote possible interventions.

focusing on understanding dementia, carer stress, and where to obtain emotional support; understanding behaviors of the person cared for and behavioral management techniques; changing unhelpful thoughts; promoting acceptance, assertive communication, and relaxation; planning for the future; increasing pleasant activities; and maintaining the skills learned. The study was not powered to find a significant change in abuse and, for ethical reasons, clinicians were made aware of abuse; thus, some carers in the control group were offered clinical and social support. Nonetheless, a nonsignificant trend in the intervention group was seen toward the reporting of less abusive behavior 4 to 8 months later.[42]

Respite Care

Previous studies have found a link between providing more care and abusive behavior.[43–45] In Western cultures, more abuse by spouses is reported, who provide most dementia care,[46,47] whereas in cultures in which adult children usually provide this care, they abuse more.[22,48] Thus, respite care to give carers a break might help in some circumstances, although without additional interventions to change the situation in which abuse is occurring, this is unlikely to resolve the abuse completely.

Improving Detection of Abuse in Psychiatric Services

When the person being abused is unable to report the abuse, health and social care professionals have an even greater responsibility to be alert for abuse and to report suspicions. Abuse is often known about by other professionals or family members, but it may go unacknowledged if they feel no better management options exist. Staff who see abuse may leave it unreported and unchallenged for many reasons, including empathy with the perpetrators, fear of recrimination, inability to recognize abuse, lack of knowledge regarding how to handle it, or belief that procedures designed to deal with it are inappropriate and punitive.[49]

Understanding that abuse by family carers is often associated with stress, it is reasonable to conceive that finding ways to increase support may enable nonabusive care at home. If professionals think that reporting abuse is likely to help the older person, they are more likely to do so. In 24-hour care facilities especially, it is likely that abuse is often witnessed. Inquiries into abuse scandals have found that abuse was known about and sometimes reported months and even years before decisive action was taken to stop it.

Only one randomized controlled trial has sought to improve professionals' management of elder abuse.[50] Findings showed that educational seminars were more effective than printed material in improving knowledge about how to manage elder abuse among nursing and social care staff in a UK psychiatry service working with older people. In a second study involving in 2 London NHS trusts,[51] 40 trainee psychiatrists completed questionnaires measuring knowledge about managing and detecting elder abuse, before and immediately after a brief group education session. They were also asked how often they considered, asked about, detected, and managed elder abuse, and their confidence in doing so. Knowledge of how to manage and detect elder abuse significantly improved after the educational intervention, and vigilance for signs of and confidence in managing abuse were also higher 3 months after the intervention. Despite this greater confidence and vigilance, the trainees were not asking older people and their carers about abuse more frequently. Those reluctant to do so reported a range of reasons in addition to lack of knowledge, such as fear of a breakdown in their therapeutic relationship or causing offense, a reluctance to ask without having evidence, and uncertainty regarding how to ask people with dementia about abuse. The intervention was brief and didactic, and seemed to change knowledge and

---

Box 2
Why professionals do not report abuse

Lack of knowledge/understanding of what constitutes abuse

Uncertainty regarding how to ask people with dementia about abuse

Inability to recognize abuse or lack of knowledge regarding how to handle it

Fear of a breakdown in therapeutic relationships

Fear of causing offense

Fear of recrimination

Fear of being wrong (reluctance to ask without strong evidence)

Empathy with the perpetrators

Belief that procedures designed to deal with the offense are inappropriate and punitive

---

awareness but not behavior. The authors suggested that incorporating a more interactive component into the intervention, including role play, communication skills training, and discussions to elicit and challenge concerns that screening for abuse might cause harm, could help change doctors' behavior so that they screen for abuse more frequently (**Box 2**).

PSYCHIATRIC CONSEQUENCES OF ABUSE AND NEGLECT

The impact of elder abuse on mental health is often more devastating, and takes longer to heal, than physical scars. In one of the few prospective cohort studies to investigate psychological outcomes in elder abuse, more than 12,000 older Australian women who were broadly representative of the national population of women aged 70 to 75 years in 1996 were followed for 12 years. Four subscales of the vulnerability to abuse measure were vulnerability, dejection, coercion and dependence. Women who scored positive on any of the first three of these scales report worse mental health over the next three years than those who did not.[52] Although numerous studies have shown a cross-sectional association between elder abuse and depression, this was the first study to show a longitudinal relationship and to confirm that abusive experiences in older people have a negative impact on mental health.[15,17–22]

SUMMARY

Abuse and neglect more frequently occur in elderly people with dementia, particularly those with significant neuropsychiatric symptoms, compared with the older general population. Elder abuse and neglect have also been associated with depression, anxiety, and harmful use of alcohol in those affected. This finding is unsurprising, because these disorders greatly increase the vulnerability of older people, through compromising cognitive and emotional abilities to avoid and respond to abuse. Those who are most dependent on others for care, especially when challenging behaviors cause the delivery of this care to be difficult and stressful, are particularly vulnerable. People who provide care to others are more likely to act abusively if they are depressed, experience anxiety, or have alcohol use disorders. Mental health services are often involved in the management of abuse, through assessing the capacity of people to decide whether to leave or report the abuse, counseling on how to handle abusive situations, and managing the psychological effects of abuse. Most abuse and neglect is undetected and unreported by health and social care professionals. Interventions to increase detection are urgently needed. This article reviews potential barriers to reporting that should be considered when designing such interventions.

REFERENCES

1. Ballard C, Oyebode F. Psychotic symptoms in patients with dementia. Int J Geriatr Psychiatry 1995;10:743–52.
2. Cooper C, Selwood A, Livingston G. The prevalence of elder abuse and neglect: a systematic review. Age Ageing 2008;37:151–60.
3. Cooper C, Selwood A, Blanchard M, et al. Abuse of people with dementia by family carers: representative cross sectional survey. BMJ 2009a;338:b155.
4. Paveza GJ, Cohen D, Eisdorfer C, et al. Severe family violence and Alzheimer's disease: prevalence and risk factors. Gerontologist 1992;32:493–7.
5. Compton SA, Flanagan P, Gregg W. Elder abuse in people with dementia in Northern Ireland: prevalence and predictors in cases referred to a psychiatry of old age service. Int J Geriatr Psychiatry 1997;12:632–5.
6. Cooney C, Howard R, Lawlor B. Abuse of vulnerable people with dementia by their carers: can we identify those most at risk? Int J Geriatr Psychiatry 2006;21:564–71.
7. Cooney C, Mortimer A. Elder abuse and dementia—a pilot study. Int J Soc Psychiatry 1995;41:276–83.
8. Homer AC, Gilleard C. Abuse of elderly people by their carers. BMJ 1990;301:1359–62.
9. Cooper C, Selwood A, Blanchard M, et al. Abusive behaviour experienced by family carers from people with dementia: the CARD (caring for relatives with dementia) study. J Neurol Neurosurg Psychiatry 2010;81:592–6.
10. Wang JJ. Psychological abuse behavior exhibited by caregivers in the care of the elderly and correlated factors in long-term care facilities in Taiwan. J Nurs Res 2005;13:271–80.
11. Goergen T. Stress, conflict, elder abuse and neglect in German nursing homes: a pilot study among professional caregivers. J Elder Abuse Negl 2001;13:1–26.
12. Pillemer K, Moore DW. Abuse of patients in nursing-homes: findings from a survey of staff. Gerontologist 1989;29:314–20.
13. Jogerst GJ, Daly JM, Dawson JD, et al. Iowa nursing home characteristics associated with reported abuse. J Am Med Dir Assoc 2006;7:203–7.
14. Cooper C, Dow B, Hay S, et al. Care workers' abusive behaviour to residents in care homes: a qualitative study of types of abuse, barriers and facilitators to good care and development of an instrument for reporting of abuse anonymously. Int Psychogeriatr 2013;25(5):733–41.
15. Cooper C, Katona C, Finne-Soveri H, et al. Indicators of elder abuse: a crossnational comparison of psychiatric morbidity and other determinants in the Ad-HOC study. Am J Geriatr Psychiatry 2006;14:489–97.
16. Shugarman LR, Fries BE, Wolf RS, et al. Identifying older people at risk of abuse during routine screening practices. J Am Geriatr Soc 2003;51:24–31.
17. Coyne AC, Reichman WE, Berbig LJ. The relationship between dementia and elder abuse. Am J Psychiatry 1993;150:643–6.
18. Dong X, Simon M, Odwazny R, et al. Depression and elder abuse and neglect among a community-dwelling Chinese elderly population. J Elder Abuse Negl 2008;20:25–41.
19. Dong X, Chen R, Chang ES, et al. Elder abuse and psychological well-being: a systematic review and implications for research and policy—a mini review. Gerontology 2013;59:132–42.

20. Dyer CB, Pavlik VN, Murphy KP, et al. The high prevalence of depression and dementia in elder abuse or neglect. J Am Geriatr Soc 2000;48:205–8.
21. Lachs MS, Williams C, OBrien S, et al. Risk factors for reported elder abuse and neglect: a nine-year observational cohort study. Gerontologist 1997;37:469–74.
22. Oh J, Kim HS, Martins D, et al. A study of elder abuse in Korea. Int J Nurs Stud 2006;43:203–14.
23. Mosqueda L, Dong X. Elder abuse and self-neglect: "I don't care anything about going to the doctor, to be honest…". JAMA 2011;306:532–40.
24. Abrams RC, Lachs M, McAvay G, et al. Predictors of self-neglect in community-dwelling elders. Am J Psychiatry 2002;159:1724–30.
25. Cisler J, Begle A, Amstadter A, et al. Mistreatment and self-reported emotional symptoms: results from the national elder mistreatment study. J Elder Abuse Negl 2012;24:216–30.
26. Cooper C, Selwood A, Blanchard M, et al. The determinants of family carers' abusive behaviour to people with dementia: results of the CARD study. J Affect Disord 2010b;121:136–42.
27. Reay AM, Browne KD. Risk factor characteristics in carers who physically abuse or neglect their elderly dependants. Aging Ment Health 2001;5:56–62.
28. Greenberg J, McKibben J, Raymond J. Dependent adult children and elder abuse. J Elder Abuse Negl 1990;2:73–86.
29. Jogerst GJ, Daly JM, Galloway LJ, et al. Substance abuse associated with elder abuse in the United States. Am J Drug Alcohol Abuse 2012;38:63–9.
30. Harris S. For better or worse: spouse abuse grown old. J Elder Abuse Negl 1996;8:1–33.
31. Cooper C, Blanchard M, Selwood A, et al. Family carers' distress and abusive behaviour: longitudinal results of the CARD study. British Journal of Psychiatry 2010;196(6):480–5.
32. Camden A, Livingston G, Cooper C. Reasons why family members become carers and the outcome for the person with dementia: results from the CARD study. Int Psychogeriatr 2011;23:1442–50.
33. Cooper C, Selwood A, Livingston G. Knowledge, detection and reporting of abuse by health and social care professionals: a systematic review. Am J Geriatr Psychiatry 2009;17:826–38.
34. Selwood A, Cooper C, Livingston G. What is elder abuse—who decides? Int J Geriatr Psychiatry 2007;22:1009–12.
35. Caciula I, Livingston G, Caciula R, et al. Recognition of elder abuse by home care workers and older people in Romania. Int Psychogeriatr 2010;22:403–8.
36. Thompson-McCormick J, Jones L, Cooper C. Medical students' recognition of elder abuse. Int J Geriatr Psychiatry 2009;24(7):770–7.
37. Hempton C, Dow B, Cortes-Simonet EN, et al. Contrasting perceptions of health professionals and older people in Australia: what constitutes elder abuse? Int J Geriatr Psychiatry 2011;26:466–72.
38. Lavoie JP, Ducharme F, Levesque L, et al. Understanding the outcomes of a psycho-educational group intervention for caregivers of persons with dementia living at home: a process evaluation. Aging Ment Health 2005;9:25–34.
39. Cooper C, Balamurali TB, Selwood A, et al. A systematic review of intervention studies about anxiety in caregivers of people with dementia. Int J Geriatr Psychiatry 2007;22:181–8.
40. Douglas IJ, Smeeth L. Exposure to antipsychotics and risk of stroke: self controlled case series study. BMJ 2008;337:a1227.

41. Livingston G, Johnston K, Katona C, et al. Systematic review of psychological approaches to the management of neuropsychiatric symptoms of dementia. Am J Psychiatry 2005;162:1996–2021.
42. Livingston G, Barber J, Rapaport P, et al. Clinical effectiveness of a manual based coping strategy programme (START, STrAtegies for RelaTives) in promoting the mental health of carers of family members with dementia: pragmatic randomised controlled trial. BMJ 2013;347:f6276.
43. Pillemer K, Suitor JJ. Violence and violent feelings: what causes them among family caregivers? J Gerontol 1992;47:S165–72.
44. Ploeg J, Hutchinson B, MacMillan H, et al. A systematic review of interventions for elder abuse. J Elder Abuse Negl 2009;21:187–210.
45. Pot AM, Dyck R, Jonker C, et al. Verbal and physical aggression against demented elderly by informal caregivers in the Netherlands. Soc Psychiatry Psychiatr Epidemiol 1996;V31:156–62.
46. Pillemer K, Finkelhor D. The prevalence of elder abuse: a random sample survey. Gerontologist 1988;28:51–7.
47. Podkieks E. National survey on abuse of the elderly in Canada. J Elder Abuse Negl 1992;4:5–58.
48. Chokkanathan S, Lee AE. Elder mistreatment in urban India: a community based study. J Elder Abuse Negl 2005;17:45–61.
49. Kitchen G, Richardson B, Livingston G. Are nurses equipped to manage actual or suspected elder abuse? Prof Nurse 2002;17(11):647–50.
50. Richardson B, Kitchen G, Livingston G. The effect of education on knowledge and management of elder abuse: a randomized controlled trial. Age Ageing 2002;31:335–41.
51. Cooper C, Huzzey L, Livingston G. The effect of an educational intervention on junior doctors' knowledge and practice in detecting and managing elder abuse. International Psychogeriatrics 2012;24(9):1447–53.
52. Schofield MJ, Mishra GD. Three year health outcomes among older women at risk of elder abuse: women's health Australia. Qual Life Res 2004;13(6): 1043–52.

The Role of Capacity Assessments in Elder Abuse Investigations and Guardianships

Erika Falk, PsyD[a],*, Nancy Hoffman, PsyD[b]

KEYWORDS

- Incapacity • Guardianships • Elder abuse and neglect • Dementia
- Capacity assessments • Capacity evaluations

KEY POINTS

- The term "capacity" is increasingly used in both legal and clinical settings.
- Capacity is decision-specific; some types of capacity primarily require the ability to decide while others also require the ability to demonstrate functional execution of tasks.
- Capacity evaluations should balance diagnostic (medical, psychological, cognitive) and functional data with assessments of risk, and values and preferences.
- The goal of a capacity evaluation is not diagnosis, but a clinical opinion about a decision-specific ability that can inform the level of protection warranted while preserving and optimizing remaining capabilities.

INTRODUCTION

Clinicians, protective services workers, and legal and law enforcement personnel must routinely decide whether an elder or dependent adult's decisions and actions can be constrained because they are impaired, or if intervention would be an unwarranted incursion on a person's rights. A person's capacity to make particular decisions or to engage in certain activities is often the determining factor in whether a situation is considered to be elder/dependent adult abuse and which type of protection is needed. Assessment of capacity is a relatively new and evolving field that integrates principles from the fields of law, medicine, and ethics.

Disclosures: None.
[a] Institute on Aging, 3575 Geary Boulevard, San Francisco, CA 94118, USA; [b] Assessment & Psychotherapy, 1330 Lincoln Avenue, Suite 110B, San Rafael, CA 94901, USA
* Corresponding author.
E-mail address: falkerika@yahoo.com

CASE EXAMPLE

Ms N. is an 88-year-old woman living alone in a single-family home in a large California city. She owns several apartment buildings in the city that she purchased when she was a medical professional working for the US Government. She came to the attention of Adult Protective Services (APS) when the fire department conducted a well-being check at the behest of a concerned neighbor; the firemen discovered severe hoarding. The Fire Department made an APS referral and APS discovered that she had appointed 5 persons as power of attorney to act on her behalf, several of whom were living rent-free in her apartment buildings and to whom she had paid considerable sums for unclear reasons. Unknown to APS at the time, Ms N. had recently been evaluated at a memory clinic, where it was found that she had mild cognitive impairment and, possibly, dementia. APS requested an additional evaluation that included an assessment of her capacity to live alone and manage her own finances. When APS and a psychologist went on a home visit to Ms N., she opened the door but refused to allow entry. She appeared thin and disheveled and was irate at the intrusion. From the threshold, piles of materials several feet high were visible and bad odors wafted from the dwelling.

The observations from home visits, allegations of financial abuse, and severity of the health and safety violations were sufficient to obtain a temporary guardianship for health care and finances while the investigation was conducted. Ms N. was briefly hospitalized in a psychiatric facility after becoming acutely distressed about the guardianship and making suicidal statements; however, she quickly stabilized without medication and was temporarily placed in a board and care. The psychologist was asked to conduct a capacity evaluation of Ms N.'s ability to live independently and to manage her finances; the purpose was to help determine if an ongoing guardianship of her person and estate was warranted. As part of the evaluation, the psychologist visited Ms N.'s home with the temporary guardian. Every area of the home was stacked high with materials, mostly new clothing with tags still attached and newspapers where her dogs would urinate and defecate. It was possible to touch the ceiling while standing on the detritus. Ms N. slept in an indentation in these materials in the living room; a single burner was used for heating canned goods. Despite her living conditions, Ms N. was found to be in robust physical health.

The psychologist evaluated Ms N. at the board and care. Her Mini Mental State Examination was 22/30 and her Independent Living Scales showed preserved functioning in most areas with the exception of memory, orientation, social adjustment, and the ability to manage her home and transportation. Scores from the Repeatable Battery for the Assessment of Neuropsychological Status (RBANS) were normal except for delayed recall, which was low average. Tests of executive functioning were normal (Clock, Trail-Making Test) and her calculation abilities were intact. Test results also suggested Ms N. was depressed, but she did not acknowledge any difficulties in functioning or any need for assistance in managing her home and finances.

The cognitive portion of the capacity assessment was consistent with the previous memory evaluation, and she was given a diagnosis of mild cognitive impairment. However, the psychologist also opined that Ms N. did in fact lack the capacity to live independently and to manage her finances, given the obvious deficits in her day-to-day functioning, poor insight, and the substantial risks to her assets and person. The court subsequently placed Ms N. under a permanent guardianship of her person and estate. The guardian began the process of cleaning out the home, and approximately $100,000 in cash and rent checks were discovered in a trash bag by the front door.

Ms N. was eventually able to move back home with part-time caregivers. Civil litigation was initiated against several of the tenants who exploited her financially.

CAPACITY: DEFINITIONS AND KEY CONCEPTS

In the broadest sense, the term capacity refers to an individual's physical or mental ability to perform an act or to make a decision, and is used in both legal and clinical settings. Formerly, it was common for capacity to denote a clinical opinion on which a legal decision about competency might be based. However, the term capacity is now used in both clinical and legal arenas.[1] The term capacity is task-specific and allows for more nuance than competency's "all-or-nothing" determination. In legal settings, capacity may refer to a judge's determination of a person's ability to make decisions or execute particular functions, or it may refer to an attorney's assessment of a client's ability to make decisions or perform certain acts. To avoid confusion, one approach is to use the terms legal capacity when referring to a legal determination and clinical capacity when referring to a clinician's determination about decision-making capacity.[2] Although a clinical capacity opinion is not a legal finding, it is often used as important evidence to inform legal proceedings, such as determining the need for guardianship.[3] One notable exception is the instance of treatment consent capacity; often a clinician's opinion is sufficient to activate the authority of a surrogate decision maker (eg, health care proxy or next of kin).[4]

Historically, capacity assessments were made by physicians, and were primarily based on a mental status interview and the presence of a diagnosis such as dementia or psychosis. Among the many problems with this approach are the following: capacity is not contingent on a medical or psychiatric diagnosis; it is task-specific and not global; decision-making ability may fluctuate; it can be affected by external factors; and it requires many different sources of data to allow a clinician to come to a reasonably well-informed opinion about a person's overall level of functioning. In the past 2 decades, capacity assessments have shifted from being a fairly minor part of legal and clinical practice to a distinct field of legal, clinical, and behavioral practice and research. The evolution of the field has led to a shifting emphasis away from diagnosis and global capacity determinations to a consideration of specific and functional abilities.[5] For example, a person with mild neurocognitive deficits may lack the capacity to manage complex financial holdings on a daily basis, but may retain the capacity to make or change a will.

An important distinction can also be drawn between decisional capacity (the ability to make a decision) and executional capacity (the ability to implement a decision). Decisional capacity is determined by 4 criteria: (1) the ability to understand the basic facts about a decision; (2) the ability to appreciate how the decision relates to one's personal situation, including one's strengths and limitations; (3) to be able to reason, rationally evaluate, and compare options and the consequences of alternative choices; and (4) to be able to make an informed decision.[6] The person must understand the implications of a decision and be able to take responsibility for the consequences of that decision. Executional capacity requires a person to be able to formulate a plan, adapt the plan in response to novel or changing conditions, and delegate tasks to appropriate others when they are physically unable to carry out the plan.[6] A person who is physically disabled and unable to execute a plan (eg, changing a wound dressing) may still retain decisional capacity (eg, decide whom to appoint to carry out the dressing change).

Capacity assessments in the context of elder abuse investigations must provide clinical, legal, and protective service professionals with relevant information. For example, an elder who has been defrauded of a significant portion of her assets who can articulate how she will respond if lottery scammers call her again (hang up, inform APS social worker, accept money management) might be unable or unwilling to carry out the plan (truly believes she will get her winnings, initially agrees to money management then refuses, is revictimized by the scammers). In this instance, the elder's ability to articulate a reasonable plan (decisional capacity) is irrelevant if she cannot, or will not, carry it out (executional capacity). Evaluators assess whether an elder is able to "articulate as well as demonstrate"[6] their decision-making capabilities.

Because capacity assessments in elder abuse investigations are often performed by clinicians (eg, physicians, psychologists) and used by legal professionals (eg, probate attorneys, district attorneys), it is helpful to note a few comparisons between legal and clinical approaches to capacity (**Table 1**). The utility of a capacity assessment is often related to how well the clinician can respond to a referral question by translating clinical findings into language that addresses the underlying legal standard in question. Legal professionals focus on "transactions," or whether a person can carry out an action (eg, make or change a will). The corollary from a clinical perspective is how well a person functions in various cognitive domains (eg, attention, memory, executive functioning).[1] Legal professionals often seek a binary yes/no, black/white response to whether a person has capacity for specific transactions. By contrast, clinicians tend to understand capacities as variable continuums, or shades of gray, between the presence or absence of capacity.[1] Finally, the law defines transactional capacity by means of simple templates that are sound conceptually, but may be difficult for clinicians to fulfill operationally. For example, the legal standards regarding testamentary capacity generally include: (1) the ability to understand the nature of a will; (2) knowledge of potential heirs and how they will be affected by a will; (3) knowledge of the nature and extent of one's assets; and (4) a general plan of distribution to heirs.[1,7,8] A clinical evaluation of a person's knowledge of potential heirs can be very challenging when the person has severe aphasia, has been married multiple times, or has a complex family system with natural, adopted, and/or step-children.

With increasing frequency clinicians are being asked to conduct an assessment of persons' capacity regarding their susceptibility to, or ability to resist, undue influence.

Table 1
Comparison of legal and clinical approaches to capacity

Legal	Clinical
Transactions: Can a person "transact" certain things, eg, make a will?	Domains: How well does a person function in various neuropsychological domains, eg, memory, executive functioning?
Binary: Is capacity present or lacking, black and white, like an on/off switch, seeks "yes" "no" answers	Continuous: Capacities are variable continuums in which there may be no bright lines
Conceptual: Offer a simple conceptual template but one that does not specify concrete tests that tap the abilities needed	Operational: Fills in the detail about operational abilities necessary to meet legal standard but must link to relevant legal standard

Adapted from American Bar Association Commission on Law and Aging & American Psychological Association. Assessment of older adults with diminished capacity: a handbook for psychologists. Washington, DC: American Bar Association and American Psychological Association; 2008. Available at: http://www.apa.org/pi/aging/programs/assessment/capacity-psychologist-handbook.pdf. Accessed December 28, 2013.

Undue influence is a concept from contract law that describes a dynamic whereby one person uses his or her power to deceptively manipulate and exploit the trust, dependency, and fear of another person, thereby gaining control over their decision making.[1,2] This dynamic is present in many instances of elder financial exploitation. Definitions of what constitutes undue influence and how it may be constrained in civil, criminal, probate, and protective service arenas are highly variable across jurisdictions. In the main, if consent to enter into a contract, transaction, or relationship is found to have been obtained through undue influence, it may be voidable. It is important that a person who retains capacity may still be victimized by means of undue influence. It is also true that cognitive vulnerabilities and factors such as isolation, dependency, or loneliness may render a person more susceptible to undue influence. Evaluations of undue influence take into consideration the vulnerabilities of the victim in addition to the behavior of the alleged abuser, the overall relational dynamics, and past or potential financial loss.

HOW IS CAPACITY ASSESSED?

A significant contribution to the synthesis of capacity research and practice are the handbooks for judges, lawyers, and psychologists produced by collaboration between the American Bar Association (ABA) Commission on Law and Aging and the American Psychological Association (APA) within the Assessment of Capacity in Older Adults Working Group. The workbooks are free and can be found at http://www.apa.org/pi/aging or www.abanet.org/aging. **Fig. 1** illustrates the conceptual

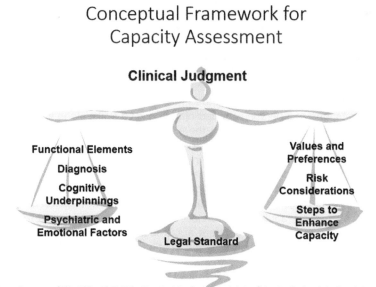

Source: Assessment of Older Adults with Diminished Capacity: A Handbook for Psychologists © American Bar Association Commission on Law and Aging-American Psychological Association

Fig. 1. Conceptual framework for capacity assessment. (*Adapted from* American Bar Association Commission on Law and Aging & American Psychological Association. Assessment of older adults with diminished capacity: a handbook for psychologists. Washington, DC: American Bar Association and American Psychological Association; 2008. Available at: http://www.apa.org/pi/aging/programs/assessment/capacity-psychologist-handbook.pdf. Accessed December 28, 2013.)

framework produced by the ABA/APA Working Group within the handbook for psychologists assessing older adults with diminished capacity. The framework focuses on issues relevant to older adults within the civil legal arena (eg, medical consent, financial capacity, testamentary capacity, driving capacity, sexual consent capacity, independent living). It is noted that questions regarding civil capacity may also arise in criminal proceedings, as when criminal or defense attorneys may inquire after a person's ability to manage his or her finances in criminal or exploitation cases. The framework stresses that a clinical judgment of capacity rests on a foundation of understanding the legal standard in question, and must balance diagnostic and functional factors against risk and values preferences. **Table 2** shows the elements of the framework for capacity assessment together with potential sources of information and resources.

There is currently no gold standard for assessing capacity in older adults, although advances in the field are leading to the development of specific tools to evaluate different types of capacity. Deficits in cognition can impair decision making and everyday functioning, as can psychiatric or emotional disturbances.[4] The challenge for the evaluator is to tie the underlying correlates of decision making into the overall finding about the capacity being assessed.[9] Therefore, all evaluations must begin by asking the referring party to clarify the referral question and type of capacity under consideration. A person can have the capacity to engage in one activity (eg, make a decision about a minor medical procedure), but not another (eg, make a decision about high-risk surgery). Each type of decision requires different cognitive abilities; a proficient evaluation will link a person's strengths and weaknesses to the specific decision for which his or her capacity is being assessed. A cognitive assessment alone will not necessarily reveal information about a person's ability to function in everyday life, but it does reveal information that may be important in understanding abuse, neglect, or undue influence in the determination of capacity.

A capacity assessment may lead to a clinical diagnosis, but the diagnosis is not usually the goal of the evaluation. The ultimate goal is to protect a vulnerable older adult from harm by determining cognitive and functional strengths and weaknesses, and offering an opinion about the ability of the elder to make a particular decision or carry out a particular act. Although a diagnosis may serve as a framework for understanding the limitations of a person with declining cognitive skills, alone it is not sufficient for a determination of capacity. To the extent possible, an evaluator should review the medical records and conduct a thorough clinical interview with this older adult. Collateral information is crucial, as many people give the impression that they function more effectively in their lives than they really do. Patients in the early stages of dementia often lack insight into the changes that are occurring in their lives, and therefore are not able to give an accurate and complete report. In cases of abuse or neglect, even an older adult who has no cognitive problems may protect the abuser out of fear of retaliation or concern about losing what little independence he or she may have. Therefore, collateral information should come from multiple sources.

Primary care physicians, nurses, and APS social workers are often the first clinicians to interact with an older adult, and may conduct an initial screening of a person's cognitive or functional status as part of their evaluation. Many physicians are now using computerized neuropsychological screening programs for basic information about a patient's cognitive strengths and weaknesses. Although these screenings can indicate the need for further evaluation,[10] they are rarely sufficient to determine a person's decision-making capacity. If a comprehensive assessment is warranted, the older adult should be referred to a neuropsychologist, geropsychologist, geriatrician,

Table 2
American Bar Association/American Psychological Association capacity assessment framework elements and information sources

Framework Element	Potential Sources of Information	Limited Specific Resources
Legal Standard: capacity assessments rest on a task that is legally defined and definitions vary between jurisdictions	Discussion with referring attorney, hospital counsel, local public guardian	The American Bar Association Commission on Law & Aging Web site may provide guidance: http://www.americanbar.org/groups/law_aging/resources/elder_abuse.html
Functional Elements: direct assessment of the specific capacity in question (eg, management of household, of finances). Often includes evaluation of activities of daily living (ADLs) (eg, grooming, dressing, eating, toileting, transferring) and instrumental activities of daily living (IADLs) (eg, managing finances, health, home/community functioning)	Specialized functional evaluation tools: eg, KELS, Independent Living Scales Screening grids (eg, Katz Index) Collateral reports from caregivers, friends/family, social services and medical providers Home visits and direct observation of tasks	Assessment of Older Adults with Diminished Capacity: A Handbook for Psychologists. Appendix B: Functional Assessments: http://www.apa.org/pi/aging/programs/assessment/capacity-psychologist-handbook.pdf Iowa Geriatric Education Center Functional Assessment Tools: http://www.healthcare.uiowa.edu/igec/tools/categoryMenu.asp?categoryID=5
Medical Diagnoses: medical diagnoses/conditions are key to consider; may be source of impairment, but may be reversible, may fluctuate	Medical records from primary care, hospital, skilled nursing. Often helpful if have records from time preceding impairment to present time- often several years	Assessment of Older Adults with Diminished Capacity: A Handbook for Psychologists. Appendix G: Medical Conditions Affecting Capacity: http://www.apa.org/pi/aging/programs/assessment/capacity-psychologist-handbook.pdf
Cognitive Underpinnings: cognitive functioning including insight and awareness of deficits; often a component of statutory standards for guardianship in many states. Cognition is influenced by many factors (eg, health status, stress, nutrition, medication) and deficits may be temporary or reversible, may fluctuate	Clinical interview and mental status examinations Record reviews, including scores from cognitive screening Cognitive screening (eg, MMSE, MoCA, SLUMS, RBANS) Neuropsychological batteries Third-party interviews/collateral reports	Assessment of Older Adults with Diminished Capacity: A Handbook for Psychologists. Appendix C: Cognitive Assessment: http://www.apa.org/pi/aging/programs/assessment/capacity-psychologist-handbook.pdf Iowa Geriatric Education Center Dementia/Delirium Assessment Tools: http://www.healthcare.uiowa.edu/iged/tools/categoryMenu.asp?categoryID=1

(continued on next page)

Table 2
(continued)

Framework Element	Potential Sources of Information	Limited Specific Resources
Psychiatric or Emotional Factors: presence of psychiatric/emotional disturbances may impair capacity if severe; also important to consider if reversible with treatment, support	Clinical interview and mental status examinations Record reviews, hospital and treatment summaries/discharges Symptom screening (eg, PHQ-9, GDS) Third-party interviews/collateral reports	Assessment of Older Adults with Diminished Capacity: A Handbook for Psychologists. Appendix D: Psychiatric and Emotional Assessment: http://www.apa.org/pi/aging/programs/assessment/capacity-psychologist-handbook.pdf SAMSHA-HRSA Center for Integrated Health Solutions: http://www.integration.samhsa.gov/clinical-practice/screening-tools
Values and Preferences: values are an underlying set of beliefs, concerns, and approaches that guide personal decisions, and preferences are preferred option of various choices that is informed by values. Extent to which current decisions are consistent with long-held values may be an indicator of capacity, but values may change. Important that mismatch between assessor and person being evaluated not be indicator of incapacity	Clinical interview Structured tools (eg, Five Wishes, Preferences for Everyday Living, POLST) Third-party interviews/collateral reports	Assessment of Older Adults with Diminished Capacity: A Handbook for Psychologists. Appendix E: Values Assessment: http://www.apa.org/pi/aging/programs/assessment/capacity-psychologist-handbook.pdf GoWish: http://www.gowish.org/ Physician Orders for Life-Sustaining Treatment: http://www.polst.org/
Risk Considerations: assessment of how risky individual decision is and what kinds of environmental supports and demands come into play. Should consider not only risk to individual under consideration but risk to others (eg, if driving)	Degree of social support: strong social support may mitigate some risk whereas lack of social support may increase risk	Hartford Institute for Geriatric Nursing (ConsultGeriRN.org) family caregiving: http://consultgerirn.org/topics/family_caregiving/want_to_know_more

Steps to Enhance Capacity: recommendations can inform the plan of care and are an opportunity for intervention	Can include anything from maximizing sensory deficits, to streamlining medications or adding caregivers	Assessment of Older Adults with Diminished Capacity: A Handbook for Psychologists. Appendix F: Interventions to Address Diminished Capacity: http://www.apa.org/pi/aging/programs/assessment/capacity-psychologist-handbook.pdf
Clinical Judgment of Capacity: considered synthesis of all framework elements, balancing structured assessments of medical/psychiatric conditions, cognitive/functional status vs risks/values/preference, and steps that could enhance capacity that culminates in answer to referral question based on legal standard	Comprehensive reports of capacity should make clear sources of information on which opinion is based, including list of test measures and results	Assessment of Older Adults with Diminished Capacity: A Handbook for Psychologists. See sample reports: http://www.apa.org/pi/aging/programs/assessment/capacity-psychologist-handbook.pdf

Abbreviations: GDS, Geriatric Depression Scale; KELS, Kohlman Evaluation of Living Skills; MMSE, Mini Mental State Examination; MoCA, Montreal Cognitive Assessment; PHQ-9, Patient Health Questionnaire; POLST, Physician Orders for Life-Sustaining Treatment; RBANS, Repeatable Battery for the Assessment of Neuropsychological Status; SLUMS, St Louis University Mental Status Examination.

Adapted from American Bar Association Commission on Law and Aging & American Psychological Association. Assessment of older adults with diminished capacity: a handbook for psychologists. Washington, DC: American Bar Association and American Psychological Association; 2008. Available at: http://www.apa.org/pi/aging/programs/assessment/capacity-psychologist-handbook.pdf. Accessed December 28, 2013.

neurologist, or geropsychiatrist (**Table 3**). Geropsychologists and neuropsychologists are in the unique position of being able to use standardized tests to assess the full range of cognitive functioning, allowing the clinician to determine an elder's strengths and weaknesses. Standardized tests help to keep the capacity evaluation from being vague and subjective.[1] Standardized tests use norms to compare the functioning of one person with that of a large sample of test-takers who represent the population for whom the test was designed. Functional abilities are also assessed (usually through interviews with informants and the use of collateral measures) and integrated into the overall picture. Independent living requires the ability to safely perform activities of daily living (ADLs) and instrumental activities of daily living (IADLs). These parameters can be assessed by asking a close friend, family member, or caregiver to complete 2 measures, the Katz Index of Independence in Activities of Daily Living and the Lawton Instrumental Activities of Daily Living Scale (see **Table 2**), both of which are readily available on the Internet. Interactions between the older adult and caregivers or other adults who may be living in the home are also important to observe and note.[11] Most elder abuse occurs behind closed doors, and the most common perpetrators are family members.[12] It is therefore important to be a good observer of

Table 3	
Clinicians working with older adults	
Primary care doctor, internist	An MD trained in the recognition and treatment of acute and chronic illnesses in patients across the life span. Often the "gatekeeper" in modern medicine
Geriatrician	A physician who specializes in the diagnosis and treatment of diseases and conditions in older adults
Neurologist	A physician who specializes in the diagnosis and treatment of diseases of the nervous system; often called on to diagnose dementia and other diseases of the nervous system
Gerontologist	A clinician who studies the social, psychological and biological issues affecting older adults. Clinician may be an MD, PhD, PsyD, RN, or Master's level
Geropsychiatrist	A psychiatrist (MD) who specializes in the diagnosis and treatment of mental illness in older adults
Forensic psychiatrist	A psychiatrist who has additional training in the application of law to psychiatry
Neuropsychologist	A clinical psychologist (PhD or PsyD) with specialized training in the use of standardized tests for the assessment, diagnosis, and treatment of clients with cognitive, neurologic, medical, developmental, or psychiatric disorders
Forensic neuropsychologist	A clinical neuropsychologist who utilizes the data from a neuropsychological evaluation to answer a legal question
Geropsychologist	A clinical psychologist (PhD or PsyD) with specialized training in the mental health of older adults; focuses on the cognitive, behavioral, and developmental changes that accompany aging
Forensic psychologist	A clinical psychologist with additional training in the relationship of psychology and the law
Nurse/RN	A clinician with a 2- or 4-year degree trained in the care of the sick or injured in a hospital or doctor's office
Social worker/LCSW	A master's level clinician with specialized training in providing social services, often to the disadvantaged

Abbreviations: LCSW, licensed clinical social worker; RN, registered nurse.

interactions in the office, such as a family member being short-tempered or belittling toward an older adult, which may be an indicator of verbal abuse at home.

Assessment of executive function is of paramount importance in addition to assessment of intelligence, memory, language, and personality.[13] The term executive function refers to a set of high-level cognitive abilities that allow a person to successfully engage in goal-oriented, purposive, self-directed behaviors, including the ability to take initiative (eg, make a doctor's appointment when a health problem is noted) and respond to novel conditions and events (eg, stock up on food during a storm).[14] A person who has intact executive functions may have significant cognitive deficits but still be independent, self-supporting, and productive.[14] However, deficits in executive functions may mean a person is no longer able to perform successfully and independently, and may have difficulty managing interpersonal relationships. Some executive function deficits are obvious, even to the untrained eye. A person may begin to neglect personal hygiene, act impulsively, or lack self-control. Other deficits may be less obvious and attributed to "laziness" or depression. These deficits include problems with the initiation of activities, managing time, lack of motivation, noncompliance with medical treatment, and difficulty with follow-through (eg, the person who can articulate how to take insulin but fails to actually do so). Common everyday tasks such as making dinner, cleaning the house, or paying bills on time may become overwhelming as the brain structures that manage planning, initiation, and sequencing are impaired. Therefore, a decline in executive function is associated with a greater risk of self-neglect.[15] Neuropsychological test data should be integrated with observations outside of the testing environment (eg, the elder's home), along with a functional assessment, to determine a person's overall level of executive function.[16]

Most older adults express a desire to "age in place,"[17] and 80% of older adults live independently in their homes.[18] Aging in place is defined by the Centers for Disease Control and Prevention as "the ability to live in one's own home and community safely, independently, and comfortably, regardless of age, income, or ability level."[19] Successful aging in place is an ongoing dynamic interaction between the older adult and their environment.[20] A person's ability to interact successfully with the environment changes with age. For instance, a home requires ongoing maintenance that an older adult may no longer be able to perform independently, and a limited income may make hiring home maintenance services cost-prohibitive. Home safety requires that a house be clean and free of obstacles that may cause falls or present a fire hazard. Appliances need to work properly and be replaced when necessary. The electrical and plumbing systems need to be kept in good working order, and the roof needs to be secure and free from leaks. The yard should be well maintained to prevent falls and/or fire hazards, and the doors and locks need to be adequate to provide safety against intruders.

Although most adults value living independently in their own homes for as long as possible, vulnerable adults may not be able to continue to live at home without assistance. Vulnerability can be understood as the inability to practice self-care and/or to maintain an adequate living environment such that personal health and safety are threatened.[21] The assessment of vulnerability is important, as older adults at risk may no longer have the ability to protect themselves from neglect and abuse; however, clues to vulnerability are not always obvious in routine medical visits.[20] Some of the signs of vulnerability include changes in a person's usual pattern: they may begin to miss appointments, look disheveled, be unclean, make mistakes with their medications, or have difficulty with scheduling. Office staff may be the first people in a doctor's office to notice a subtle change. Although most routine clinical evaluations take place in the medical office or hospital, home visits offer the unique opportunity to assess the functional capacity of the older adult. Capacity assessments are essential evaluations to determine how successfully older adults can interact with their chosen environment.[11] An elder's "fit" with their environment (both the social and the physical environments) will have an influence on the determination of capacity.[22]

ROLE OF CAPACITY ASSESSMENTS IN ELDER ABUSE INVESTIGATIONS

Definitions of what constitutes elder abuse, and when a person may meet eligibility criteria for intervention from APS or law enforcement, vary widely between jurisdictions. Capacity assessments may help determine if intervention is warranted and, if so, what supports may be needed. One important guiding principle of APS is the right for individuals to refuse services.[23] However, APS, clinicians, and law enforcement often struggle with the following dilemma as stated by Linda Farber-Post, clinical ethicist and educator: "Honoring the wishes of a person with capacity demonstrates respect for the individual. Honoring the wishes of a person without capacity is a form of abandonment. The distinction, insofar as it can be reliably made, is critical."[6] While it is true that decisions about capacity are legal judgments enforced by the states, in practice most determinations of impaired or diminished capacity are made in the community by clinicians, APS workers, attorneys, and others who work with older adults.[6] In the case of Ms N., APS had to make a determination about whether Ms N.'s wishes that she be left alone be heeded. Was Ms N. a rugged individualist whose decision to refuse help was consistent with her dearly held value of independence? Did she understand her situation and could she live with the consequences? The issue was not only that Ms N. had a severe hoarding problem, or mild cognitive impairment, or some financially dubious relationships, but rather that she was unable to appreciate that she had the problems and take steps to correct them. It was APS's assessment of Ms N.'s entire situation, and their determination that she lacked sufficient capacity to practice appropriate self-care, that guided the decision to file for the temporary guardianship.

Some states have enhanced penalties for crimes committed against older adults, and in others elder abuse is not considered a crime; rather, abusive behavior toward an older adult can be prosecuted only if it fits within the definition of another crime, such as assault, theft, or fraud.[24] The following are examples of criteria for an act to be classified as elder abuse in various states: (1) the victim must have a debilitating illness or condition that compromises his or her independence or judgment; (2) a special relationship of trust, confidence, or dependency must exist with the abuse; (3) the act is intentional (thus excluding acts that are passive, or committed by a person considered incapable of intent); (4) the conduct results in injury, physical pain, or impairment; and (5) the act is an ongoing versus a single instance of abuse.[25] In some instances, therefore, a capacity evaluation may help elucidate whether the person in question is in a protected class warranting protective services or legal intervention because of vulnerability (eg, has dementia).

Table 4 shows the relationship between categories of elder abuse/neglect and the types of decision-specific capacities that may be at issue during an investigation. For example, financial exploitation can take many forms: it can range from a caregiver siphoning off grocery funds each week to deceptive annuity sales practices. One must be aware that there is no single capacity that underlies financial exploitation. Rather, those investigating an instance of elder financial exploitation may seek a capacity assessment to help determine whether the elder has or lacks a decision-specific capacity. For example, for an elder who was financially exploited by a handyman when he charged her multiple times for the same service, the specific decision-specific capacity may be her ability to enter into a contract. If she is found to have deficits that suggests she was of "unsound mind" at the time she entered into the contract, the contract may be legally voided. In some jurisdictions, damages may be awarded. Just as many cases of elder abuse involve multiple types of abuse, a capacity assessment may involve multiple types of capacity to be addressed. For example, in the case of Ms N., the referral question involved her ability to both continue to live independently and manage her finances.

Capacity assessments in elder abuse investigations are also used to help guide the type of intervention or support that may be warranted. Low social support among older adults is correlated with abuse, and high social support may be a protective factor.[26] In the case of Ms N., it was clear that the only people in her life were those who were financially dependent on her, from the tenants who lived rent-free to the boutique owner who sold her clothing she would never wear. Addressing her loneliness by finding caregivers who were appropriately monitored and increasing pleasurable activities (eg, getting her dog groomed) was important in helping her separate from many financially exploitive relationships. Uncovering and treating medical and psychological conditions and linking to appropriate services can enhance capacity and improve the quality of life for many older adults. For example, a woman with a long history of self-neglect who was isolated because she was embarrassed by her rotting teeth was able to get dental care, which improved her mood and self-esteem. A timely home-safety evaluation, whereby bathing equipment and a commode are installed, may well prevent falls and keep a person who is aging in place free from abuse.

Finally, capacity assessments can also guide law enforcement and protective services in determining how much a victim may be able to participate in an investigation or legal process. In many types of neurocognitive disorders, particularly Alzheimer dementia, verbal and social skills may remain intact when memory and other cognitive domains are compromised. This situation may make it difficult to assess the accuracy of a person's report of abuse, and a capacity evaluation may help quantify the nature and extent of the person's cognitive deficits to assist investigators. In another example, a capacity evaluation that identifies that an adult has a neurodevelopmental disorder (formerly called mental retardation) and was not able to understand the implications of signing over the deed to a home his mother left him, can assist prosecutors in charging the case under elder abuse/dependent adult statutes and in understanding his strengths and challenges as a witness.

ROLE OF CAPACITY ASSESSMENT IN GUARDIANSHIPS

Guardianships, also known as conservatorships, were designed to protect the interests of incapacitated adults, and older adults in particular. Guardianship is a relationship whereby a state court gives one person or entity (the guardian) the duty and power to make personal and/or property decisions for another (the ward).[27] Although there is variation from state to state, in general the guardian of a person possesses some or all power with regard to personal affairs (health and welfare) of the individual, while a guardian of the estate possesses some or all powers with regard to the real and personal property of the individual (guardians of the estate may also be referred to as fiduciaries). Guardianships are considered to be an option of last resort when other measures to protect persons and their interests have failed or prove to be unworkable.[27]

The court can order either a full or limited guardianship for an incapacitated person. Under full guardianship, wards lose the right to manage their own finances, buy or sell property, make medical decisions for themselves, get married, vote in elections, and

Table 4
Categories of elder abuse and types of capacity evaluations commonly requested

Category of Elder Abuse/Neglect	Types of Capacity Assessments Commonly Requested	Scope/Nature of Abilities Assessed[a]	Most Common Uses of Assessment	Examples
Financial exploitation	Ability to manage finances	Broad; involves cognitive and functional skills	APS investigating if abuse occurred; guardianship proceedings; powers of attorney to "spring" into effect	Elder repeatedly falling victim to lottery/telemarketing scams; unable to manage routine financial matters
	Ability to contract	Narrow; primarily a cognitive task	APS investigating if abuse occurred; guardianship proceedings; civil and criminal elder abuse proceedings	Appoints power of attorney who appropriates assets; enters into annuity that rewards seller and not buyer; marries exploiter
	Testamentary capacity	Narrow; primarily a cognitive task	APS investigating if abuse occurred; guardianship proceedings; civil and criminal elder abuse proceedings	Siblings fighting about recent change in mother's will favoring one child over another (will contest)
	Susceptibility to and/or ability to resist undue influence	Broad and highly variable depending on state laws; often involves evaluation of cognition and relational/situational variables	APS investigating if abuse occurred; guardianship proceedings; civil and criminal elder abuse proceedings	Sweetheart scams; caregiver isolates victim and threatens to abandon her if she doesn't give her a car
Self-neglect	Ability to consent to medical treatment	Narrow; primarily a cognitive task	Medical professionals making treatment disposition; APS investigating if intervention warranted; guardianship proceedings	Elder rejects in-home nursing care and wounds become life-threateningly infected
	Ability to live independently	Broad; involves cognitive and functional skills	Medical professionals making treatment disposition; APS investigating if intervention warranted; guardianship proceedings	Person has long history of unabated hoarding and unable to leave dwelling but refuses help

Neglect by others/abandonment	Ability to live independently	Broad; involves cognitive and functional skills	Criminal elder abuse proceedings; APS investigating type of intervention warranted; medical professionals making treatment disposition; guardianship proceedings	Bed-bound elder's daughter leaves mother unattended for days while at casino
Physical abuse	General cognitive assessment (not a civil capacity); possibly ability to live independently	Cognitive: ability to report abuse; accuracy of recollection; ability to assist in investigation and/or participate in prosecution. Functional: ability to execute a safety plan	Criminal elder abuse proceedings; APS investigating type of intervention warranted; medical professionals making treatment disposition; guardianship proceedings	Elder with mild dementia is physically assaulted by daughter
Isolation	Rare, but if so, likely susceptibility to and/or ability to resist undue influence or ability to live independently	Broad and highly variable depending on state laws; often involves evaluation of cognition and relational/situational variables	APS investigating type of intervention warranted; guardianship proceedings	Son intercepts mother's mail and all phone calls and keeps family and other visitors away
Sexual abuse	Sexual consent	Narrow; primarily a cognitive task	Criminal elder abuse proceedings; ombudsman investigation; care facility investigation	Care facility resident having sexual relationship with another resident
Emotional/psychological abuse (often co-occurs with other types of abuse)	Possibly susceptibility to and/or ability to resist undue influence	Broad and highly variable depending on state laws; often involves evaluation of cognition and relational/situational variables	APS investigating if abuse occurred; guardianship proceedings	Daughter berates mother, calls her names, threatens to keep grandchildren away unless she gives in to demands

[a] Adapted from Moye J, Marson D. Assessment of decision-making capacity in older adults: an emerging area of practice and research. J Gerontol B Psychol Sci Soc Sci 2007;62:4.

enter into contracts. For this reason, limited guardianships, whereby the guardian's powers and duties are limited so that the ward retains some rights (depending on their level of capacity), tend to be preferred.[27] Guardians may be family members, private professionals, or publicly funded guardians. After the initial investigation, if the person is found to be incapacitated, the judge appoints a guardian and writes an order describing the duration of the guardianship. The court has the authority to expand or reduce guardianship orders, remove guardians for failing to fulfill their responsibilities, and terminate guardianships to restore the rights of wards who have regained their capacity.[27]

Within the context of guardianships, capacity evaluations help courts determine whether a person meets the legal threshold for someone requiring protection. This aspect is particularly important in cases where deficits may be subtle and the risks are high, or in cases where the guardianship is contested. In some types of financial abuse, subtle cognitive deficits may have outsized effects on financial decision making.[28] Consider the case of a man in his 90s who had successfully and actively managed a large stock portfolio throughout his adult life, but in past months had started making risky investments that resulted in the loss of a substantial portion of his wealth. On cognitive screening, he did not seem impaired and dismissed his recent losses as bad luck or lacking in importance. On further evaluation, he was found to have marked deficits in executive functioning, and a collateral interview with his long-time stock broker revealed that his recent pattern of investing was radically different from his norm. In contested guardianship cases, as when siblings are arguing about who should have control of mother's finances, capacity evaluations, particularly if they are court-ordered and neutral regarding the source of payer, can provide data about a person's susceptibility to undue influence, testamentary capacity, ability to manage finances, and other factors critical in determining whether protection is warranted.

With the trend toward limited guardianship, one of the most important purposes of a capacity evaluation is to identify a person's strengths and preserved areas of ability. For example, if Ms N. had valued driving, she might have undergone a thorough driving evaluation through the Department of Motor Vehicles. In theory, if she had passed the functional and written examinations, she could retain her driver's license, with the possibility of recommendations to curtail her ability to drive at night, on freeways, over long distances, or in unfamiliar settings. Many fiduciaries may manage a ward's larger assets but leave the person in control of household expenses to the extent manageable. For example, a woman in her late 70s was the repeat victim of international lottery scams despite many attempts at remedies short of guardianship (eg, money management). She was mortified that she had been adjudged to lack the capacity to manage her finances, although she was not under guardianship of her person. Sensitive to her feelings, her guardianship stipulated that her retirement portfolio be managed by the guardian, and she was able to manage her other monies at her discretion.

SUMMARY

Capacity evaluations play an important role in determining whether a situation can be considered elder/dependent adult abuse and which type of intervention is warranted. Capacity evaluations must integrate multiple sources of data and focus on functional abilities. Understanding the legal standard underlying a decision-specific capacity is key in making a clinical opinion relevant in legal settings. Capacity evaluations for guardianships can help to identify preserved abilities and make recommendations to enhance decisional and functional capacities that promote the dignity and independence of victims of elder abuse and neglect.

REFERENCES

1. American Bar Association Commission on Law and Aging & American Psychological Association. Assessment of older adults with diminished capacity: a handbook for psychologists. Washington, DC: American Bar Association and American Psychological Association; 2008. Available at: http://www.apa.org/pi/aging/programs/assessment/capacity-psychologist-handbook.pdf. Accessed December 28, 2013.
2. American Bar Association Commission on Law and Aging & American Psychological Association. Assessment of older adults with diminished capacity: a handbook for lawyers. Washington, DC: American Bar Association and American Psychological Association; 2005. Available at: http://www.apa.org/pi/aging/resources/guides/diminished-capacity.pdf. Accessed December 28, 2013.
3. Moye J, Butz S, Marson D, et al. A conceptual model and assessment template for capacity evaluations in adult guardianship. Gerontologist 2007;47(5):591–603.
4. Moye J. Clinical frameworks for capacity assessment. In: Qualls S, Smyer M, editors. Changes in decision-making capacity in older adults: assessment and intervention. Hoboken (NJ): John Wiley & Sons; 2007. p. 177–89.
5. Moye J, Marson D. Assessment of decision-making capacity in older adults: an emerging area of practice and research. J Gerontol B Psychol Sci Soc Sci 2007;62(1):3–11.
6. Naik A, Lai J, Kunic M, et al. Assessing capacity in cases of self-neglect. Geriatrics 2008;62:26.
7. Mart E, Alban A. The practical assessment of testamentary capacity and undue influence in the elderly. Sarasota (FL): Professional Resource Press; 2011.
8. Grisso T. Evaluating competencies: forensic assessment and instruments. New York: Kluwer Academic/Plenum Publishers; 2007.
9. Sullivan KA. Civil capacity instruments: research trends and recommendations for future research. In: Demakis GJ, editor. Civil capacities in clinical neuropsychology. New York: Oxford University Press; 2012. p. 206–27.
10. White RF, James KE, Vasterling JJ, et al. Neuropsychological screening for cognitive impairment using computer-assisted tasks. Assessment 2003;10(1):86–101.
11. Falk E, Landsverk E, Mosqueda L, et al. Geriatricians and psychologists: essential ingredients in the evaluation of elder abuse and neglect. J Elder Abuse Negl 2010;22:281–90.
12. Mellor J, Brownell P. Elder abuse and mistreatment. New York: Routledge; 2006. p. 133.
13. Demakis GJ. Introduction to basic issues in civil capacities. In: Demakis GJ, editor. Civil capacities in clinical neuropsychology: research findings and practical applications. New York: Oxford University Press; 2012. p. 3–16.
14. Lezak M, Howieson DB, Loring DW. Neuropsychological assessment. 4th edition. New York: Oxford University Press; 2004. p. 611.
15. Dong X, Simon MA, Wilson RS, et al. Decline in cognitive function and risk of elder self-neglect: findings from the Chicago healthy aging project. J Am Geriatr Soc 2010;58(12):2292–9.
16. Dugbartey AT, Rosenbaum JG, Sanchez PN, et al. Neuropsychological assessment of executive functions. Semin Clin Neuropsychiatry 1999;4(1):5–12.

17. Nicholas Farber, Douglas Shinkle, Jana Lynott, et al. Aging in place: a state survey of livability policies and practices. Washington, DC: AARP Public Policy Institute; 2011. Available at: http://assets.aarp.org/rgcenter/ppi/liv-com/ib190.pdf. Accessed January 2, 2014.

18. Houser A, Fox-Grange W, Gibson MJ. Across the states: profiles of long-term care and independent living. Washington, DC: AARP Public Policy Institute; 2009. Available at: http://assets.aarp.org/rgcenter/il/d19105_2008_ats.pdf. Accessed December 26, 2013.

19. Healthy places terminology. In: Healthy places. 2013. Available at: http://www.cdc.gov/healthyplaces/terminology.htm. Accessed December 29, 2013.

20. Fausset CB, Kelly AJ, Rogers WA, et al. Challenges to aging in place: understanding home maintenance difficulties. J Hous Elderly 2011;25(2):125–41.

21. Naik AD, Pickens S, Burnett J. Vulnerable elders: when it is no longer safe to live alone. JAMA 2007;298:1448–50.

22. Naik AD, Kunik ME, Cassidy KR, et al. Assessing safe and independent living in vulnerable older adults: perspectives of professionals who conduct home assessments. J Am Board Fam Med 2010;23(5):614–21.

23. Adult Protective Services Association. About NAPSA: NAPSA (or APS) code of ethics. Available at: http://www.napsa-now.org/about-napsa/code-of-ethics. Accessed January 19, 2014.

24. United States Government Accountability Office. Elder justice: stronger federal leadership could enhance national response to elder abuse. Washington, DC: US Government Printing Office; 2011 (GAO Publication No. 11-208).

25. Nerenberg L. Elder abuse prevention: emerging trends and promising strategies. New York: Springer Publishing Company; 2008.

26. Acierno R, Hernandez M, Amstadter A, et al. Prevalence and correlates of emotional, physical, sexual and financial abuse and potential neglect in the United States: the national elder mistreatment study. Am J Public Health 2010; 100(2):292–7.

27. National Guardianship Organization. Guardianship of the elderly: past performance and future promises. Available at: http://www.guardianship.org/reports/Guardianship_of_the_Elderly.pdf. Accessed January 26, 2014.

28. Triebel M, Martin R, Griffith H, et al. Declining financial capacity in mild cognitive impairment: a 1-year longitudinal study. Neurology 2009;73:928–34.

Care of the Victim

Lidia Vognar, MD[a], Lisa M. Gibbs, MD[b],*

KEYWORDS

- Elder abuse • Victim • Adult protective services

KEY POINTS

- Elder abuse cases are expected to rise as the population ages.
- Health care professionals need to be familiar with providing ongoing care to elder abuse victims.
- Health care professionals need to be familiar with the legal system as it pertains to elder abuse victims.
- Victims of elder abuse have significant medical consequences including increased mortality and morbidity.

INTRODUCTION

Elder abuse has long been an underrecognized topic; however, at present, there is a sense of urgency to identify and elevate elder abuse as a topic of utmost importance. For health care providers, much emphasis has been given to recognizing and reporting elder abuse. However, these essential steps are the beginning of a process of caring for patients who are survivors of elder abuse. The care of the victim must be recognized as an equally important topic for research and education.

Definition

...he was non ambulatory and incontinent of bowel and bladder; his skin was caked with dirt and his carpet was soaked of urine; he had open ulcers on his legs; feces was on the floor; and his room was filled with roaches... (excerpt from Adult Protection Service case report, May 2012)

This is elder abuse, a problem that was first described in the 1970s as granny battering, a problem that has grown over the decades, and a problem that is expected to continue growing as the older adult population increases from 35 million to 72 million by 2030.[1]

Disclosures: None.
[a] Division of Geriatric and Palliative Medicine, Alpert School of Medicine, Brown University, 593 Eddy Street, Providence, RI 02903, USA; [b] Division of Geriatric Medicine and Gerontology, Department of Family Medicine, University of California, Irvine, 101 The City Drive, Orange, CA 92868, USA
* Corresponding author.
E-mail address: lgibbs@uci.edu

Defined by the National Research Council as "intentional actions that cause harm or a serious risk of harm to an older adult by a caregiver or other person who stands in a trust relationship to the elder, or failure by a caregiver to satisfy the elders' basic needs or to protect the elder from harm,"[2] elder abuse depicts a horrifying national health problem that can further be differentiated into six types of abuse: (1) physical, (2) emotional, (3) sexual, (4) financial, (5) neglect, and (6) self-neglect.

An estimated 1 to 2 million older adults living in the United States are victims of elder mistreatment annually.[3] More specifically, a study of cognitively intact older adults 60 years of age and older showed that 4.6% suffered from emotional abuse, 1.6% from physical abuse, 0.6% from sexual abuse, and 5.2% from financial abuse; in total, 11% reported being abused in the past year.[4]

Recent data show that elder mistreatment is not only detrimental to the individual being victimized but also to social, law, and health systems. Elder mistreatment has been associated with increased emergency room services; risk for nursing home placement; all-cause mortality[4]; and according to a recent prospective epidemiologic study, an increased rate of hospitalization.[5] Economic costs of elder mistreatment are also significant, with an estimated contribution of more than 5.3 billion dollars to the annual health care expenditure in the United States.[6]

Victims of Elder Abuse

There are presently about 39 million individuals older than age 65 and the US Census Bureau projects that number to rise to more than 62 million by 2025.[7] As of 2003, there were an estimated 1 to 2 million victims of elder abuse each year.[2] The oldest of the seniors, 80 years and older, are being abused and neglected at two to three times the proportion of all other senior citizens.[8] Women (67%) are also far more likely than men (32%) to suffer from abuse.[8] Such factors as longer life expectancy, increased dependency of elders on caregivers, fewer family members living in the same geographic regions, caregivers being elderly themselves, and an increased incidence of substance abuse and mental illness all predispose older adults to victimization.[9] Most perpetrators (90%) have a relationship with their victims: 33% are adult children, 22% are other family members, 16% are strangers, and 11% are spouses and intimate partners.[10] More than half of the alleged perpetrators of elder abuse were female (53%), as noted in the last National Center on Elder Abuse Study in 2004. Elder abuse transcends race, religion, and socioeconomic status and is encountered across all health care and community settings. As such, care of the victim falls not only to health care professionals but many different professionals, including agents from adult protective services (APS), law enforcement, and other community-based service programs.[11]

Health Care Response: Reporting

Given the clear prevalence of elder mistreatment, a busy clinician who sees between 20 and 40 patients daily could encounter at least one victim of elder mistreatment[12] during that time. However, according to an APS survey, health care professionals submitted only 11.1% of elder abuse reports; more specifically, physicians accounted for only 1.0% of reported cases. This is irrespective of the fact that virtually all states mandate reporting of suspected elder abuse by health care professionals.[4,13]

Aside from reporting issues, another major concern is that physicians and other health care providers who do not recognize elder abuse are ineffective at addressing the consequences of abuse in patient care. According to the American Medical Association, physicians may be the only person outside the family that an older adult sees regularly and as such, are in a key position to recognize and report elder mistreatment.[14] However, a survey of almost 400 family and internal medicine physicians showed that 63% had never asked their patients about elder abuse and only 23% believed elder abuse to be a significant problem in their own patient populations.[15]

Elder abuse has not historically been a formal part of medical education curriculum and poor case detection and reporting by health care professionals has often been explained by lack of sufficient knowledge of elder mistreatment definitions, types, risk factors, signs and symptoms, and the reporting process.[14,16] In the same survey mentioned previously, 98% of physicians stated that there should be more education on elder mistreatment, 96% thought education should be included in medical training, and 80% believed they had not been trained to diagnose elder mistreatment.[15] Unpublished data from a pilot study done by Lidia Vognar, MD in 2013, at the Durham Veterans Affairs (VA) Medical Center also showed poor baseline knowledge of elder abuse among health care professionals, including social workers, geriatric pharmacists, and internal medicine residents. Furthermore, respondents identified a lack of knowledge of how to intervene once elder abuse was identified.

Elder abuse education is not consistent or highly prioritized in many primary care residency programs[17] even though it is believed that exposure to elder abuse education should begin in medical school and continue throughout residency training.[3,18] Accreditation Council for Graduate Medical Education, the accrediting organization for medical residencies, requires geriatric training for all family and internal medicine residents; however, it does not specify the nature and quantity of exposure to elder abuse education, nor does it explicitly require geriatric training to provide elder abuse education.[3,19] However, geriatric fellowship training guidelines for elder abuse training are being developed as part of the Next Accreditation System. This change will provide uniformity to the highly variable training of even geriatricians in elder abuse.

The American Medical Association Council, however, recommends that physicians be able to institute measures needed to prevent further injury to the elder abuse victim, provide medical evaluation and treatment of injuries resulting from abuse and neglect, remain objective and nonjudgmental, attempt to establish or maintain a therapeutic alliance with family, and report all suspected cases in accordance with local statutes.[20]

Health Care Response: Working with Other Disciplines

Elder abuse cases tend to be peppered with multiple medical conditions, cognitive impairment, functional disabilities, and psychosocial issues; because of the highly complex nature of these cases, it is most helpful to have allied professional resources available. For the practitioner in private practice, APS social workers are essential, not only in terms of investigating the alleged abuse, but also by offering the client and family appropriate resources. Physicians in group practices or larger health systems may also have access to social workers and case management nurse specialists. In the VA setting, elder abuse cases are first investigated by VA social workers and, if substantiated, are further referred to state agencies, such as the Department of Social Services or APS. Health professionals can also proactively help patients by referring for necessary evaluations, including occupational and physical therapy for functional and gait assessments, and to a geriatrician, neurologist, or psychologist for cognitive testing to evaluate one's capacity for decision making.

A team approach is effective in the management of elder abuse cases involving older adults with multiple comorbidities. Clinically, comprehensive geriatric assessment teams should be used because they asses functional, medical, and social status, and develop further recommendations for care of the victim. Alternatives include a referral to a geriatrician for consultation. Outside of the health care setting, other teams include multiple agencies. Currently, there are five of the most well-developed teams, known as Forensic Centers, in the country. Forensic Centers may include physicians, nurses, social workers, APS caseworkers, law enforcement officers, prosecutors, clergy, and representatives from financial institutions.[21] Although the direct patient care provider does not refer to this team, it is helpful to know when these resources are available in one's area.

A societal response to elder abuse also includes improved education for other disciplines. Research has also shown that preprofessionals from other disciplines, including nursing, social work, law enforcement, APS, financial sectors, and community-based aging services, also do not receive adequate, if any, education on elder abuse. Police officers believed they lacked knowledge about elder abuse and did not feel prepared to deal with victimized elders. Social workers, even from APS, believed they needed a stronger skill set to work with victims of elder abuse, and the amount of required APS training was found to differ considerably among states.[1,22,23] Learning about each other's fields is a critical component to the education needed for effective intervention. For instance, nonmedical responders often use a resource of basic medical information focusing on the assessment of older adults called the Pocket Doc.[24]

Clinical Response

If suspicion for elder abuse arises during a clinical encounter, a general interview of the victim and alleged perpetrator should be performed separately in a comfortable and safe environment. The interview should be carried out with objective, nonjudgmental language and open-ended questions. It is imperative to remember and understand that victims are often reluctant to speak about being abused for many reasons. These may include love and protection of the perpetrator, mistrust of the system, denial, embarrassment, shame, or fear of retaliation by the perpetrator.[25] A thorough physical examination should follow with appropriate documentation of all abnormal findings. Photographs of physical findings are instrumental in tracking resolution of injury and are valuable to law enforcement officers. An intervention strategy with a coordinated plan across several disciplines should address the individual victim's need for treatment, education, and prevention.[26]

Safety of the patient is the first concern. Whether in the office, hospital, emergency room, or nursing facility, any discharge of an alleged victim must be prefaced with a safety evaluation. In many cases, the patient should not return home because of unsafe environmental conditions, inadequate or incompetent caregiving, or inability to care for one's self. Asking about weapons in the home is an essential part of the safety assessment. If one does not have proper access to food, shelter, and safety, is in danger of physical injury, or does not have the capacity to call for emergency assistance, alternative plans should be developed.

Cases of elder abuse where the victim has a cognitive impairment often require a capacity evaluation. Capacity evaluations are beneficial because they provide information about the intensity of caregiving needed for the victim; whether he or she requires guardianship; and whether the victim is able to reject offered services, such as APS intervention or other community-based services. All APS recommendations are voluntary and if a victim meets capacity, they have a right to decline services. If they do not meet capacity, they then may need a guardian or conservator.[27] In addition, a capacity evaluation may also help investigators determine if elder abuse occurred. This is especially important in cases of financial abuse, where an abuser asks or forces a victim to sign over assets. In some cases, it is possible to determine whether the victim had capacity when they signed legal paperwork.

If victims of elder abuse do not have capacity for decision making, and are at risk of hurting themselves or others, or of being hurt by others, APS caseworkers have the ability to obtain mental health warrants or emergency removal orders in some states. These orders usually require judicial approval and entail involuntary admission into a psychiatric or medical hospital. In other programs, mental health professionals or law enforcement may place a victim on a 5150 psychiatric hold and arrange for admission to the hospital. A 5150 hold provides a period of up to 72 hours for assessment, evaluation, and crisis intervention. This time period may be extended by health care recommendation and judicial intervention, but requires that ongoing assessment and evaluation be performed to justify a continued hold.[28]

After the initial report to APS and a safety assessment has been completed, health care providers may find that other interventions are needed. For instance, legal services may be needed to terminate an existing power of attorney or pursue a civil action to recoup lost assets.[27] If appropriate, instructing patient and families to contact banks or other financial institutions may stop further abuse while the case is being investigated by APS and, if involved, law enforcement. Of note, many employees of the financial industry are now mandated reporters, depending on individual state law.[29]

Careful discharge planning is important to ensure that the victim is being discharged to a safe, abuse-free environment, and that a short- and long-term plan is in place. Patients who are victims of neglect are at risk of being discharged home to neglectful caregivers unless all parties, including health care providers and case managers, are apprised of dangerous situations. Involving case managers, nurses, and social workers early during an inpatient admission allows for other care plan options to be considered. Similarly, if victims are participants in senior centers or daycare settings, staff at those programs should be informed so that they may intervene and protect their clients if needed. Discharges from nursing facilities should be carefully monitored.

Caregivers who are unable to safely take care of patients at home, may, nonetheless, request their discharge from long-term care because of financial reasons. They may use the elders' pension or social security funds for themselves rather than to pay for care in the facility. In these cases, caregivers should be questioned about their ability to offer the same level of care that a nursing home provides. If suspicions arise, physicians may report to the ombudsman while the patient is still in the facility and APS if the patient has already been discharged. Some of the most severe elder abuse neglect cases have been discovered by investigators in such instances (**Fig. 1**).

ELDER ABUSE SHELTERS

Discharge planning may also require emergency placement for elder abuse victims. There are very few shelters available for older adults. Although the shelter model has been used extensively for victims of domestic abuse, most do not meet the needs of the older population, who may have unique needs, including additional help with activities of daily living and instrumental activities of daily living. In response to this growing need, elder abuse shelters are starting to be developed across the nation.[30]

Elder abuse shelters may be located within existing nursing homes that have agreed to provide short-term emergency housing and health care services to victims who are often referred by emergency room staff, police officers, and social service agents.[30]

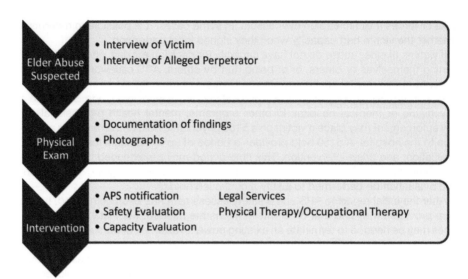

Fig. 1. Care of the victim of elder abuse.

Elder abuse shelters may also be freestanding. They allow multidisciplinary team members time to assess and adequately address cases of elder abuse while keeping the victim in a safe and protected environment.[31] Examples include the Hebrew Home in Riverdale, New York which was established in 2005, and Crest View Senior Communities in Minnesota, which has most recently replicated the Hebrew Home shelter model with great success.

CARING FOR THE VICTIM: LEGAL SYSTEM

Care of the elder abuse victim often requires legal intervention. State statutes protecting the elderly population did not exist until 1977. The first federal government legislation to address elder abuse was called Title XX of the Social Service Block Grant, which allocated funds for states to establish protective service programs for victims of elder abuse. By 1985, more than 44 states had enacted legislation concerning the care and protection of older adults. At present, all 50 states have legislation addressing domestic and institutional elder abuse, and have created systems to address elder abuse.[13] The statutes vary from state to state with regard to definitions of age at which a victim is covered, the definition of elder abuse, classification of criminal versus civil acts, reporting requirements, and remedies for abuse.[27] The protective services program, now called APS, was specifically created to help older individuals or persons with disabilities that are in danger of being mistreated or neglected and are unable to protect themselves. All health care professionals should be familiar with their own local APS agencies because APS can be a resource for a multitude of services for the victim and family if appropriate.

APS ethical principles for clients include the following[32]:

- Right to safety
- Right to retain civil and constitutional rights
- Right to decisions that may not mimic societal norms as long as they do not cause harm to others
- Right to accept or refuse all services for all adults

All adults are presumed to have decision-making capacity unless a court adjudicates otherwise. APS practice guidelines include the following[32]:

- Recognizing that the interests of the adult are the main concern of any intervention
- Respecting the individual's right to confidentiality
- Appreciating cultural, historical, and personal values
- Involving the adult in the development of a service plan
- Maximizing adults' independence as much as possible
- Using community-based services rather than institutionally based services whenever possible

APS caseworkers can intervene with services if the alleged victim wishes but also can intervene if the victim does not have capacity but is in imminent danger to self or others.[25] Emergency cases where there is imminent danger of harm to self or others have an urgent response time and nonemergent cases are seen anywhere from 1 to 14 days from the time of the report, depending on the local APS guidelines. Removal of victims from their homes is rarely done and only in the most severe of cases. In fact, APS social workers are mandated to offer the least invasive or restrictive options first. APS interventions may include arranging for housing services; emergency housing; cleaning services; home repairs; home modifications; obtaining medical services; referring to health care professionals; applying for health care benefits; addressing personal needs, such as food delivery, food stamps, or securing caretakers; providing service coordination; and serving as client advocates.

Legal interventions, such as involuntary admissions to psychiatric and inpatient medical wards, obtainment of guardianship or conservatorship, or removal of the elder from their home, are the most restrictive actions that APS can take and are only used when less invasive actions have failed or are not appropriate. These cases represent only about 7% of all interventions.[25] APS investigates all cases and within 30 to 60 days deems a case substantiated, unsubstantiated, or indeterminate based on their findings.

Also of importance to health care professionals are the mandatory reporting laws that exist in all 50 states, and the District of Columbia, for confirmed cases. Forty-three states mandate reporting of suspected cases and 30 states have penalties for failing to report elder abuse, making it of utmost importance for health care professionals to know the law in one's own particular state.[13] Under the mandatory reporting law, anyone who makes a report, testifies in court, or participates in a required evaluation is immune from civil or criminal liability, unless such person acts in bad faith or with malicious purpose.[13] Reporters are not expected to obtain proof of abuse, but rather to report suspicions of abuse and allow state agencies and caseworkers to investigate the allegations.[33]

GUARDIANSHIP AND OTHER LEGAL ISSUES

On an individual level, victims may need a plethora of legal services including powers of attorney assignment or arranging for guardianship or conservatorship of person or estate. It is not uncommon for older adults to retain the right to make decisions about personal care while requiring guardianship over financial affairs. Older adults or their families may turn to their health care provider for additional information or services. Health care professionals should be familiar with elder law attorneys as a potential resource. Some cases may require attorneys who are experienced in cases of financial abuse. Obtaining guardianship should only be reserved for the most serious of cases when victims do not meet capacity and are in danger of harm from themselves or others. Temporary guardianships can be obtained via the judicial system quickly when there is an emergent case. There are also limited guardianships, when the court limits the guardian's authority to matters beyond the wards ability to decide, and plenary guardianship, which leave the ward, or victim, with no ability to make personal or financial decisions on his or her own behalf. This is only appropriate if the individual is totally incapable of managing his or her personal or financial affairs; is decided by the court; and is usually petitioned by a state agency, such as APS.[13]

FINANCIAL ABUSE

Although all types of abuse are egregious and presented elsewhere in this issue, financial abuse is very common and health care providers should be aware of the signs. Presenting clues may be nonspecific and may include nonadherence to medications, worsening medical conditions, missed appointments, new financial concerns, depression, and functional decline. Financial abuse or exploitation is simply defined as "...the unauthorized use of funds and property..." and can include fraud, embezzlement, undue influence, and misuse of guardianship/conservatorship and powers of attorney.[34]

According to a recent MetLife Market Institute study, financial abuse costs victims about $2.9 billion[30] and can be very distressing to the victim and family members. It often entails complicated legal proceedings that may seem intimidating to those victimized and their families.

Health care professionals should be familiar with financial abuse to educate and provide victims with resources when appropriate. For instance, appropriate legal counsel may advise ways to stop the abuse and recover some assets. Financial exploitation may be prosecuted as actions for theft, burglary, forgery, mail fraud, possession of stolen property, extortion, and embezzlement. Most of these crimes are considered felonies and carry a fine and jail time.

Of note, physicians are commonly asked to complete financial forms for patients that authorize changes in payee status. This would allow payee representatives to receive the patient's social security or pension funds. If one is not sure of his or her patient's capacity to sign over this right to a payee, an interview alone with the patient, potentially followed by a referral for cognitive capacity, may be helpful. Other ways to help patients to protect their rights and assets may be to suggest oversight from a geriatric care manger, from a designated representative payee for all government benefits, or from shared powers of attorney so no one person can act alone.

MEDICAL CONSEQUENCES OF ABUSE

Elder abuse has serious implications on the overall health and well-being of elders who are victimized. Older adults have fewer options for resolving or avoiding abusive situations because of age, health, and limited resources, making this population more vulnerable and less able to recover from victimization. A single incident of mistreatment is more likely to trigger a downward spiral leading to loss of independence, a serious complicating illness, and even death.[35]

According to the Centers for Disease Control and Prevention, clinical signs of elder abuse can be categorized as physical and psychological. Physical signs include injuries, such as bruises, lacerations, persistent pain, nutrition and hydration deficiencies, sleep disturbance, exacerbations of existing chronic diseases, and increased susceptibility to new illnesses. Psychological signs include fear, anxiety, posttraumatic stress disorder, and depression.[36]

A victim's quality of life is often adversely affected by increasing dependence for activities of daily living, a sense of helplessness, social isolation,[37] and an increased risk for institutionalization. Victims of elder abuse have a higher 10-year mortality and morbidity than elders who have not been mistreated[4,37,38] and elder abuse is associated with higher use of emergency department services and higher hospitalization rates.[5] A higher prevalence of depression in victims of elder abuse compared with patients referred for other reasons was noted in a study by Dyer and Pavlik.[39] It is also estimated that the annual health care expenditures from elder abuse are more than $5.3 billion.[6]

ADDITIONAL SERVICES AND RESOURCES FOR ELDER ABUSE VICTIMS

There are many other collaborations and teams available to address elder abuse. Many professional agencies are developing collaborations regionally and nationally.[40] This information is presented so that health professionals are familiar with the entire elder abuse response system.

Multidisciplinary Teams

These teams consist of representatives from medical, social, and legal specialties that work closely with APS on complex cases. Alleged abuse cases are presented to the team for recommendations. Interventions may include medical evaluations for acute issues and capacity assessments, evaluation for guardianship, educating patients and families, troubleshooting, and offering possible services that may be of benefit.

Legal Intervention Teams

These teams address the legal issues that often arise in elder abuse cases. Often, victims have suffered abuse, neglect, and/or exploitation and need protection and advisement on financial management, probate, and guardianship.

Criminal Justice System

This system includes law enforcement officers who are first responders and investigators of elder abuse cases, and prosecuting attorneys who initiate charges against offenders and pursue prosecution in the criminal court system.

Civil Justice System

This system includes family, estate planning, tax, and probate lawyers who can seek court orders and guardianships; initiate lawsuits for theft, assault, and battery, conversion, breach of contract, and negligence; and appoint power of attorney agents and establish trusts.

Fiduciary Abuse Specialist Teams

Fiduciary abuse specialist teams have been developed to address financial exploitation cases. Members include law enforcement, APS, banking industry representatives, forensic accountants, elder law lawyers, probate investigators, and mental health professionals.

Elder Fatality Review Teams

Elder fatality review teams review deaths of elder persons for evidence of elder abuse involvement. Some teams focus on current active investigations, whereas others focus on education and policy.

Agencies on Aging

These are local agencies that were established under the Older Americans Act to provide information for older adults regarding community-based services, in home services, assistance with housing, and support of elder rights.

National Center for Elder Abuse

This national center was funded by the US Administration on Aging and serves as a national resource for national and state statistics and other pertinent and useful information on elder abuse.

Clearinghouse for the Abuse Neglect of the Elderly

This is the nation's largest archive, and houses published research, training resources, and government documents on elder abuse.

The American Bar Association Commission of Law and Aging

This organization provides legal guides and online brochures related to elder abuse (www.americanbar.org).

SUMMARY

Care of the victim and survivor of elder abuse is an area that needs further education and research. Health professionals are essential in addressing elder abuse, not only by recognizing and reporting, but also by being available to social workers, law enforcement, and court systems if medical expertise is needed. The health care professional's response also includes knowledge of the medical consequences of abuse over time and addressing major medical conditions, such as depression and functional decline. Continuity of care over time is also critical and may serve as one of the victim's few support systems because many will have lost contact with abusive family members and caregivers. An awareness of how other disciplines address abuse is also valuable because an effective response to elder abuse transcends many disciplines, including medicine, social work, state and federal agencies, and law enforcement.

REFERENCES

1. Policastro C, Payne B. Assessing the level of elder abuse knowledge pre- professionals possess: implications for the further development of university curriculum. J Elder Abuse Negl 2014;26:12–30.
2. Bonnie R, Wallace R. Elder mistreatment: abuse, neglect and exploitation in an aging America. Washington, DC: The National Academies Press; 2003.
3. Wagenaar D, Rosenbaum R, Herman S. Elder abuse education in primary care residency programs: a cluster group analysis, family medicine. Fam Med 2009; 41:481–6.
4. Mosqueda L, Dong X. Elder abuse and neglect, "I don't care anything about going to the doctor, to be honest...". JAMA 2011;306:532–40.
5. Dong X, Simon M. Elder abuse as a risk factor for hospitalization in older persons. JAMA Intern Med 2013;173:911–7.
6. Choo WY, Othman S, Francis DP, et al. Interventions for preventing abuse in the elderly (Protocol). Cochrane Database Syst Rev 2013;1:CD010321.
7. McCoy K, Hansen B. Special report: havens for elderly may expose them to deadly risks. USA Today 2004;1A.

8. Available at: www.bjs.gov. Accessed June 10, 2014.

9. Sengstock M, Hwaleck M, Petrone S. Services of aged victims: service types and related factors. J Elder Abuse Negl 1990;1:37–56.

10. National Center on Elder Abuse. The National Elder Abuse Incidence Study: final report. Washington, DC: Westat, Inc; 1998.

11. Sengstock M. Elder abuse: identifying and assisting the victim. Mich Fam Rev 1996;2:77–92.

12. Halphen J, Varas G, Sadowsky J. Recognizing and reporting elder abuse and neglect. Geriatrics 2009;64:13–8.

13. Koenig R, DeGuerre C. The legal and governmental response to domestic elder abuse. Orlando (FL): Elsevier Saunders; 2005. p. 383–98.

14. Schmeidel A, Daly J, Rosenbaum M, et al. Health care processionals' perspectives on barriers to elder abuse detection and reporting in primary care settings. J Elder Abuse Negl 2012;24:17–36.

15. Kennedy R. Elder abuse and neglect: the experience, knowledge, and attitudes of primary care physicians. Fam Med 2005;37:481–5.

16. Alt K, Nguyen A, Meurer L. The effectiveness of educational programs to improve recognition and reporting of elder abuse and neglect: a systematic review of literature. J Elder Abuse Negl 2011;23:213–33.

17. Wagenaar D, Rosenbaum R. Elder abuse: education in residency programs: how are we doing? Acad Med 2009;84:611–8.

18. Hazzard WR. Elder abuse: definitions and implications for medical education. Acad Med 1995;70:979–81.

19. American Medical Association, Accreditation Council for Graduate Medical Education. Available at: www.acgme.org. Accessed June 5, 2014.

20. Elder abuse and neglect. Council on Scientific Affairs. JAMA 1987;257:966–71.

21. Schneider D, Mosqueda L, Falk E, et al. Elder abuse forensic centers. J Elder Abuse Negl 2010;22:255–74.

22. Almogue A, Weiss A, Marcus E, et al. Attitudes and knowledge of medical and nursing staff toward elder abuse. Arch Gerontol Geriatr 2010;51:86–91.

23. National Committee for the Prevention of Elder Abuse. Available at: www.preventelderabuse.org. Accessed June 5, 2014.

24. Mosqueda L. Geriatric pocket doc: a resource for non-physicians. 2nd edition. Irvine (CA): Program in Geriatrics; 2012.

25. Dyer C. Community approaches to elder abuse. Orlando (FL): Elsevier Saunders; 2005. p. 429–47.

26. Dong X. Medical implications of elder abuse and neglect. In: Lorusso M, editor. Clinics in geriatric medicine elder abuse & neglect. Orlando (FL): Elsevier Saunders; 2005. p. 293–331.

27. American Bar Association. Commission on legal problems of the elderly: report to the house of delegates. Washington, DC: American Bar Association; 2002.

28. Welfare and institutions code 5150-5155. Available at: www.legalinfo.legislature.ca.gov. Accessed June 13, 2014.

29. Available at: http://www.napsa-now.org/wp-content/uploads/2012/04/Mandatory-Reporting-Chart.pdf. Accessed June 17, 2014.

30. Leonard K. Nursing homes begin to offer shelter for elder abuse victims. US News World Rep 2013. March 18, 2013. Available at: http://health.usnews.com/health-news/best-nursing-homes/articles/2013/03/18/nursing-homes-begin-to-offer-shelter-for-elder-abuse-victims.

31. Heck L, Gillespie G. Interprofessional program to provide emergency sheltering to abused elders. Adv Emerg Nurs J 2013;35:170–81.

32. Ethical Principles and Best Practice Guidelines for APS. Available at: www.ncea. aoa.gov. Accessed June 10, 2014.
33. National Committee on Elder Abuse. Available at: www.ncea.aoa.gov. Accessed June 8, 2014.
34. Reed K. When elders lose their cents: financial abuse of the elderly. Orlando (FL): Elsevier Saunders; 2005. p. 365–82.
35. Burgess AW, Hanrahan NP, Baker T. Forensic markers in elder female sexual abuse cases. Clin Geriatr Med 2005;21:399–412.
36. Available at: www.cdc.gov. Accessed June 14, 2014.
37. Lachs MS, Williams CS, O'Brien S, et al. The mortality of elder mistreatment. JAMA 1998;280:428–32.
38. Lachs MS, Williams CS, O'Brien S, et al. Adult Protective Service use and nursing home placement. Gerontologist 2002;42:734–9.
39. Dyer C, Pavlik V. The high prevalence of depression and dementia in elder abuse or neglect. J Am Geriatr Soc 2000;48:205–8.
40. Keilitz S, Uekert B, Jones T. Prosecution guide to effective collaboration on elder abuse. Madison, (WI): National Clearinghouse on Abuse in Later Life; 2012.

Health Professionals' Roles and Relationships with Other Agencies

Mary S. Twomey, MSW*, Christine Weber, MSG

KEYWORDS

- Interdisciplinary teams • Elder abuse prevention • Elder abuse intervention
- Health professionals

KEY POINTS

- This article describes the social service and law enforcement agencies that are integral to elder abuse work (eg, Adult Protective Services).
- Terms frequently used by social workers, law enforcement, and other nonmedical professionals who work in the elder abuse response system are defined.
- Roles for health professionals within interdisciplinary teams are described.

INTRODUCTION

Health care professionals' participation in addressing elder abuse is critical. Many opportunities exist to improve the lives of individuals and communities affected by elder abuse. Many, if not most, cases of elder abuse evaluation involve an assessment of the victim's physical, cognitive, functional, and psychological well-being. Without timely and sufficient medical expertise, many victims will not receive the attention they deserve.

It is estimated that 10% of older Americans experience some type of abuse,[1] and it is likely that most health care professionals in clinical care encounter elder abuse victims. Health care professionals are generally aware of their legal mandate to report suspected elder abuse to the proper authorities. Nevertheless, fewer than 1% of all

Disclosure Statement: The authors have no relevant financial relationships to disclose.
Division of Geriatric Medicine and Gerontology, Center of Excellence on Elder Abuse and Neglect, University of California, Irvine, 101 The City Drive, South, Building 200, Suite 835, Orange, CA 92868, USA
* Corresponding author.
E-mail address: marytwomey1@gmail.com

Clin Geriatr Med 30 (2014) 881–895
http://dx.doi.org/10.1016/j.cger.2014.08.014
0749-0690/14/$ – see front matter © 2014 Elsevier Inc. All rights reserved.
geriatric.theclinics.com

abuse reports to Adult Protective Services come from physicians.[2] Reporting suspected abuse, while vitally important, is only one of several actions that physicians and other health professionals can take in addressing elder abuse. As the elder justice field has evolved, the opportunity for health professionals to assist elder abuse victims has expanded.

However, health professionals' full participation in elder justice efforts requires familiarity with the current system that serves elder abuse victims. Such awareness includes an understanding of the various agencies that work together to ensure safety and to pursue justice for the victims of abuse. In addition, knowledge regarding the differences in professional culture and even vocabulary is helpful in interdisciplinary endeavors.

This article describes the social service and law enforcement agencies that are integral to elder abuse work. In addition, terms frequently used by social workers, law enforcement, and other nonmedical professionals who work in the elder abuse response system are defined. The goal of this article is to inform the reader and to inspire health professionals to take increased action on behalf of elder abuse victims.

RESPONDING TO ELDER ABUSE: AN INTERDISCIPLINARY APPROACH IS CRUCIAL

Originally used successfully in child abuse cases, interdisciplinary teams (IDTs) are groups of professionals from diverse disciplines who come together, usually monthly, to provide comprehensive assessment and consultation in elder abuse cases.[3] Experience shows that a coordinated interdisciplinary approach that includes social workers, law enforcement, medical professionals, mental health professionals, attorneys, and others yields the best outcomes for the victims of abuse by providing additional resources (eg, psychological evaluations, physician review of medications).[4] The teams review cases of suspected or known elder abuse, neglect, and self-neglect referred to them by team members. The IDT's goals are to provide advice, resources, and new perspectives to the agencies working on the cases.[5]

In addition to better outcomes for the victims, professionals working on elder abuse cases within an IDT also relate better outcomes. For example, in one study, 97% of those who referred cases to an elder abuse IDT indicated that the team was helpful in confirming abuse, documenting impaired capacity, reviewing medications and medical conditions, facilitating the conservatorship process, persuading the client or family to take action, and supporting the need for law enforcement involvement.[6]

Professional disciplines that are typically represented on elder abuse teams include Adult Protective Services (APS), the Long-Term Care Ombudsman, the civil and criminal justice systems, health and social services, and mental health. Optimally, other agencies or individuals who may also be able to participate as members or as consultants include:

- Animal care and control
- Area agency on aging
- Community care licensing
- Seniors legal aid
- Disability services

- Domestic violence program
- Forensic nurse
- Forensic pathologist
- Medicaid fraud investigators
- Public guardian/public administrator/public conservator
- Sexual assault program

The IDT model reflects a "one-stop-shop" where the "consumer" is an agency with a complex elder abuse case who requests the assistance of other agencies with expertise in elder abuse. A mutual team meeting allows for increased efficiency. The team process also encourages deeper understanding and building of relationships between individuals within these agencies.

The following case illustrates the systems and agencies that typically address elder abuse. As the case unfolds, the reader will be oriented to "who's who" and the roles that each agency plays in the case. This case was initially reported to APS.

Sheriff

The Sheriff's office received a call about an 80-year-old woman, Jane Jones, whose neighbor heard the daughter screaming at her mother a few nights ago. A Sheriff responded to the home but when the older woman came to the door, she stated that nothing was wrong. The Sheriff reports that the woman was very thin, disheveled, and seemed confused. In the background, he could hear a woman's voice asking who was at the door. The older woman insisted that nothing was wrong so the officer left. The Sheriff took down the names of both the elder and her daughter and ran both names through the database. It turns out the daughter had been released from jail a month ago where she had spent 60 days for petty theft and methamphetamine use. The officer was concerned enough that he made a report to APS for suspected elder abuse or neglect.

Adult Protective Services

The APS worker made an unannounced home visit yesterday morning. The older woman was home alone. Her home was cluttered and her refrigerator lacked edible food. The older woman reported having high blood pressure, problems with her sugar, and something wrong with her lungs. She did not know the names of any of her medicines and could not remember the last time she had taken any medications. She appeared drawn and thin. The older woman reported that everything was "OK" at home. When pressed she said that her daughter sometimes had "a bad temper."

WHO'S WHO IN ELDER ABUSE

A summary of who's who in elder abuse is divided into 2 tables. **Table 1** details professionals from social service provider agencies typically involved in elder abuse. **Table 2** lists the professionals from the legal/law enforcement agencies that are typically involved.

Table 1
Who's who in elder abuse: social service providers

Agency	Who Are They?	What Do They Do?
Adult Protective Services (APS)	Social workers, case workers	In most states, mandated reports of suspected elder abuse are made to APS. APS workers are the first responders to alleged victims of abuse, neglect, and exploitation and self-neglect. Services are provided to ensure the safety and well-being of elders and adults with disabilities in danger of being mistreated or neglected. APS balances the client's right to self-determination with their mandate to protect the vulnerable adult. Clients with capacity have the "right to folly"
		Interventions provided by APS include, but are not limited to:
		• Receiving reports of adult abuse, exploitation or neglect
		• Investigating these reports
		• Case planning
		• Monitoring and evaluation
		In addition to casework services, APS may provide or arrange for the provision of medical, social, economic, legal, housing, law enforcement or other protective, emergency or supportive services
		Most APS programs serve both older and younger vulnerable adults. In some states, APS is responsible only for cases involving older adults (eligibility may be based on age, incapacity or vulnerability of the adult). A few APS programs serve only younger adults, ages 18–59 y[7]
		Resource: For a listing of state APS programs, go to: www.napsa-now.org
Domestic violence service providers	Domestic violence advocates and trained volunteers	Domestic violence services are provided in the community for victims who have been abused within the context of an intimate partner relationship (eg, 2 people who are dating, married, living together). 85% of intimate partner violence in the USA is perpetrated against women.[8]
		Domestic violence services may include:
		• Counseling
		• Legal advocacy
		• Case management
		• Information and referrals
		• Community education and outreach
		• Support groups
		Resource: For a listing of domestic violence programs in the USA, call: National Domestic Violence Hotline 800-799-SAFE (7233); 800-787-3224 TTY; www.thehotline.org
		Resource: For information about programs serving victims of abuse in later life, go to www.ncall.us

Long-term care ombudsman	Social workers, trained volunteers, others	A trained and designated volunteer or professional long-term care ombudsman works to resolve complaints made by or on behalf of residents of long-term care facilities (eg, skilled nursing facilities, assisted living facilities). Many complaints involve inadequate care (30% of all complaints), and abuse, neglect, or exploitation (7% of all complaints)[9] Long-term care ombudsmen are dedicated to enhancing the lives of long-term care residents by: • Advocating for residents rights and quality care • Educating consumers and providers • Resolving residents' complaints • Providing information to the public *Resource: To find an ombudsman's office go to http://www.theconsumervoice.org/*
Mental health services	Psychiatrists, psychologists, social workers	Community-based mental health agencies provide mental health services to community-dwelling older adults. Services may include: • Access to outpatient clinics • Community crisis evaluation services • Drug and alcohol prevention education • Listings of licensed housing and residential care facilities • Home visitations to underserved adults • Preventive health care for older adults In some communities, emergency mental health services may respond to older adults who need crisis intervention
State licensing of long-term care facilities	Social workers, nurses	States require that certain kinds of facilities that provide housing and services for vulnerable adults acquire a license to provide these services. A state department is responsible for ensuring that the licensee meets all state and federal requirements. The state receives complaints about poor care in these facilities. It is the mission of the licensing entity to promote the health, safety, and quality of life of each person in community care facilities through the administration of an effective regulatory enforcement system When a facility fails to protect a resident's health or safety, or when a facility is unwilling or unable to stay in compliance with licensing laws and regulations, corrective action is taken by the licensing agency. Enforcement is typically maintained through: • Fines and civil penalties (these may vary according to the violation) • Administrative legal actions • Compliance plans • Probationary license • Temporary suspension of license • Revocation of license *Resource: See http://www.law.cornell.edu/cfr/text/42/483.13 for more information about federal law related to facilities and abuse and neglect of residents*

Table 2
Who's who in elder abuse: legal services and law enforcement

Agency	Who Are They?	What Do They Do?
Civil attorneys	Attorneys, paralegals	Civil elder law encompasses many different fields of law, several of which are germane to elder abuse cases, particularly cases of financial exploitation. Some of these include: • Conservatorships and guardianships • Estate planning, including planning for the management of one's estate during life and its disposition on death through the use of trusts, wills, and other planning documents • Probate • Administration and management of trusts and estates • Long-term care placements in nursing home and life care communities • Nursing home issues including questions of patients' rights and nursing home quality of care • Elder abuse and fraud recovery cases[10] *Resource: To find an elder law attorney, go to:* https://www.naela.org/
Courts	Judges, Attorneys, Court investigators, Court mediators	Courts play a critical role in protecting the rights and the safety of older adults and persons with disabilities Elder abuse cases may be heard in many kinds of courts including criminal, civil, probate, and family law. Some court systems have created specialty courts for elder abuse cases or for all cases in which an elder is the victim or petitioner[11] *Resource: For more information about the courts and elder abuse go to:* http://www.eldersandcourts.org/
Law enforcement	Police officers, sheriffs	Police, sheriff, and other peace officers are often called when safety is endangered or a crime committed. Although mistreatment of elders and adults with disabilities, like other forms of family violence, has traditionally been viewed as a family problem, criminal justice systems are developing ways to better address elder abuse and neglect as a criminal issue In addition to preparing cases for prosecution, law enforcement agencies also work with social services providers, community sentinels, and other local resources to protect the safety and welfare of elders and adults with disabilities: • Arrest perpetrators • Enforce restraining orders • Perform "well-being" checks • Provide assistance to APS in conducting investigations[12]

(continued on next page)

Table 2 *(continued)*		
Agency	**Who Are They?**	**What Do They Do?**
Legal aid	Attorneys, paralegals	The Older Americans Act funds free legal services for people older than 60. Elder abuse cases often require the services of a civil attorney to assist with acquiring protective orders, and petitioning the Probate Court for matters related to guardianship. *Resource: For a list of free legal services for seniors go to:* http://www.aoa.gov/AoARoot/AoA_Programs/Elder_Rights/Legal/Index.aspx
Victim Services	Social workers, others	Usually housed within the court or prosecutor's office, Victim Services advocates assist individuals and families with: • Navigating the criminal justice system • Advocacy • Crime victim compensation • Crisis intervention and counseling *Resource: Office for Victims of Crime:* www.ovc.gov/

INTERVENING IN THE ELDER ABUSE CASE: IMPORTANT TERMINOLOGY

As the IDT continues its discussion of the alleged elder abuse case of Mrs Jones, other team members bring their expertise to bear. **Table 3** provides guidance regarding terminology for the common abbreviations used by each agency.

Mental Health

What about a referral to Community-Based Adult Services? It would be good for Mrs Jones to get out of the house and interact with others. Would she be eligible for other day programs?

Public Guardian

Have you checked to see if the daughter has any power of attorney? I can check with the Probate Court to see if the daughter is Mrs Jones' guardian. I know she is not under our jurisdiction currently, but if the daughter is guardian and is not taking good care of Mrs Jones, we could look at taking her case in our office.

Legal Aid

I'd like to know if she would be interested in getting a restraining order. We could help her with this. If the daughter is threatening her, that's grounds enough for a restraining order in our state.

Mental Health

Has anyone done a cognitive or psychological evaluation of Mrs. Jones? Do you think she has any dementia or depression? We could send someone out to talk with her and do an evaluation. Do you think there is any undue influence involved in this case?

Adult Protective Services

The social worker did a field test for cognition. Mrs Jones scored 22 out of 30. It was difficult to know if her low score is due to dementia or something else. She couldn't

Table 3
Terms encountered in elder abuse cases

Term	Definition
AAA	Area Agency on Aging: a county agency or nonprofit agency that receives Older American's Act funds to provide services to older people in the community. Some typical services include home-delivered meals, legal assistance to the elderly, and information and referral
ADLs/IADLs	Activities of Daily Living include: • Bathing and showering • Bowel and bladder management (including recognizing the need to relieve oneself) • Dressing • Eating • Feeding (setting up food and bringing it to one's mouth) • Functional mobility (moving from one place to another while performing activities) • Personal hygiene and grooming (including brushing/combing/styling hair) • Toilet hygiene (completing the act of urinating/defecating)[13] Instrumental activities of daily living (IADLs) are not necessary for fundamental functioning, but they let an individual live independently in a community: • Housework • Taking medications as prescribed • Managing money • Shopping for necessities • Use of telephone or other form of communication • Use of technology (as applicable) • Transportation within the community[14]
Agent	The person who acts on the principal's behalf through a power of attorney or durable power of attorney agreement
Capacity	Capacity is the ability to make informed decisions. It is contextual and may fluctuate over time, situation, and task. Please compare with the term "competence" (though these 2 terms are related, they are often mistakenly used as synonyms, which is not correct)

CBAS (formerly Adult Day Care/Adult Day Health Care)	Designed to keep older adults and adults with disabilities living and thriving in the community, Community-Based Adult Services (CBAS) offers nonresidential day programs to eligible older adults and/or adults with disabilities to restore or maintain their optimal capacity for self-care. CBAS services include: an individual assessment; professional nursing services; physical, occupational and speech therapies; mental health services; therapeutic activities; social services; personal care; meals; nutritional counseling; and transportation to and from the participant's residence and the CBAS center. CBAS replaced Adult Day Health Care (ADHC) services, which were an optional benefit under the Medicaid Program through February 2012[15]
Competency	The mental ability to understand and make decisions about a specific problem or issue. Competency is a legal status determined by the courts. All adults are presumed to be competent unless adjudicated otherwise by a court
District Attorney	The District Attorney, also known as the Prosecutor, brings charges against the alleged abuser in the criminal court
Elder Death Review Team	Elder Death Review Teams evaluate elder death cases for abuse and neglect. Teams may be convened by the Medical Examiner, Coroner, District Attorney, or another public entity. Some teams meet to determine the feasibility of prosecution. Others focus only on systemic issues raised by the cases. Team membership typically consists of public agencies involved in the investigation of elder abuse cases, and may also include geriatricians, psychologists, and forensic experts[16]
EPO	Emergency Protective Order: a legal document executed by a judge that restricts contact between an alleged abuser and the "protected person." An EPO is in effect for a short period of time (generally 5–7 d). Protected individuals may seek a full restraining order through the courts so that protection continues past the expiration of the EPO
Family Court	Restraining orders against abusers are typically adjudicated through the Family Court
Fiduciary	A person in a position of authority whom the law obligates to act in good faith and solely on behalf of the person he or she represents. Examples of fiduciaries are agents under powers of attorney, executors, trustees, guardians, and officers of corporations[17]
Financial Abuse Specialist Team (FAST)	FAST teams focus on complex financial elder abuse cases. Teams may comprise of public agencies (Adult Protective Services, law enforcement, Public Guardian, LTC Ombudsman), or public-private partnerships, which include private practitioners from the fields of law, real estate, and banking. Teams typically meet monthly and discuss 1 to 3 cases[18]

(continued on next page)

Table 3
(continued)

Term	Definition
Forensic Center	An elder abuse Forensic Center differs from the more common interdisciplinary team (IDT) in several key ways Forensic Centers include a greater array of disciplines and is a more focused, action-oriented collaboration than the traditional IDT. Forensic Centers must include at least one physician and psychologist The Forensic Center team is task-oriented and each member of the team provides a unique service based on their agency affiliation. Meeting on a weekly basis (vs monthly for a traditional IDT), a plan of action is determined by the collective team and team members assist in actually carrying out recommendations[19]
Guardianship (also called Conservatorship in some states)	Guardianship is a relationship created by state law in which a court gives one person (the guardian) the duty and power to make personal and/or property decisions for another (the ward). The appointment of a guardian occurs when a judge decides the ward is not competent to make decisions. Through the imposition of a guardianship, an individual loses fundamental rights and a surrogate is given the responsibility and power to make decisions about health care, living arrangements, finances, and property. There are 2 kinds of general guardianships: guardians of the person and guardians of the estate or finances. In many cases, both kinds are appointed. In addition, in some states, guardianship orders may be tailored to address the specific needs of the ward. Tailored or limited guardianships have the advantage of leaving intact those rights that the ward can still exercise without oversight (eg, a guardian of the estate may be appointed by the court to manage a person's stock portfolio, but the court may allow the ward to continue to control a bank account)[20]
IADLs	Instrumental Activities of Daily Living. See ADLs above
In-Home Support Services (IHSS)	State or county program that provides in-home support services for people who need assistance to stay at home. These services include actions such as housekeeping, cooking, and assistance with bathing
IPV	Intimate Partner Violence (also known as domestic violence): usually described as a pattern of abusive behavior in any relationship that is used by one partner to gain or maintain power and control over another
Involuntary mental health commitment	Legal mechanism authorized under state law that allows specific professionals (eg, police, emergency mental health system) to hold someone against their will in a psychiatric hospital because they are judged to be a danger to themselves or others, or are "gravely disabled" as a result of a psychiatric illness. Typically, the initial involuntary hold is for a short period of time. To extend this, a court hearing must be held

Long-term care facilities	Long-term care facilities include board and care homes, assisted living facilities, and nursing homes. Board and care homes, which can also be called residential care facilities or group homes, are the smallest type of facility with usually 20 or fewer residents. Assisted living facilities range in size from as few as 20 residents to 120 or more. For both board and care and assisted living, residents will have either private or shared rooms. Residents will also receive help with ADLs and have staff available around the clock. Unlike a nursing facility, these 2 types of facilities usually do not provide nursing and medical care
	Nursing homes, also called skilled nursing facilities, provide a wide range of health and personal care services. In addition to the assistance with ADLs and 24-h staffing, they provide health care and rehabilitation services such as physical, occupational, and speech therapy. A stay at a nursing home can be temporary (for example, to recover from surgery) or permanent. All 3 types of facilities are starting to offer special arrangements for people suffering from Alzheimer disease and other types of dementia[21]
	Resource: To find a long-term care facility near you, go to: www.eldercare.gov
Power of Attorney (POA)	A legal document through which a "principal" gives power to an "agent" to act on the principal's behalf. In a standard POA, an agent's authority ends if the principal revokes that authority, if the principal dies, or if the principal loses decision-making capacity and cannot revoke the agent's authority. The law does this to protect the incapacitated principal who is no longer able to monitor an agent and take action if the agent abuses his/her authority
	In addition to the standard POA, there are 2 other kinds of POAs: durable and springing. In a durable POA, the agent remains in force even if the principal loses the legal capacity to revoke the agent's authority. In a springing POA, the agent does not assume authority until a later time or when a certain event that is specified occurs (eg, when 2 doctors have determined that the person is incapacitated)[21]
Principal	The person who authorizes another person to act on his or her behalf through a POA[22]
Probate Court	Guardianship (also called conservatorship in some states) proceedings are typically adjudicated in the Probate Court. Other matters related to elder abuse handled in the Probate Court include trust disputes and will contests
Psychological evaluation	A psychological evaluation typically assesses various domains (appearance, attention, memory) through observation and communication during a clinical interview. An example of one tool typically used is the MoCA, the Montreal Cognitive Assessment
Restraining order (also called protective order)	A restraining order is a legal document that restricts contact between an abuser and a "protected person"
Undue influence	Sometimes likened to "brainwashing," undue influence is when an individual who is stronger or more powerful gets a weaker individual to do something that the weaker person would not have done otherwise. The stronger person uses a variety of techniques over time to gain power and compliance; they may isolate the weaker person, lie, promote dependency, or induce fear and distrust of others[23]

remember when she had last eaten or taken any medications, so that could be causing some of her confusion. She had pill bottles everywhere, but the pills were all mixed up. She is not able to independently perform many of her activities of daily living or instrumental activities of daily living. We feel a psychological evaluation would be very useful in this case.

Another area of concern to the worker was that a neighbor told her that Mrs Jones has recently signed over her house, which she owns free and clear, to the daughter. The daughter was bragging about it to the neighbor. I'm afraid that we aren't just looking at neglect but also financial abuse.

Table 4
Health professionals' expertise in elder abuse prevention and intervention

Role	Explanation
Review medications	Many elders take multiple medications. By reviewing the client's medication list, one can clarify what the medications are for, identify interactions and adverse effects, and determine medication adherence
Review medical records	Medical professionals review the victim's medical records for evidence of abuse and neglect, and offer supporting documentation to social services and law enforcement
Medical assessments	Medical evaluations can take place in several locations: the victim's home, the hospital, the facility where he/she is a resident, or at a medical office. Evaluations may include a physical examination and/or a cognitive evaluation. The assessment will focus on the concern as expressed by members of the IDT (ie, allegations of neglect, allegations of physical abuse)[24]
Psychological assessments	Psychological assessment of the alleged victim of abuse is the service most frequently requested by the other members of the IDT.[6] The psychological assessment may be global in nature or may explore a narrow question of whether the alleged victim had the capacity to undertake a particular course of action, such as signing away certain rights, conveying property, or entering into marriage
Facilitate communication with other MDs	Health care professionals often serve to communicate with other providers in the community, such as alleged victims' personal physicians
Training	Medical professionals have important knowledge that is essential to social workers, law enforcement, and other team members in their work with abused elders. All engaged professions should have basic medical knowledge of cognitive impairment, dementia, as well as some chronic illnesses, and functional status. Such training can occur within the context of the IDT meeting or can be conducted separately
Provide expert testimony in court	A medical professional may be asked to provide expert testimony on a case of elder abuse relating to their own patient or as a consultant elder abuse expert. For example, a pharmacist may be asked to testify about the possible risks of taking 2 medications concurrently or a physician might be asked to testify about how Alzheimer disease affects one's capacity to make decisions. Many health professionals who serve on IDTs will provide expert testimony as part of their contribution to the team's work

District Attorney

If we are going to bring charges against the daughter for elder neglect and financial abuse, we'll need to know if Mrs Jones had the capacity to sign over her home to the daughter.

Every field has its jargon and shorthand, and elder abuse is no exception. **Table 3** defines some of the terms that come up frequently when discussing elder abuse cases.

THE ROLE OF THE MEDICAL PROFESSIONAL IN INTERDISCIPLINARY CASE CONSULTATION

Medical professionals are necessary team members in an interdisciplinary evaluation of abuse. Many, if not most, cases involve an assessment of the victim's physical, cognitive, and/or psychological well-being, as well as a determination of the vulnerabilities that place one at risk of abuse. Medical expertise is also needed to evaluate the medical aspects of abuse and neglect, such as in traumatic injuries, physical findings of neglect, and cognitive status (**Table 4**).

As the case unfolds, the addition of a physician and a psychologist to the elder abuse IDT enhances the services to the victim and the other service providers.

Psychologist

I can accompany the APS social worker to the victim's home and conduct a psychological evaluation. That should help us figure out whether Mrs Jones had the capacity to sign over her house to her daughter.

Physician

If APS can create a list of the medications found at her home, I can let you know what Mrs Jones was being treated for and whether she has been taking her medications. Please ask APS to include information about dose and frequency. I can also go out with the psychologist and do a medical evaluation for neglect or physical abuse. I hope that will give all of us a better sense of Mrs Jones' physical and cognitive status.

SUMMARY

Elder abuse cases often present with complex issues, necessitating the determination of physical, cognitive, and psychological abilities of victims. Interventions for elder abuse victims typically involve several social service, legal, and law enforcement agencies. Medical professionals' participation significantly enhances these interdisciplinary efforts. Their involvement adds value to both the victim and the other professionals by providing essential information about the client's health and/or mental health, interpreting medical evidence, and explaining how the health care field works. There are 5 official Elder Abuse Forensic Centers throughout the United States, and many other agencies have other formal affiliations with medical professionals. A toolkit for starting these types of collaborations can be found at *Creating an Elder Abuse Forensic Center: Philosophy into Action* (DVD and manual) (http://www. centeronelderabuse.org/publications.asp).

REFERENCES

1. Acierno R, Hernandez M, Amstadter A, et al. Prevalence and correlates of emotional, physical, sexual and financial abuse and potential neglect in the United States: the national elder mistreatment study. Am J Public Health 2010; 100(2):292–7.

2. Teaster P. A response to the abuse of vulnerable adults: the 2000 survey of state Adult Protective Services. Available at: http://www.ncea.aoa.gov/Resources/Publication/docs/apsreport030703.pdf. Accessed March 19, 2014.

3. Teaster P, Nerenberg L, Stansbury K. A national look at elder abuse multidisciplinary teams. J Elder Abuse Negl 2003;15(3/4):91–107.

4. Navarro AE, Gassoumis Z, Wilber K. Holding abusers accountable: an Elder Abuse Forensic Center increases criminal prosecution of financial exploitation. Gerontologist 2013;53(2):303–12.

5. Twomey M, Jackson G, Li H, et al. The successes and challenges of seven multidisciplinary teams. J Elder Abuse Negl 2010;22(3–4):291–305.

6. Mosqueda L, Burnight K, Liao S, et al. Advancing the field of elder mistreatment: a new model for integration of social and medical services. Gerontologist 2004; 44(5):703–8.

7. National Adult Protective Services Association. Get help. Available at: http://www.napsa-now.org/get-help/how-aps-helps/. Accessed March 20, 2014.

8. U.S. Department of Justice. Crime data brief: Intimate partner violence, 1993–2001. Available at: http://www.bjs.gov/content/pub/pdf/ipv01.pdf. Accessed June 2, 2014.

9. Administration on Aging. 2010 national ombudsman reporting system data tables. Available at: http://www.aoa.gov/aoa_programs/elder_rights/Ombudsman/National_State_Data/2010/Index.aspx. Accessed May 29, 2014.

10. National Academy of Elder Law Attorneys, Inc. NAELA question and answer brochure. Available at: https://www.naela.org/Public/Library/Brochures/Consumer_Brochure/Public/Library/Brochures/Consumer_Brochure.aspx?hkey=fc71f2d2-4aad-434e-8b48-715026be0f12. Accessed March 10, 2014.

11. National Center for state courts. Court guide to effective collaboration on elder abuse. Available at: http://www.eldersandcourts.org/Elder-Abuse/~/media/Microsites/Files/cec/Court Collaboration.ashx. Accessed March 17, 2014.

12. National Center on elder abuse. Law enforcement. Available at: http://www.ncea.aoa.gov/Stop_Abuse/Partners/Law_Enforce/index.aspx. Accessed March 12, 2014.

13. Roley S, DeLany JV, Barrows CJ, et al. Occupational therapy practice framework: domain & practice. Am J Occup Ther 2008;62(6):625–83.

14. Bookman A, Harrington M, Pass L, et al. Family caregiver handbook. Cambridge (MA): Massachusetts Institute of Technology; 2007.

15. U.S. Department of Health and Human Services. Regulatory review of adult day services: final report. Available at: http://aspe.hhs.gov/daltcp/reports/adultday1.pdf. Accessed March 10, 2014.

16. American Bar Association. Elder abuse fatality review teams: a replication manual. Washington, DC: American Bar Association; 2005.

17. Consumer Financial Protection Bureau. What is a fiduciary? Available at: http://www.consumerfinance.gov/askcfpb/1769/what-fiduciary.html. Accessed March 10, 2014.

18. National Center on Elder Abuse. Financial abuse specialist teams. Available at: http://www.ncea.aoa.gov/Stop_Abuse/Teams/FAST/index.aspx. Accessed March 17, 2014.

19. Mosqueda L, Twomey M, Chen E, et al. Creating an elder abuse forensic center: philosophy into action. Available at: http://www.centeronelderabuse.org/EAFC_manual.asp. Accessed March 20, 2014.

20. The Center for Elders and the Courts. Basics: guardianship definitions and types. Available at: http://www.eldersandcourts.org/Guardianship/Guardianship-Basics.aspx. Accessed March 19, 2014.

21. National Institutes of Health. Senior health. Long-term care: facility-based care. Available at: http://nihseniorhealth.gov/longtermcare/facilitybasedservices/01. html. Accessed May 29, 2014.

22. Stiegel LA. Durable power of attorney: it's a crime too. A National Center on elder abuse factsheet for criminal justice professionals. Available at: http://www.ncea. aoa.gov/Resources/Publication/docs/DurablePowerOfAttorneyAbuseFactSheet_ CriminalJusticeProfessionals.pdf. Accessed March 12, 2014.

23. National Committee for the prevention of elder abuse. Mental capacity, consent and undue influence. Available at: http://www.preventelderabuse.org/ elderabuse/issues/capacity.html. Accessed March 17, 2014.

24. Falk E, Landsverk E. Geriatricians and psychologists: essential ingredients in the evaluation of elder abuse and neglect. J Elder Abuse Negl 2010;22:281–90.

Index

Note: Page numbers of article titles are in **boldface** type.

Clin Geriatr Med 30 (2014) 897–902
http://dx.doi.org/10.1016/S0749-0690(14)00108-6
0749-0690/14/$ – see front matter © 2014 Elsevier Inc. All rights reserved.

geriatric.theclinics.com

United States Postal Service

Statement of Ownership, Management, and Circulation
(All Periodicals Publications Except Requestor Publications)

1. Publication Title	2. Publication Number	3. Filing Date
Clinics in Geriatric Medicine	0 0 0 - 7 0 4	9/14/14

4. Issue Frequency	5. Number of Issues Published Annually	6. Annual Subscription Price
Feb, May, Aug, Nov	4	$280.00

7. Complete Mailing Address of Known Office of Publication (Not printer) (Street, city, county, state, and ZIP+4®)

Elsevier Inc.
360 Park Avenue South
New York, NY 10010-1710

Contact Person
Stephen R. Bushing
Telephone (Include area code)
215-239-3688

8. Complete Mailing Address of Headquarters or General Business Office of Publisher (Not printer)

Elsevier Inc., 360 Park Avenue South, New York, NY 10010-1710

9. Full Names and Complete Mailing Addresses of Publisher, Editor, and Managing Editor (Do not leave blank)

Publisher (Name and complete mailing address)

Linda Belfus, Elsevier Inc., 1600 John F. Kennedy Blvd., Suite 1800, Philadelphia, PA 19103-2899

Editor (Name and complete mailing address)

Jessica McCool, Elsevier Inc., 1600 John F. Kennedy Blvd., Suite 1800, Philadelphia, PA 19103-2899

Managing Editor (Name and complete mailing address)

Adrianne Brigido, Elsevier Inc., 1600 John F. Kennedy Blvd., Suite 1800, Philadelphia, PA 19103-2899

10. Owner (Do not leave blank. If the publication is owned by a corporation, give the name and address of the corporation immediately followed by the names and addresses of all stockholders owning or holding 1 percent or more of the total amount of stock. If not owned by a corporation, give the names and addresses of the individual owners. If owned by a partnership or other unincorporated firm, give its name and address as well as those of each individual owner. If the publication is published by a nonprofit organization, give its name and address.)

Full Name	Complete Mailing Address
Wholly owned subsidiary of	1600 John F. Kennedy Blvd., Ste. 1800
Reed/Elsevier, US holdings	Philadelphia, PA 19103-2899

11. Known Bondholders, Mortgagees, and Other Security Holders Owning or Holding 1 Percent or More of Total Amount of Bonds, Mortgages, or Other Securities. If none, check box ☐ None

Full Name	Complete Mailing Address
N/A	

12. Tax Status (For completion by nonprofit organizations authorized to mail at nonprofit rates) (Check one)
The purpose, function, and nonprofit status of this organization and the exempt status for federal income tax purposes:
☐ Has Not Changed During Preceding 12 Months
☐ Has Changed During Preceding 12 Months (Publisher must submit explanation of change with this statement)

PS Form 3526, August 2012 (Page 1 of 3 (Instructions Page 3)) PSN 7530-01-000-9931 PRIVACY NOTICE: See our Privacy policy in www.usps.com

13. Publication Title	14. Issue Date for Circulation Data Below
Clinics in Geriatric Medicine	August 2014

15. Extent and Nature of Circulation			Average No. Copies Each Issue During Preceding 12 Months	No. Copies of Single Issue Published Nearest to Filing Date
a. Total Number of Copies (Net press run)			497	529
b. Paid Circulation (By Mail and Outside the Mail)	(1)	Mailed Outside-County Paid Subscriptions Stated on PS Form 3541. (Include paid distribution above nominal rate, advertiser's proof copies, and exchange copies)	246	221
	(2)	Mailed In-County Paid Subscriptions Stated on PS Form 3541 (Include paid distribution above nominal rate, advertiser's proof copies, and exchange copies)		
	(3)	Paid Distribution Outside the Mails Including Sales Through Dealers and Carriers, Street Vendors, Counter Sales, and Other Paid Distribution Outside USPS®	65	82
	(4)	Paid Distribution by Other Classes Mailed Through the USPS (e.g. First-Class Mail®)		
c. Total Paid Distribution (Sum of 15b (1), (2), (3), and (4))			311	303
d. Free or Nominal Rate Distribution (By Mail and Outside the Mail)	(1)	Free or Nominal Rate Outside-County Copies Included on PS Form 3541	82	113
	(2)	Free or Nominal Rate In-County Copies Included on PS Form 3541		
	(3)	Free or Nominal Rate Copies Mailed at Other Classes Through the USPS (e.g. First-Class Mail)		
	(4)	Free or Nominal Rate Distribution Outside the Mail (Carriers or other means)		
e. Total Free or Nominal Rate Distribution (Sum of 15d (1), (2), (3) and (4))			82	113
f. Total Distribution (Sum of 15c and 15e)			393	416
g. Copies not Distributed (See instructions to publishers #4 (page #3))			104	113
h. Total (Sum of 15f and g)			497	529
i. Percent Paid (15c divided by 15f times 100)			79.13%	72.84%

16. Total circulation includes electronic copies. Report circulation on PS form 3526-X worksheet.

17. Publication of Statement of Ownership
If the publication is a general publication, publication of this statement is required. Will be printed in the November 2014 issue of this publication.

18. Signature and Title of Editor, Publisher, Business Manager, or Owner

Stephen R. Bushing — Inventory Distribution Coordinator

Date
September 14, 2014

I certify that all information furnished on this form is true and complete. I understand that anyone who furnishes false or misleading information on this form or who omits material or information requested on the form may be subject to criminal sanctions (including fines and imprisonment) and/or civil sanctions (including civil penalties).

PS Form 3526, August 2012 (Page 2 of 3)

Moving?

Make sure your subscription moves with you!

To notify us of your new address, find your **Clinics Account Number** (located on your mailing label above your name), and contact customer service at:

Email: journalscustomerservice-usa@elsevier.com

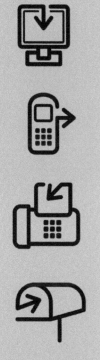

800-654-2452 (subscribers in the U.S. & Canada)
314-447-8871 (subscribers outside of the U.S. & Canada)

Fax number: 314-447-8029

Elsevier Health Sciences Division
Subscription Customer Service
3251 Riverport Lane
Maryland Heights, MO 63043

*To ensure uninterrupted delivery of your subscription, please notify us at least 4 weeks in advance of move.